Universalising Healthcare in India:
From Care to Coverage

Universalising Healthcare in India: From Care to Coverage

Editors
Imrana Qadeer
K.B. Saxena
P.M. Arathi

AAKAR

Universalising Healthcare in India: From Care to Coverage
Edited by Imrana Qadeer, K.B. Saxena, P.M. Arathi

First Published 2019
Second Edition 2025

ISBN 978-93-5002-588-8

Published by
AAKAR BOOKS
28 E Pocket IV, Mayur Vihar Phase I
Delhi 110 091 India
aakarbooks@gmail.com

Laser Typeset at
Arpit Printographers, Delhi

Printed at
D.K. Fine Art Press, Delhi

This collective work is dedicated to

Pushpa M. Bhargava,

A scientist with a social vision

Foreword

The provision of comprehensive public healthcare was regarded as an important duty of the welfare state that was established in India after its independence. This was spelt out in the Constitution of India in its chapter on the 'Directive Principles of State Policy'. Article 47 in this chapter stated that the state 'shall regard ... the improvement of public health as among its primary duties'. Given the fact that several of the provisions under the Directive Principles have been elevated to the status of fundamental rights in large part due to the creative interpretation of the Constitution by the superior courts of India, it was expected until a few years ago that the provision of public health would also acquire the status of a legally enforceable right under the Indian Constitution. In fact, several civil society organisations in India have been working to this end. The Directive Principles also include political and socio-economic measures that go to determine the quality, adequacy, and effectiveness of public health services. Article 39-A provides that 'the citizens ... have the right to adequate means of livelihood'. Article 45, which has now become a fundamental right, under Article 21-A, enjoined upon the state to endeavour to provide free and compulsory elementary education within a period of ten years after the commencement of the Constitution. Another important primary duty prescribed for the state in Article 47 is raising people's standard of living. Availability of minimum income is a precondition for availing of health services. And finally, in a welfare state, the provision of social services has to be universal, inclusive, just, and equitable. This is the crux of Article 38 (1) & (2) of the Directive Principles.

The Government of India adopted a number of measures in the macro-economic domain as well as in social sectors, including health, in order to give effect to these provisions. The most prominent among them was the scheme of providing comprehensive primary health services to the people. Therefore, when the Alma Ata Declaration on comprehensive primary healthcare (CPHC) was adopted in 1978, India embraced it wholeheartedly and in totality. The Alma Ata Declaration included ensuring fulfilment of socio-economic conditions conducive to comprehensive primary healthcare. It regarded preventive and promotive measures of public health to be more important than the curative ones. It had built into it the elements of inclusiveness and universality.

It is implicit both in the Indian Constitution and the Alma Ata Declaration that comprehensive primary healthcare is a public good which must be provided by the government. This is mainly because it is in the nature of a right for the securing of which the state is constitutionally and legally accountable. Moreover, every citizen is entitled to this right. This implies that comprehensive primary healthcare must be universalised. This can be done only by the state as it is beyond the capacity of the private sector to do so. Further, the provision of such primary health services is related to the whole host of socio- economic factors such as enhancement of income, its equitable distribution, ensuring livelihood security, and providing related goods and services like food, nutrition, water, housing, etc. This requires a coordinated, holistic, and planned strategy, which the state alone is in a position to design and implement.

The Alma Ata Declaration turned out to be the highest point reached in building an international consensus on the objectives and attributes of a public health system. Since then there has been continuing and progressive erosion of the values enshrined in the declaration. The erosion is reflected mainly in the policy changes relating to primary healthcare that have taken place at the national level. In India, the concept of comprehensive primary health services gave way to selective primary health services. In the next stage, it was confined to essential care. And recently, the concept that has come to dominate the field is universal healthcare.

Universal healthcare is neither 'universal' nor in the nature of 'care'. It is not universal because it leaves out millions who are struggling to eke out a living at or just above the poverty line. It is not in the nature of 'care' because it is not motivated by ethics or public purpose but by profit motive.

The departure from the concept of CPHC has been characterised by the gradual retreat of the state from investment in health services, the consequent privatisation of these services and provision on public–private partnership basis, switchover to the state subsidisation of private health services, and the inadequacy and ineffectiveness of the regulatory system in the private health sector. As a result, equity and justice have fallen by the wayside. The goal of universalisation of CPHC has been discarded, as private providers have no incentive to cater to the needs of the poorest and those living in remote areas.

These developments in India have coincided with the decline of the United Nations (UN) system of organisations, including the World Health Organisation (WHO). Starting from the mid-1980s, there has been a virtual ban on an increase in the regular budgetary resources of these organisations. In fact, there has been a continuing decline in this component of their budget in real terms. As a consequence, they have now come to rely overwhelmingly on voluntary resources of financing including that by the World Bank (WB), multinational corporations, bilateral arrangement within the multilateral framework, and voluntary contributions by member states. Another feature of the enfeeblement of UN organisations has been that they have been effectively prevented from discharging their norm setting and negotiating roles. On the other hand, the World Bank has suffered no such constraint. It has gone ahead and created its own capacities in social sectors like health and education at the cost of the specialised agencies like WHO, UNESCO whose well-recognised capacities in their areas of expertise have been virtually dismantled. The World Bank has unabashedly used its resources and leverage to promote products, processes, and technologies in the health and other fields, all geared to meet the needs of the multinational corporations, elite and well-to-do sections of population.

WHO's last contribution in the domain of public health was the formulation in 1982 at the expert level, of its Essential Drugs Policy. However, when it was discussed for possible adoption at the inter-governmental level in the World Health Assembly in 1983, the multinational corporations and the governments of the countries, where they are located, exercised strong pressure against it. As a result, member countries including those from the Third World were obliged to agree to the adoption of an innocuous resolution urging and providing incentives to physicians to promote the essential drugs, rather than accepting the Essential Drugs Policy as a legal obligation.

An important component of India's public health policy during the 1970s was the adoption of a legal framework and a policy for making drugs available to the people in adequate quantities and at affordable prices. The two-prong strategy adopted for this purpose was the enactment of the Patent Act of 1970 and the adoption of the Drug Policy of 1978. The 1970 Patent Act was universally regarded as the best legislation in operation in the world, combining the public purpose of ensuring the supply of drugs in sufficient quantities and at affordable prices, with the provision of incentives for innovation in the pharmaceutical industry. Through the implementation of this strategy, India emerged as a major international player in the global drug and pharmaceutical market, so much so that the well-known global non- governmental agency, Medecins Sans Frontieres (MSF), characterised India as 'the pharmacy of the world' (see the chapter by Biswajit Dhar and Reji Joseph in this volume).

The revised Patent Act adopted by India in the first decade of the twenty-first century brings the 1970 legislation in conformity with the World Trade Organisation (WTO) Agreement on Trade related aspects of intellectual property rights (TRIPS), while at the same time retaining its unique features, i.e. flexibility to grant compulsory licences and laying down a rigorous criterion for patentability. These are precisely the provisions which were challenged by international pharmaceutical giants in Indian law courts which, however, upheld them as being consistent with the Indian laws. In spite of this, these corporations and their government protagonists have not relented from their pressures to get these provisions eliminated. There are indications that the Government of India may yield to these pressures and revise its latest patent laws to suit the interest of these global companies. At a Global Exhibition on Services held in New Delhi, the Prime Minister of India stated on 2 April 2015 that India's patent laws should be brought on par with global standards. Bringing our patent laws on par with global standards simply means aligning them with those of the advanced countries, particularly the USA. There is in fact only one global standard on intellectual property rights and that is provided in the WTO's TRIPS Agreement. India's patent laws are fully compatible with this agreement.

The Government of India has also agreed to remain engaged in a dialogue on this issue with the USA, in a bilateral working group on patents. We have thus consented to remain subjected to continuous pressure on this issue by the USA. There are newspaper reports that in the discussion in the group, the Indian delegation has assured to its interlocutors that the contentious issues under discussion would not be applied in practice.

If the current drift in the Indian health system is allowed to continue, it would soon get totally alienated from the interest of the majority, especially marginalised sections in the country. It is therefore imperative to reverse this trend. This will be possible only by going back to the comprehensive and holistic approach to public health conceived and sought to be put in place during the early post-independence period. For this, it would be necessary to prevent the ongoing decay and decline of the public health institutions and strengthen and expand them. Foremost among them should be the comprehensive primary healthcare centres. The entire country should be covered by such centres. These centres and other health institutions in the country can be run effectively only by doctors, other health workers, nurses, and health administrators. Institutions for training these cadres in the required numbers need to be set up on a large scale. The responsibility for running health services and related institutions should be entrusted to trained health administrators. It is important to delink the governance of the national health system from the domination and influence of politicians and general administrators. Finally, the government should institute a system of effective regulation of the health sector in all its aspects. Universalisation of comprehensive primary health services should be made a legal right, and a time limit should be set for realising this goal. The above measures call for a radical policy shift and allocation of resources that is several times larger than is currently being made available to the health sector. In this context, it is important to bear in mind that the public expenditure on health in India is only slightly more than one per cent of its GDP as contrasted with 2.4% in China, 4.9% in Brazil, and 10% or above in several developed countries. In fact, so far as public expenditure in health is concerned, India is moving in the reverse direction. Allocations in the national budget for the Health Ministry and on such related items as the Integrated Child Development Services (ICDS), food security, the Rural Employment Guarantee Scheme, etc., have either been reduced or left stagnant in real terms during the last few years. The frequent public statements at the high political level that enhancement of the budget provision for the social sectors will depend on higher growth in GDP and larger collection of revenues amount to callous disregard of and indifference towards the fundamental rights of the people.

This book *Universalising Healthcare in India: From Care to Coverage* covers most of the current issues of public health in India. It contains in-depth analyses of these issues, mostly based on empirical studies. Its first part traces the history and explains the concepts and practices of comprehensive primary healthcare in India and globally. It then describes the transition to universal health coverage (UHC) and brings out its main features and consequences for the welfare of the people. It has also chapters on health insurance schemes and one on the extent and implications of the privatisation of medical education in India. The book contains several chapters on the socio-economic determinants of health, such as drinking water, housing, food security, and decline in calorie intake. It has chapters on the degree of the penetration and limitations of private–public partnership in the health sector. It also has a chapter bringing out the ineffectiveness and inadequacy of the regulatory framework prevailing in the Indian health sector in general and the drug industry in particular. There are three chapters dealing with the wrong choices made under the influence of profit-driven multinational companies, in the selection of the technology packages for immunisation in the country. All these chapters are set in the backdrop of an exhaustive chapter giving the trajectory of the development strategies and policies followed by the country since independence. The chapters of the last section provide a glimpse of the context in which public health services operate as well as the contemporary challenge of handling the COVID-19 pandemic.

This book thus makes an important contribution to the knowledge available on the subject of public health and provides a number of important policy guidelines. It is a must read for policy-makers and practitioners in the field of health, for civil society organisations working in this domain, and for scholars and experts in this subject.

February 2021

Muchkund Dubey
President
Council for Social Development
New Delhi, India

Acknowledgements

The idea of this book emerged from a seminar on, 'Strengthening of Public Sector Health Systems for Universal Access to Health Coverage', organised by the Council for Social Development in 2012. The initial plan of publishing all the papers as a volume evolved into enlarging the scope of the debate by inviting additional papers on newer themes emerging due to the rapidly changing political, economic, and administrative scenario along with policy shifts and their implications for universal health coverage and care.

While working on this collection, we interacted with and learned from many concerned public health scholars, researchers, and activists who gave us new insights. We have tried to capture the transitions in public health in India through different lenses and from different vantage points within a broader frame of what we consider is public health. We hope that it helps understand better the amnesia that seems to have pervaded not only the professional and the political class about the history of public health in our very diverse and dynamic country, as also those who are being fed with the elitist bio-medical perspective limited to hi-tech interventions, at the cost of a balanced view on healthcare. We are therefore very grateful to the contributors and to the Council for Social Development for supporting the idea of expanding the volume and helping in the final publication of this collection.

We would also like to thank *Social Change*, the journal of the Council for Social Development and Sage, for permitting us to include some of the papers published in the journal in 2013. Two more papers published in 2019 and 2020 have formed the basis of two chapters in this edition. These papers have been revised and updated by the authors. Special thanks to Aakar and Springer, our publishers, for working on the second edition of the book and to Andy Naorem for designing the cover page for the book. We greatly appreciate the help extended by Rachel A. Varghese and Indira Chakravarthi for the first round of copy editing and comments.

Our biggest challenge was to decide where the book should end as events overtook us with the first edition. Finally, the volume was closed with a decision that we address the contemporary changes till before the publication of the new health policy of 2017. This policy and the subsequent events demanded further expansion to the scope of the book as the promise of shifting health rights from Directive Principles to fundamental rights in the Constitution and to strengthen the public health service system to be inclusive in the 2015 draft policy—that once brought hope—still remains a mirage. This book is all about understanding the root cause of these floundering promises.

Imrana Qadeer
K. B. Saxena
P. M. Arathi

Introduction: The Idea of Universal Healthcare—Its Passage Through Time

Universal healthcare is often presented to the public as something new and innovative, a project uncluttered by externalities and non-medical issues. Despite recognising its complexities, some believe that it should have a strong gatekeeping framework that does not allow patients to seek hospital-based care and that it is much more narrowly focused on what the healthcare system itself can provide directly (Mor & Kalita, 2014). State obligation for universal healthcare and ensuing financial responsibility in other words get conveniently curtailed. This kind of gatekeeping in fact opens the gates for private providers to take over secondary and tertiary level care and excludes even the broader social determinants from core healthcare. The World Health Organisation (WHO) over time shifted to the use of the term coverage; it sees universal health coverage (UHC) not as something new, but as a minor elaboration of what was there before, of comprehensive primary healthcare (CPHC), a shift that simply makes certain features of primary healthcare more accessible, by encouraging a better use of available resources (WHO, 2005). This shift, however, was not a natural progression, but a response to the demands of the World Bank (WB), which has recently become a major player and source of finance for global healthcare, importing into healthcare its larger agenda of financial reforms (World Bank, 1987: 7–18).

While welfare and overall development have been acknowledged by the WHO to be crucially important to health, it has preferred instead to play up the importance of more medical determinants, like timely access to health services (promotion, prevention, cure, and rehabilitation) (WHO, 2010). Only a well-functioning health financing system determines whether health services can exist, they argued, and, 'whether people can afford to use these health services when they need them' (WHO, 2010: 7). This has allowed the state to retreat from its commitment to provide free CPHC to all. The idea that a health service was intrinsically dependent on welfare and overall development, as visualised in the Alma Ata Declaration (WHO, 1978), fell by the wayside, and the private sector was brought into the healthcare system in the name of efficiency, without the rules of partnership being properly laid out. The use of the notion of universal similarity in the words primary healthcare and UHC often confuses readers between 'care' or 'coverage'. Thus, these words create an initial impression that the state is still in charge of providing and extending these services.

These confusions were perpetuated in India by the Draft National Health Bill 2009, which defined itself as a bill to provide for protection and fulfilment of rights in relation to health equity and justice including those related to all the underlying determinants of health as well as healthcare and for achieving the goal of healthcare for all (Qadeer & Chakravarthi, 2010). However, what it failed to spell out was that it was set to ensure only access (coverage) and not necessarily at all the three levels of public sector services. The focus of the UHC was less on ensuring comprehensive care and more on clinical coverage through public as well as private institutions. Health problems were not tackled in terms of basic health needs or epidemiological assessment, but on the basis of available technologies. The bill defined 'affordability' as an individual's capacity to pay, and the state needs only be concerned with those who could not afford care (the below poverty line population). Its responsibility even for access was thus reduced, while a significant section of the lower middle class was left to purchase or wait for coverage.

This is a sharp departure from the constitutional understanding that health, a Directive Principle of State Policy, should in time move over to become one of the fundamental rights. The specificities of the UHC, as projected by the bill, were very different from the original concept of primary healthcare as a need-based comprehensive primary-level service covering more than just clinical care and supported by secondary and tertiary care. A strong inbuilt referral support within the different levels of care of the national health services was a component of primary healthcare. It had been conceptualised as the core of a development process that was to be self-reliant and participatory, based on scientifically sound and socially acceptable technologies (WHO, 1978). Why then did the WHO change its position between 1978 and 2005, and why did it choose the words 'universal coverage'?

Universal coverage with health services is an old ambition, one born in the post-Second World War period in European countries. Its new incarnation, the contemporary UHC, is a product of the global health agenda of more recent years. The journey from 'care' to 'coverage' is a long one for the developed and the developing countries, meandering through their respective political economies, and reflecting the threads of inequality that bind them. Also revealed in this transition are the shifts within the WHO.

The Background of Universal Healthcare

In the Western countries, over the eighteenth and the early nineteenth centuries, health services were available either as charity from voluntary institutions or on payment to providers. The late nineteenth and the early twentieth century saw the evolution of other modes of payment, such as small mutual benefit societies like the workers' contributory funds, later joined by some employers, and limited national as well as private insurance for special groups. Disease, destitution, and widespread epidemics however forced local bodies to intervene in ways that were considered preventive, such as isolation, institutionalisation, and fumigation and other sanitary measures. Poor Laws (1838) and the British Public Health Act (1848) also came into being during this period (Rosen, 1958).The Second World War brought together these fragmented providers for the first time in Britain through the national health services (NHS). While Britain evolved the tax-based NHS, Germany and France adopted insurance-based systems. In France, the private sector was very powerful in shaping the health services, while in Canada the tilt was towards state-led systems. Germany moved away from compulsory insurance due to a conflict between insurance organisations and doctors' organisations on the issue of protection of the autonomy of panel physicians under the compulsory insurance. This conflict was resolved only with the introduction of the social security system that gave equal rights to all doctors to participate as well as to practise (Labisch, 1997: 35–54).

Most of the developed countries, at the time of their industrial revolutions, through working class movements and liberal politicians like Bismarck and Chadwick, built significantly strong sanitary, water, housing, food, and other welfare systems. Post-war reconstruction over the 1940s, and the pressure of a growing middle class, further augmented these services through state interventions. The state's attempt to provide UHC was in addition to the then existing private practitioners and in partnership with them. It was also backed by high economic growth rates for over a century, in addition to the wealth that came in from Asian and African colonies. This partnership was regulated by the state. The simultaneous growth of medical services, the economy, and the welfare sector hid the crucial role of welfare services in public health till the mid-twentieth century. It was then pointed out by researchers that the early declines in mortality actually preceded the discovery of antibiotics and were linked to the role of increased food availability and better sanitary facilities (McKeown et al., 1975). By the first half of the twentieth century, however, welfare facilities became available to the majority in the West, and the wide use of antibiotics also helped in controlling infectious diseases. The importance of overall socio-economic development, rather than medical interventions, in terms of their impact on general health was thus not obvious, except to a small number of academics. Within the WHO too, these two perspectives continued to be regarded as competing with the social welfare approach not receiving the importance it deserved. Technology, institutional growth, and professionals were generally credited as the prime movers for improved health.

It is interesting that while Canada closely integrated its economy over time with the United States (USA), its welfare state opted for experiments in UHC and had one of the most vibrant Federal Laws, the Universal Medical Care Insurance Act of 1968. The movement for universal health insurance in the USA, on the other hand, was repeatedly defeated in congress as it was portrayed as giving in to socialism, a loss of freedom for individual doctors and patients, and it was considered to entail high costs due to the large number of people covered (Palmer, 1999). The USA conceded only to insurance for the elderly and for the poor, which kept a large population out of state coverage till the twenty-first century.

In Europe, the state's commitment to a social contract that ensured a certain degree of equity, distributive justice, and expansion of infrastructure allowed the emergence of UHC and universal care, as the state was able to provide a basic quality of care besides monitoring and regulating the private partners. The British NHS was the inspiration for the European countries and others to build health coverage for large populations through different patterns of infrastructure, personnel, and different mixes of public and private services. Though the experience of each of these countries with UHC varied, it is important to point out two things. Firstly, most of the Western European states focused on medical care and technology-based preventive services. Secondly, because of their early success in the economic and welfare spheres, while welfare services and economic growth were theoretically recognised as important to the health of the population, in policy and practice, health services remained quite separate from welfare planning.

Within these developed countries, healthcare moved towards corporatisation, with intensification of cost containment through financially motivated information management systems. Designed to limit wide variation in practice by professionals to suit individual needs, power shifted from autonomous practitioners to corporate healthcare managers, giving priority to administrative and bureaucratic controls. These health maintenance organisations (HMOs) were forced into mergers, consolidation, and oligopoly, raising the costs of care, favouring private insurance systems, the corporatisation of the pharmaceutical industry, and the use of more costly and more invasive technology.

This led to the emergence of the industrial–medical complex (Feinglass & Salmon, 1990; Geyman, 2003), which reduced access to services due to high costs in developed countries and brought a need to capture medical markets in the developing world to combat their own economic crisis. The one thing it certainly did not contemplate as a solution was UHC for the developing world. Interestingly, as the expansion of state insurance was a key slogan for Barack Obama's election, his Affordable Healthcare for Americans Act, 2010, had to be diluted and re-framed as the Patient Protection and Affordable Care Act for Americans 2010, because of strong opposition in Congress, before it could be passed by the House of Representatives (Qadeer & Chakravarthi, 2010).

The World Health Organisation: Transformations Within

The initial mandate for WHO (1948–58) was international monitoring of epidemics and their control and cross-border management of the spread of infectious diseases. It then expanded into training of health personnel in underdeveloped countries. Major donors of WHO favoured technology-based vertical programmes for eradication of diseases, like malaria and small pox. This model of international help without any social reforms appealed to the USA between 1958 and 1968, as this pushed for modernisation and allowed global technology markets and their influence in the developing world to grow (Packard, 1997; Brown et al., 2006). Despite this,

WHO gained reasonable global respectability due to its success in eradicating small pox over 1968–78 in the developing nations. The changed political circumstances of its members emerging from their colonial past to constitute the United Nations Conference on Trade and Development (UNCTAD) and demand fair trade and greater investment in development, gave WHO a new impetus. There was a difference of opinion about the best approach to health for a long time within WHO. One was purely based on technology, while the other emphasised socio-economic development. The new members from poor countries pressed for the second option, socio-economic development, and subsequently, the Alma Ata Declaration on CPHC was passed in 1978.

The very next year, the Rockefeller Foundation organised a conference in Bellagio with assistance from WB and the participation of the United States Agency for International Development (USAID), Ford Foundation and the UNICEF to promote selective as opposed to CPHC. The 1970s was also the time when the World Bank recognised the importance of investing in health projects, for which it established its own Nutrition Population and Health Unit (Ruger, 2005). Its influence on WHO became crucial, as the organisation was obliged to depend upon external funding, most of which came from the World Bank.

In 1982, the World Health Assembly voted for a freeze on the WHO budget, and in 1985 the World Bank gave only 20% of its assessed share to the UN bodies to show its disapproval of the WHO's Essential Drug Policy: the bank, on the other hand, now had its own drug lobby (Brown et al., 2006). Within WHO, some considered this move a threat from the World Bank (Newell, 1988) as it trapped WHO in financial dependence and conditions imposed by the external donors on its operations (Walt, 1993). Such views, however, were soon hushed up as the bank pushed for privatisation of healthcare and rolling back of investments in the public sector in the name of efficiency, macro-stability, and trade liberalisation. The financial pressure on WHO was visible from the fact that by 1986–87, its external funds were US $ 437 million, and its regular membership funding was now only US $ 543 million. By 1990, external funding overtook the regular funds by US $ 21 million, and the two Director Generals, Dr. Gro Harlem Brundtland and Dr. Margaret Chan, both accepted the strategy of external partnerships with the major stakeholders for global health.

This resulted in the emergence of new multilateral alliances between corporates in the drug industry, private financial institutions, international non-governmental organisations (NGOs), the Global Alliance for Vaccines and Immunisation (GAVI), the Bill and Melinda Gates Foundation (BMGF), and UN organisations such as Global Fund to fight HIV, AIDS, tuberculosis, and malaria, on the one hand, and governments on the other. These partners had a major role in setting the agenda for WHO and the globe, and they focused on technological solutions like universal immunisations, Stop TB 2001, and Rollback Malaria (Brown et al., 2006).

Margaret Chan claimed that the private partnerships that initiated the drive to reach the health-related Millennium Development Goals (MDGs), 'unleashed the best of human creativity' (Clarke, 2014: 17–21). The truth, however, was that by 1990, the World Bank controlled WHO by holding 54% of its total budget (Brown et al., 2006) and revealed its agenda through its report, *Investing in Health* (World

Bank, 1993: 8–11), which pushed technology packages, population control, user fees, and promoted the private sector as efficient (without providing any evidence to support this), and called for a rollback of investment in the public sector (Ibid.). In 1997 Dr. Uton Muchtar Rafei, the regional director of WHO for the South East Asian region welcomed partnerships between the private, NGO, and public sector and talked of pooling their vast resources to overcome the increasing disparities in health (Rafei, 1997).

By the turn of the century, WHO became an instrument of the new health sector reform agenda. In 2001, it came out with the report of the Macroeconomic Commission that argued for investing in health to promote economic growth, presuming that economic growth per se would improve health without taking the issue of distribution into account (Commission on Macroeconomics and Health, 2001). This myth was exposed as the much acclaimed Indian growth rate, despite touching 8–9% over the 1990s was actually accompanied by a decelerating decline in infant mortality and persistence of regional, rural urban, and social disparity. India's declines in maternal mortality over this period also remained much less as compared with other South Asian countries (Rao and Kurian, 2012) and improvements in health indicators occurred only in states where distributive justice was already greater (Deb, 2012). Moreover, food intake, especially for the poorer quintiles of the Indian population, declined as we see in the figures for calorie intake over the last twenty years (Qadeer et al., 2016).

None of this stopped WHO from moving ahead with its new partners. In the World Health Assembly 2005, the WHO for the first time endorsed a resolution on UHC. In 2009, donors announced a commitment and new financing strategy to generate US $ 5.3 billion to support it (Bump, 2010). During the conception of UHC, as it emerges from the debates, the key thrust was pooled international resources for health financing systems (insurances, taxation, with or without user fee), and for health service coverage (promotive, preventive, curative, and rehabilitative) for countries whose gross domestic product (GDP) fell short of the required levels for this sort of coverage (up to US $ 55 per capita per month). UHC was supposed to reduce financial risk and offers a service package (that was left vague). It was supported by a logic that was not really based on any historical evidence, but only theoretical assumptions. Expansion through partnerships in finance and provision, according to these assumptions, would help fill the three-dimensional gap and increase security; it would reduce cost sharing for users, help add providers, and extend coverage to the uninsured.

Unfortunately, all these assumptions were only in theory, never substantiated, as the private partner's need for financial support dominated the deal, while they did not necessarily share the aims and objectives of the public sector providers within the imaginary cube. While the coverage through any kind of insurance does not go beyond 25% of the total population, 5% of this is for government servants and private insurance (Purohit, 2014). By 2011, though Rashtriya Swathya Bima Yojana

(RSBY) had covered 27.8% of the below poverty line (BPL) families[1], even with the entry of additional insurance and providers, the cost share did not necessarily decline (Selvaraj et al., 2015). Even though the present average coverage at present is around 50%, there is little hope of reaching out to the remaining BPL and just above BPL households in the near future. This financial model also did not explain why public financing has had to shrink so much, and why it could not be expanded without bringing in all these new partners, since we see the same countries easily finding the funds to support an arms race and encourage luxury consumption (Stuckler et al., 2010; Sengupta, 2013). Countries that accepted reforms realised its problems and opted for course correction, such as Brazil and South Africa, which increased the role of public sector provisioning. Though WHO literature keeps insisting that UHC is essentially no different from the primary healthcare of the Alma Ata Declaration (WHO, 2010), clearly the two are not the same thing at all.

WHO's transit from universal care through CPHC to universal coverage via UHC is thus the story of its conceptual and ideological shift under pressure from its financiers, and its caving is until it retained only the original words, losing the essence of primary healthcare, and letting UHC become a vehicle for neoliberal reforms. The experience of health sector planning in the developing world has to be seen within the changing context of international support to global priorities in health. These new priorities bring together the 'stakeholders' as in business to pool their finances, intervene, and capture the medical markets in developing countries to promote their self-interest in trade. The ambit of this trade spans from healthcare services to drugs, medical instruments, information technology, insurance systems, personnel training, and even loans and aid. This, as Brown et al. (2006) point out, marks the shift in perspective from international to global health, where monetary efficiency, profit maximisation, and commodification of health overtake concerns for people's health. The old terminology may have been preserved, but the intent has changed from assistance and cooperation to control and market penetration.

Healthcare Strategies for the Other Half: International to Global

When the world capitalist system was hit by its second economic crisis in the 1970s, the competition between the developed economies was replaced by cooperation under the leadership of their global financial institutions. These proposed offering aid and loans at rates below global market rates and insisted on structural adjustments of national economies and health sector reforms (HSR). Most peripheral economies were persuaded to accept these reforms, while the developed countries opted for a few austerity measures affecting job markets and wages, while maintaining their heavy investment in welfare. Even so, while protecting their health sector, they ended

---

[1] This is based on the Tendulkar Committee's estimate of BPL households being 37.6% of the total in 2011 (Dror and Vellakal 2012).

up accepting severe structural changes that left it completely transformed, as we see with the NHS in Britain (Leys & Player, 2011). The USA, on the other hand, not only protected its investment in health but also managed, to some degree, to expand its national insurance coverage in the face of opposition from the private lobby. The private sector demanded greater freedom and financial coverage as partners in the UHC schemes, and their demands were met. European countries, the USA, and Australia continued to invest 8–14% of their gross national product (GNP) in the health sector (WHO, 2015: 146–155).

With the collapse of the USSR and the end of the Cold War, the ideological resistance to HSR took a big hit. International financial institutions of the metropolis, through conditional lending and loans, could now influence the trajectories of peripheral economies even as they earned profits. In the process, many countries on the periphery were forced to limit their welfare sectors and hand them over to open markets where the developed world could invest. It was this possibility of transforming the welfare sectors of the peripheral countries and entering into their medical markets that became a more attractive option for the developed nations. The World Bank's shifting concern from wealth to well-being under Robert McNamara thus created a basis for the UHC strategy.

The original concept of CPHC had envisaged meeting community health needs through participatory, appropriate technology-based primary-level care that the country and community could afford, and which was supported fully by the higher levels of health services and by state finance (WHO, 1978).This mutated into selective primary healthcare (SPHC) in the 1980s, and the first formal call for a change to a techno-centric approach that would marginalise the social dimensions of public health. By the 1990s, notions such as 'social security net', 'international standards', and even later, 'information society' were coined for middle-class consumption, and in the year 2000, the UN Summit announced its MDGs. Among its eight objectives were the eradication of poverty and hunger and providing education and health. The last, but by no means the least, was global partnerships for development. These have been replaced by Sustainable Development Goals (SDGs)[2] with renewed commitment to partnerships but, with little reflection on the failures of MDGs.

It was under these global partnerships for development that several pledges and declarations were made to pool resources for the benefit of the world's poor. It emphasised market strategy and claimed to move beyond financial aid to UHC as an overarching goal, the co-financing of a global public good through international global partnerships. In essence, though UHC was defined as 'access to healthcare', 'a right not to be denied', and 'equitable services' assured by an open market system (Ruger, 2005), it took the notion of services back to vertical technology-based programmes, borrowed or purchased from other countries at high prices: services like immunisation programmes, drugs, private insurance systems, and managed care programmes (Bump, 2010).

---

[2] The eight MGDs have been expanded to 17 SDGs that focus on symptoms, without asking why MGDs failed and are still devoid of the courage to touch the core political economy issues (Sustainable Development Goals Fund 2014).

The strategy was to deepen the links between public and private sectors, international donors and national governments of the recipient countries, and shift finance to private players for technological interventions. The World Bank's *World Development Report* in 1993 offered packages that were guides to help break up 'public good' (government health services) into marketable and non-marketable components and transform them into commodities: in the process transforming the integrated public health system. State-led insurance, wherever possible, was to provide low-cost packages for the poor to contain social unrest and to make state financing highly profitable. Balancing corporate interests, elite demands for personalised hi-tech services, and meeting some needs of the rest of the population became major objectives, and interest in welfare and poverty reduction at the global level was revived. Primary healthcare, as Bump (2010) and Low (2012) argue, had been something organic and domestic, with deep roots in the community, while UHC was something entirely new, set in motion by external forces with their own set of interests.

This raises several ethical issues as to the nature of this 'social contract' with the international collective that invests in medical service but takes no responsibility for distributive justice and ignores social concerns. It has not reviewed or studied the impact of earlier international initiatives brought from outside into developing countries, such as communicable disease control programmes, family planning, reproductive health, and child survival (Banerji, 1985; Bump, 2010). It was, in fact, the failure of these isolated interventions that led to the demand for a change in primary healthcare, and the question remains: Why are the developing countries falling back into this trap? Stuckler et al. (2010) show how the corporate and private sectors within these countries have welcomed these reforms while trade unions, nurses, and other health workers have opposed them, demanding a return to state responsibility. They point out that "the WHO must decide as an international agency whether it casts itself firmly in support of this fundamentally political process' (Stuckler et al., 2010: 6). This demand is too late, as the WHO has already thrown in its lot with the neoliberal camp.

The Universalisation of Healthcare in India

The growth of modern health services in British India was guided by the colonial government's interests: the health of the army and British civilians, the need to appease the elite, its own economic interests, as well as containing dissent such as the Mutiny of 1857. These compelled setting up positions for sanitary commissioners and stringent public health laws such as the Military Cantonment Act of 1864 and the Contagious Disease Act of 1897 for compulsory isolation in epidemics like the plague. Thus, the prime focus of sanitary reforms and protection was on maintaining the cantonment area or on very oppressive sanitary measures during epidemics for the common people (Harrison, 1994: 60–97). This narrow strategy of the colonial government was then scrutinised by the League of Nations which, in the 1920s, pressed for public health interventions, disease control, and care of migrants in the wake of large population movements as an aftermath of the First World War. The Empire too understood the importance of actually mobilising the support of local populations to ward off the possibility of political challenge. With the Indian Council Act of 1909 (Morley-Minto Reforms), health and education were transferred to the provincial governments along with financial responsibility for the two sectors. More Indians were taken into the Indian Medical Services, and local elites were encouraged to invest in setting up health institutions. The public health policy of 1914 talked of paying attention to rural healthcare, but the financial burden was shifted to provincial governments (Qadeer, 2001). Thus, by the 1920s, when spaces for public health were opened up in the presidency areas (Ramanna, 2012), it was already evident that services were inadequate, simply from the skewed distribution of drugs, vaccines, sanitary services and availability of institutions and personnel (Qadeer, 2005). The then prevailing vision of public health in Britain was certainly not applied in the colony either in terms of the sanitary reforms or population-level interventions for infectious disease (epidemic) control. Given that, even in Britain, the role of economic and welfare development (food availability and sanitary facilities, water supplies and housing) was underplayed, measures like these were far too radical to be a part of any agenda for health in the colonial context. The continuing epidemics and the famine records of British India (Zurbrigg, 1992) make it very clear that UHC was nowhere on the agenda. The focus was on British economic interest, the need to gather knowledge, handle international pressures, and elicit some local support for governance.

In the year 1937, the Bandung Conference on health and hygiene proposed that the vast rural populations be provided with basic healthcare and hygiene. The International Division of the Rockefeller Foundation played a key role here. Despite Selskar M. Gunn's proposed broad-based developmental approach to public health developed through his work in China (which is considered the basis for the later Alma Ata Declaration), and which he carried out as an employee of the Rockefeller Foundation, the Foundation pushed for a techno-centric approach to create a scaffolding for services in the colonies (Brown & Fee, 2008). As Bump notes, 'The Bandung Conference was a high watermark for advocates of social medicine and integrated approaches to health and development, but not all delegates supported this view. Paul Russell, also of the Rockefeller Foundation, was one of the principal advocates for narrow, technological interventions targeted at weak points in the transmission cycles of specific diseases. Within the Foundation—a dominant force in international health—Russell's view had the weight of history and experience on its side. Predating the Foundation, the Rockefeller family had made its first philanthropic foray into health with a campaign against hookworm in the American South beginning in 1909'. (Bump, 2010: 29)

This approach, Bump argues, was 'also much better suited to a private foundation with global ambitions because it depended very little on a knowledge of local culture, did not require a long-term presence, and could be managed by a small number of experts' (Ibid). The Second World War consolidated Russell's approach, as the fear of an economic crisis, the need for European reconstruction, resource shortages, the glamour of technologies like Dichloro Diphenyl Trichloroethane (DDT) with proven short-term success in mosquito control, all further strengthened the technology-based developmental strategy. The penetration of the markets of the developing countries by the capitalist market economies could become a security for capitalists in the developed countries. The aim of providing assistance to health programmes in developing countries to promote good will and influence policies thus became the seed for the evolution of international health (Packard, 1997). An added force in favour of modernisation and technical assistance came from the nascent educated middle class and the nationalists, who either demanded their share in governance for better development or political rights for the Indian people.

These internal pressures also led to the setting up of the Committee on Health Survey and Development in 1942, to provide basic health services to all irrespective of their paying capacity. The report of this committee was called a blueprint for India's health planning, and it specified clearly that the ill health of people was rooted in poverty and the miserable conditions they lived in (Government of India (GoI), 1946: 4–11). Yet, even when hunger and poor living conditions and lack of economic opportunities were recognised as critical for health, it did not discern the close links between the pattern and pace of India's future overall development and its implications for health and the growth of health service infrastructure. The two were treated as independent of each other: one for removing poverty and the other for improving health.

Strangely enough, this history repeats itself in the late twentieth and early twenty-first century. Despite repeated evidence from different parts of the globe, isolated, independent planning for health remained a part of that phase of international health where international bodies (USAID, Ford and Rockefeller Foundations) and the WHO influenced policies and programmes in India through their experts in advisory positions. Consultancy, aid, and technical assistance that appeared important for health to the leaders of developing countries at that point of time became a way of influencing leaders like Nehru, Nasser, Bandaranaike, and Sukarno who had worked for solidarity in the Third World and mutual cooperation and internationalism built on self-reliance, openness, and national integrity. The glamour of technology and its success in other places gave these leaders hope, and the majority of them continued to depend on international advice, especially from the WHO.

In India and other parts of South Asia, while the primary health centre network within districts was inspired by the Bandung Conference (1937), vertical disease control programmes and the family planning programme came later in the 1950s under the influence of the Rockefeller Foundation, USAID, and Ford Foundation organisations, which played a key role in narrowing down strategies of disease and population control to technology-based interventions that depended on international aid (Banerji, 1985; Bump, 2010).This shows the power of the belief that borrowed technology, irrespective of the level of development of the region to which it is transferred, can be a shortcut to health for its people. The international health advocates clung to this assumption even more strongly when inadequate land reforms, limitations of the green revolution, skewed industrialisation, stagnation of the manufacturing sector, and India's failure to break into the export market did not bring the expected economic growth. The mismatch between domestic production and needs of the majority, slow growth rates, poverty, and inequity persisted, and a narrow focus on caste-based reservations and Scheduled Caste (SC) and Scheduled Tribes (ST) welfare allowed the political leadership to ignore the other social structures that went hand in hand with economic exploitation. Thus, in the 1980s, India remained a signatory to the Alma Ata Declaration, but initially SPHC, then essential care and later primary-level care (Qadeer, 1999), replaced CPHC, in the belief that that one does not have to wait for poverty reduction or improved social opportunities to achieve health. The urban focus of health services, neglect of rural areas, failure of vertical programmes (except for small pox and polio in a very technical sense as only the polio virus was to be eliminated, not paralysis), corruption, inefficiencies, and the strong involvement of the private sector became hallmarks of the decline in health services (Prasad, 2006; Saxena, 2006).

When the capitalist crises of the 1970s hit the economy and the pressure to retreat from welfare increased, the Sixth Five Year Plan opened medical care to the Non-Governmental Organisation (NGO) and private sector, giving universal coverage by the state a final burial. By 1990, the rollback of health sector investment was to the extent of 0.9% of the GDP (Rao & Kurian, 2012). It was blindly accepted that there was no alternative to structural adjustment, and a range of systemic reforms were introduced along with a social security net. The year 2015 was then set as the year by which the MDGs were to be achieved. In India, it was the National Rural Health Mission (NRHM) that was to achieve its health goals, even though the required resources and the infrastructure and necessary administrative reforms were not in place to take it forward (GoI, 2011). Thus, none of these strategies were able to protect the poor, and the systemic distortions, inequities, and high costs of healthcare continued.

At this point then, could the UHC as proposed in the Draft National Health Bill 2010, really have worked? Was it any different from the turnkey projects adopted in the past, like malaria eradication, leprosy control, national filarial control programme, etc., which came in without any assessment of their feasibility in the Indian context and their technical effectiveness? Perhaps universality is a myth needed by the medical industry, controlled as it is by the international and national corporate organisations and their professionals. They are the ones who have gained from this new incarnation of primary healthcare, where coverage through private partnerships (with public institutions or public insurance) is the key, without ever raising issues about the definitions and content of UHC and the role of the state in it.

The Twelfth Five Year Plan went so far as to separate UHC and NRHM into two distinct programmes. For the Planning Commission experts, UHC was a means of expanding medical markets, and NRHM was simply meant for primary-level care (GoI, 2012). Now even environmental sanitation, drinking water supply, and other welfare services have become targets for the expanded technology markets, without any concern for issues of social justice for sanitation workers and structural constraints (Ramanathan & Wilson, 2015). The role of global health experts has been to push the approach of investing in health primarily through public–private partnerships (PPPs), and technology-focused medical care (which paid no attention to social and economic equity and challenges of generating employment) (WHO, 2001), through a convergence of global fund for investment in selected areas of healthcare, for which technology is available (Lancet Commission, 2013) and by shaping research in a way that it is subservient to these new guidelines of an economic rationale (WHO, 2013). The spirit of these changing national and international perspectives was imbibed by the national health policy 2017 that retracted from declaring health as a right and the responsibility of the state towards free and universal primary healthcare. It opted for targeted services and strategic purchasing from the private sector, considering it more efficient and a part of the health service system despite its divergent objectives. This assumption has been proven false globally.

The questions this book asks are: Can the present model of UHC in India be the answer to universal access/coverage and provisioning of quality basic healthcare? Is there any evidence of its advantages for the majority? And what specific challenges does it pose for the future in the Indian context? It has five sections that deal with the historical context and politics of the debates around UHC in India; strategies of the Indian state to address the present crisis of public health in the country and its limitations; an analysis of how the present policies on pharmaceutical industry and vaccines aggregates the crisis; some missing links in universalising health and importance of social determinants of health. It ends with a postscript that weaves the sections together, looks at the contemporary official hard financial data to unravel conscious overlaps of terminology that promote misconceptions, and camouflages the sickness of our present health financing system. It hopes for a genuine search for an alternative way of thinking to strengthen the public health sector.

The chapters in Part I debate the idea, concepts, history, and practice of UHC in India. Imrana Qadeer, in her chapter, exposes the inevitability of transformation of the concept of CPHC, by global markets that reconstruct healthcare from services to commodities. The official strategies in India to implement UHC are analysed to underline the neoliberal logic used by the government to expand health markets and promote UHC at the cost of CPHC. Indira Chakravarthi illustrates how neoliberal policies provide both the ideology and the mechanisms by which markets are created and expanded nationally and internationally in the health sector. Examining the current status of the corporate private sector in the healthcare industry and using experiences of mixed systems of healthcare with corporatisation from abroad, she cautions against such developments in India. Her analysis of largest private players in India illustrates how the International financial corporation contributes to the growth of private healthcare. Her evidence shows that markets and competition in healthcare systems have neither achieved universality nor cost control and regulation in the private sector. Indranil Mukhopadhyay, differentiating between concepts of 'health for all' and 'universal coverage', argues that the insurance-based financing and managed care approach based on private partnership can result in further consolidation of capital at the expense of people's money, hampering the principle of universality. This, he argues, is an outcome of the shift in the role of government from a provider to a major purchaser of services, while it continues to finance the health sector. Prachinkumar Ghodajkar unpacks the complex construct of quality in healthcare that is influenced by several tangible and intangible dimensions, including an individual patient's interest and larger social concerns regarding healthcare systems.

He conceptualises 'quality' and its different dimensions and determinants, especially in public health by taking up an analysis of different health planning and policy documents to comprehend the conceptualisation of quality in public health planning. This leads him to identify the contradictions within the present model of UHC. Archana Diwate goes beyond the explanations of financial pressure on the state by neoliberal international forces to promote market penetration into the health sector to explain its privatisation. She unravets the local sociopolitical and economic reasons behind privatisation of medical education by exploring the regional political economy that brings surpluses out of agriculture for diversification and higher profits. This social dynamics in itself limits the potential of expanding UHC through the resources—institutional as well as professional—of private medical colleges that multiply mainly in urban and developed areas.

Part II mobilises evidence that reveals the dark side of the strategies chosen for UHC, which promote shift of state subsidies to the private sector and its unregulated penetration of the health sector. Sylvia Karpagam and her co-authors bring forth empirical evidence to challenge PPP as a model for tertiary care. Their chapter critiques the Planning Commission's reference to Rajiv Gandhi Super Specialty Hospital, Raichur, as evidence for a good PPP model. It critiques the evaluation report by the Government of Karnataka and points out the limitation of this PPP model, such as the absence of third-party evaluation, poor utilisation rates, lack of measurable benefits to the BPL population, poor governance, and accountability system. Bijoya Roy explores the extent of proliferation of PPP, their types, and structural complexities. She also examines the available evidence on these arrangements with respect to their access, quality, and operational aspects, to illustrate that the complexity of monitoring, lack of efficiency, and transparency makes PPPs an unviable model even from a financial angle. The impact of totally unregulated and callous commercialisation in the public sector through PPPs is discussed through P. M. Arathi's study of sterilisation camps. She rightly argues that the state has to be responsible for the gross negligence that is often committed. The deaths in sterilisation camps, the chapter argues, have to be viewed in the context of global propaganda of population explosion despite slowing of growth rates and national policies favouring fragmentation and neglect of public healthcare delivery systems, an aggressive population control strategy, and an unregulated but protected private sector. Rajib Dasgupta, Sulakshana Nandi, and co-authors present the findings of a qualitative study on RSBY, based on provider perspective across diverse category of hospitals such as public, not-for-profit, and private. They highlight design-related issues in implementation of the scheme that neglects the nature and compulsion of different categories of institutions and explain the shortfalls in RSBY. Likewise, Sunita Reddy and Immaculate Mary provide critical reflections on a community health insurance scheme known as the Arogyasri scheme. Skewed towards curative tertiary care, it is a big drain on the state exchequer with questionable sustainability as it undermines and underutilises the existence of the larger public sector. It has led to a shift in priorities to provisioning of curative services at the cost of preventive, promotive, and rehabilitative services.

Part III explores issues in the domain of availability of drugs and pharmaceuticals. Biswajit Dhar and Reji Joseph explain how the nature of the patent regime was an important factor for the growth of the generic industry and tracks the recent developments in the Indian generic industry. They address the challenge of re-energising bulk drug production, effective integration of small and medium sector drug production, a public-supported venture fund to finance pharmaceutical innovations, integration of pharmaceutical industry with academic institutions, and a proper price control system in place to govern the market. Jacob Puliyel critiques current vaccine policy and the ensuing shifts in monitoring and regulatory process highlighting their inadequacies. He prescribes an economic model for the evaluation of vaccines in his chapter. Pushpa Bhargava shows how we make wrong choices of vaccines when better alternatives are available with relevant examples. He highlights the problems of the profit-driven private sector and inadequate and ineffective regulatory framework in the context of the Indian drug industry. S. Srinivasan and Malini Aisola describe the activities of the booming export pharmaceutical companies and emphasise the importance of medicine pricing and access by critically analysing government reports. Public–private partnership in immunisation kills the universality of preventive care model, argues Y. Madhavi, in her chapter shows a need for evidence based policy. By doing a situational analysis of vaccines in India, she argues that the market forces and international organisations are distorting national vaccine needs by extrapolating other country experiences, overstating disease burden for vaccine preventable diseases, and pushing new vaccine without a proper cost–benefit analysis.

Part IV focuses on some crucial social determinants of health and UHC. Through a historical analysis of India's political economy, K. B. Saxena examines key developmental issues and a range of related policies in India. He questions the ability of these policies to eliminate what the WHO Commission on SDH calls 'the toxic combination': a combination of bad policies, poor social and economic programmes, and unfair economic arrangements in addressing wide-ranging inequities in health. In its historical analysis, the chapter marks the changing role of state and market, transitions in agrarian relationships, trends in wages, and conditions of work. It argues that the economy would need to integrate redistribution and environmental protection to ensure developmental goals and to address health inequities.

Water distribution should be based on principles of equality, conservation, and sustainability, argues Dunu Roy and his co-authors. They critically evaluate the shifts in urban governance in the implementation of the Jawaharlal Nehru National Urban Revival Mission (JNNURM) and 'Smart Cities' and show how the proposed increase in revenues and efficiency is based on the underlying principles of legal, financial, and structural 'reforms', rationalising higher user charges, attracting external funding, private investments and partnerships in setting up hi-tech services as well as governance. The two strategies differ, but, only in the degree of aggression and dependence on foreign direct investment (FDI). They argue that the uneven distribution of safe and adequate drinking water for marginalised social groups, who are ill-equipped economically to cope with health hazards, is increasing. Sourindra M. Ghosh examines the explanations for declining calorie intakes between 1993–94 and 2010–11 by examining the intricate relationships between monthly per capita expenditure

(MPCE), total calorie/food, and expenditure on food to argue that the shifts over time are neither the outcome of declining basic needs (work pressure) for the majority, nor improved quality of food, but are linked to purchasing capacity of people, which impacts their ability to access food as they have to make difficult choices between competing needs including health. Given the importance of access to food, this dynamics has serious implications for population health. Abhay Shukla and P. M. Arathi emphasise the importance of people's participation in health service functioning and implementing programmes. The paper uses the experience from Maharashtra on the community-based monitoring system as part of NRHM within the framework of deepening democracy. It envisages people's participation as a process of expanding democracy, altering power structures in the public health system, challenging the power of health bureaucracy, and promoting people's collective power to shape health-related decision-making.

These parts are finally tied together by a postscript that summarises the reasons for the historical transition from one type of approach towards primary healthcare to another. It explores who the beneficiaries of this transition are in India and unravels how the state as a steward adopts mechanisms of data analysis and accounting that rationalise its choices. Universality and equity in health, it argues, are not the functions of the private sector but the prime responsibility of the state. The potential and possibilities lie buried in India's experience. The contradiction lies in the very nature of the state, which has for long ignored the much needed democratic correctives for realising universal and comprehensive primary healthcare.

References

Banerji, D. (1985). *Health and family planning services in India: An epidemiological, political and socio-cultural analysis and a perspective*. Lok Paksh.

Brown, T. M., & Fee, E. (2008). The Bandoeng conference of 1937: A milestone in health and development. *American Journal of Public Health, 98*(1), 42–43.

Brown, T. M., Cueto, M., & Fee, E. (2006). The World Health Organisation and the transition from 'International' to 'Global' public health. *American Journal of Public Health, 96*(1), 62–72.

Bump, J. B. (2010). *The long road to universal health coverage: A century of lessons for development strategy*. Rockefeller Foundation. Accessed May 20, 2015. http://www.paho.org/forocoberturagt2014/wp-content/uploads/2014/08/DIM-The-Long-Road-to-UHC.pdf

Clarke, L. (2014). *Public-private partnerships and responsibility under international law: A global health perspective*. Routledge.

Deb, S. (2012). Social development index in India. In Z. Hasan & M. Hasan (Eds.), *India: Social development report 2012: Minorities at the margin*. Council for Social Development, Oxford University Press.

Dror, D. M., & Vellakkal, S. (2012). Is RSBY India's platform to implementing universal hospital insurance? *The Indian Journal of Medical Research*, 135, 56–63.

Feinglass, J., & Salmon, J. W. (1990). Corporatisation of medicine: The use of medical management information systems to increase the clinical productivity of physicians. *International Journal of Health Services: Planning, Administration, Evaluation, 20*(2), 233–252.

Geyman, J. P. (2003). The corporate transformation of medicine and its impact on costs and access to care. *The Journal of the American Board of Family Practice, 16*(5) (September 1), 443–454.

Government of India. (1946). *Report of the health survey and development committee, volume II*. Manager of Publications.

Government of India. (2011). *Report of the working group on national rural health mission (NRHM) for the twelfth five year plan (2012–2017)*. Accessed December 27, 2015. http://planningcommission.nic.in/aboutus/committee/wrkgrp12/health/WG_1NRHM.pdf

Government of India. (2012). *Twelfth five year plan (2012–2017) social sectors, Volume III*. Sage.

Harrison, M. (1994). *Public health in British India: Anglo-Indian preventive medicine 1859–1914*. Cambridge University Press.

Labisch, A. (1997). From traditional individualism to collective professionalism: State, patient, compulsory health insurance, and the panel doctor question in Germany, 1883–1931. In M. Berg & G. Cock (Eds.), *Medicine and modernity public health and medical care in nineteenth and twentieth century Germany*. Cambridge University Press.

Lancet Commission. (2013). Global health 2035: A world converging within a generation. Accessed May 15, 2015. http://globalhealth2035.org/

Leys, C., & Player, S. (2011). *The plot against the NHS*. Pontypool. Merlin Press.

Low, O. G. (2012). *From ideals to implementation: Explaining the global transition to universal health coverage*. Undergraduate Thesis. Barnard College. https://academincommons.columbia.edu/…/Olivia_Low_Barnard_Thesis

McKeown, T., Record, R. G., & Turner, R. D. (1975). An interpretation of the decline of mortality in England and Wales during the twentieth century. *Population Studies*, *29*(3), 391–422.

Mor, N., & Kalita, A. (2014). Missing links in universal healthcare. *The Hindu*, November 21.

Newell, K. W. (1988). Selective primary healthcare: The counter revolution. *Social Science and Medicine*, *26*(9), 903–906.

Packard, R. M. (1997). Malaria dreams: Postwar visions of health and development in the third world. *Medical Anthropology*, *17*(3), 279–296.

Palmer, K. S. (1999). *A brief history: Universal healthcare efforts in the US*. Accessed April 6, 2015. http://www.pnhp.org/facts/a-brief-history-universal-healthcare-efforts-in-the-us

Prasad, S. (2006). Health security: A fractured dialogue. In S. Prasad & C. Sathyamala (Eds.), *Securing health for all dimensions and challenges*. Institute of Human Development.

Purohit, B. (2014). Community based health insurance in India: Prospects and challenges. *Health*, *6*(11), 1237–1245.

Qadeer, I., Sourindra M. G., & Arathi, P. M. (2016). India's declining calorie intake: Development or distress?. *Social Change*, *46*(1), 1–26.

Qadeer, I. (1999). Primary healthcare from adjustment to reform. In K. Seetha Prabhu & R. Sudarshan (Eds.), *Reforming India's social sector poverty, nutrition, health and education*. Social Science Press.

Qadeer, I. (2005). Continuities and discontinuities in public health: The Indian experience. In A. K. Bagchi & K. Soman (Eds.), *Maladies preventives and curatives: Debates in public health in India* (pp. 117–156). Tulika Books.

Qadeer, I. (2001). Impact of structural adjustment on concepts in public health. In I. Qadeer, K. Sen & K. R. Nayar (Eds.), *Public health and the poverty of reforms: The South Asian predicament* (pp. 117–156). Sage Publications.

Qadeer, I., & Chakravarty, I. (2010). The neo-liberal interpretation of health. *Social Scientist*, *38*(5–6), 49–61.

Rafei, U. M. (1997). *Partnerships: A new health vision*. WHO.

Ramanathan, U., & Wilson, B. (2015). Locating health in the movement against manual scavenging. In I. Qadeer (Ed.), *India: Social development report 2014: Challenges of public health* (pp. 81–89). Council for Social Development. Oxford University Press.

Ramanna, M. (2012). *Healthcare in Bombay presidency, 1896–1930*. Primus Books.

Rao, M., & Kurian, O. C. (2012). India's health: Not shining. In Z. Hasan & M. Hasan (Eds.), *India: Social development report 2012: minorities at the margin*. Council for Social Development, Oxford University Press.

Rosen, G. (1993). *A history of public health* (Revised Expanded ed.). JHU Press.

Ruger, J. P. (2005). The changing role of the world bank in global health." *American Journal of Public Health*, *95*(1), 60–70.

Saxena, K. B. (2006). Governance and the health sector. In S. Prasad & C. Sathyamala (Eds.), *Securing health for all dimensions and challenges*. Institute of Human Development.

Sengupta, A. (2013). Universal health coverage: Beyond rhetoric. Occasional Paper 20, *Municipal services project*. Accessed December 18, 2014. http://www.alames.org/documentos/uhcamit.pdf

Selvaraj, S., Anup, K. K., & Mukhupadhyay, I. (2015). Publically financed health insurance schemes in India: How effective are they in providing financial risk protection? In I. Qadeer (Ed.), *India social development report 2014: Challenges of public health*. Oxford University Press.

Stuckler, D., Andrea B. Feigl, Sanjay Basu, and Martin MacKee. 2010. "The Political Economy of Universal Health Coverage." (Background Paper) *First Global Symposium on Health Systems Research*. Montreux. November 16–19. Accessed April 9, 2015. http://healthsystemsresearch.org/hsr2010/images/stories/8political_economy.pdf

Sustainable Development Goals Fund. (2014). *From MDGs to SDGs*. December 17. Accessed May 10, 2014. http://www.sdgfund.org/mdgs-sdgs

Walt, G. (1993). WHO under stress: implications for health policy. *Health Policy*, *24*(2), 125–144.

World Bank. (1987). *Financing health services in developing countries/: An agenda for reform*. World Bank.

World Bank. (1993). *World development report 1993: Investing in health*. Oxford University Press.

World Health Organisation. (1978). *Primary healthcare: Report of the international conference on primary healthcare Alma-Ata, USSR*, September 6–12. WHO.

World Health Organisation. (2001). *Macroeconomics and health: Investing in health for economic development: Report of the commission on macroeconomics and health. 20 December*. WHO.

World Health Organisation. (2005). *Technical briefs for policy makers number 1: Achieving universal health coverage: Developing the health financing system*. WHO. Accessed January 1, 2016. http://www.who.int/health_financing/pb_1.pdf

World Health Organisation. (2010). *World health report: Health systems financing: The path to universal coverage*. WHO. Accessed April 7, 2015. http://www.who.int/whr/2010/10_summary_en.pdf

World Health Organisation. (2013). *Research for universal health coverage: The world health report 2013*. August. WHO. Accessed May 25, 2016. http://apps.who.int/iris/bitstream/10665/85761/2/9789240690837_eng.pdf

World Health Organisation. (2015). *World health statistics*. WHO. Accessed May 2, 2015. http://apps.who.int/iris/bitstream/10665/112738/1/9789240692671_eng.pdf

Zurbrigg, S. (1992). Hunger and epidemic malaria in Punjab, 1868–1940. *Economic and Political Weekly*, *27*(4), PE2–PE26.

Contents

Editors and Contributors

About the Editors

Imrana Qadeer is a distinguished professor at the Council for Social Development, New Delhi, India. She is a well-known public health expert. Before joining CSD in 2012, she was a professor in Jawaharlal Nehru University, where she taught for 35 years and then served as a J. P. Naik senior fellow at the Centre for Women's Development Studies. Her area of interest includes organisational issues in health services in South Asia with a special focus on India, social epidemiology and political economy of health, and women's health and research methodology with an emphasis on interdisciplinary research methodologies. She has also worked with the Ministry of Health and Family Welfare, the Planning Commission, Population Commission, and the advisory and monitoring bodies for the National Rural Health Mission.

K. B. Saxena is a distinguished professor at the Council for Social Development, New Delhi, India. He was a teacher of Political Science in the University of Delhi before he joined the Indian Administrative Service in 1964 and held important government positions such as Joint Secretary, Land Reforms; additional Chief Secretary, Government of Bihar; Secretary in the Ministries of Welfare, Rural Development and Health, Government of India. He was the principal adviser to the Planning Commission as well. He prepared the report on Atrocities against Scheduled Castes for the National Human Rights Commission and has contributed a number of articles and papers and edited several books.

P. M. Arathi is an assistant professor, School of Indian Legal Thought, Mahatma Gandhi University, Kottayam, Kerala, India. She holds a masters in law specialising in healthcare law. She has been an assistant professor in law (FIP Substitute) at Government Law College, Thrissur, Kerala, and a research assistant on a collaborative project of the London School of Economics and Jawaharlal Nehru University on spousal violence in India. She also worked as an assistant professor at the Council for Social Development, New Delhi, India.

Contributors

Malini Aisola All India Drug Action Network (AIDAN), New Delhi, India

Vasudha Akshintala Hazards Centre, New Delhi, India

P. M. Arathi School of Indian Legal Thought, Mahatma Gandhi University, Kottayam, Kerala, India

Pushpa M. Bhargava Centre for Cellular and Molecular Biology, Hyderabad, India

Indira Chakravarthi Nehru Memorial Museum and Library, New Delhi, India

Rajib Dasgupta Centre of Social Medicine and Community Health, Jawaharlal Nehru University, New Delhi, India

Biswajit Dhar Centre for Economic Studies and Planning, Jawaharlal Nehru University, New Delhi, India

Archana Diwate SATHI, Pune, India

Elangovan Gajraj National Institute of Clinical Excellence (NICE), London, England

Samir Garg State Health Research Centre, Chattisgarh, India

Prachinkumar Ghodajkar Centre of Social Medicine and Community Health, Jawaharlal Nehru University, New Delhi, India

Sourindra Mohan Ghosh Centre for Economic Studies and Planning, Jawaharlal Nehru University, New Delhi, India

Reji K. Joseph Central University of Gujarat, Gandhinagar, India

Kanica Kanungo Public Health Resource Network (PHRN), New Delhi, India

Sylvia Karpagam Urban marginalized communities, Karnataka, India

Y. Madhavi National Institute of Science, Technology and Development Studies, New Delhi, India

Reeti Mahobe Ambedkar University Delhi, New Delhi, India

Immaculate Mary Academics, i4 Connect Foundation, Hyderabad, India

Indranil Mukhopadhyay School of Government and Public Policy, O. P. Jindal University, Sonipat, India

Ganapathy Murugan Executive Director, Public Health Resource Network (PHRN), New Delhi, India

Sulakshana Nandi Co-convener of Public Health Movement, New Delhi, India

Madhurima Nundy Institute of Chinese Studies, New Delhi, India

Jacob Puliyel Paediatrics Department, St. Stephens Hospital, New Delhi, India; National Technical Advisory Group on Immunization (NTAGI), Government of India, New Delhi, India

Imrana Qadeer Council for Social Development, New Delhi, India

Sunita Reddy Centre of Social Medicine and Community Health, Jawaharlal Nehru University, New Delhi, India

Bijoya Roy Centre for Women's Development Studies, New Delhi, India

Dunu Roy Hazards Centre, New Delhi, India

Sangeeta Sahu Ambedkar University Delhi, New Delhi, India

K. B. Saxena Council for Social Development, New Delhi, India

Ruchika Sharma Hazards Centre, New Delhi, India

Abhay Shukla SATHI, Pune, India;
National Convener of People's Health Movement, New Delhi, India;
National Rural Health Mission, New Delhi, India

Dipa Sinha Ambedkar University Delhi, New Delhi, India

S. Srinivasan LOCOST (Low Cost Standard Therapeutics), Vadodara, India;
All India Drug Action Network (AIDAN), New Delhi, India

Akhila Vasan Activist with the Karnataka Janaarogya Chaluvali, Karnataka, India

Abbreviations

ACCP	Alliance for Cervical Cancer Prevention
ACE	Angiotensin-Converting Enzyme
ACIP	Advisory Committee on Immunisation Practices
ADB	Asian Development Bank
ADIP	Accelerated Development and Introduction Plans
AEFI	Adverse Events Following Immunisation
AHEL	Apollo Health Enterprises Ltd
AIDAN	All India Drug Action Network
AIIMS	All India Institute of Medical Sciences
AIMA	All India Management Association
AMC	Advance Market Commitments
AMRUT	Atal Mission for Rejuvenation and Urban Transformation
ANM	Auxiliary Nurse Midwife
APL	Above Poverty Line
ART	Antiretroviral Therapy
ASHA	Accredited Social Health Activists
AWW	Anganwadi Worker
BCG	*Bacillus Calmette–Guérin*
BCSIA	Belfer Center for Science and International Affairs
BD	Becton Dickinson
BIS	Bureau of Indian Standards
BJP	Bharatiya Janata Party
BMGF	Bill and Melinda Gates Foundation
BOOT	Build, Own, Operate, and Transfer
BOT	Build, Operate, and Transfer
BPL	Below Poverty Line
BVP	Bessemer Venture Partners
CAG	Comptroller and Auditor General of India
CAGR	Compound Annual Growth Rate
CBMP	Community-Based Monitoring and Planning
CCEA	Cabinet Committee on Economic Affairs

CES	Consumption Expenditure Survey
CGHS	Central Government Health Scheme
CHC	Community Health Centres
CHOICE	Choosing Interventions that are Cost Effective
CHW	Community Health Worker
CII	Confederation of Indian Industry
CIMS	Chhattisgarh Institute of Medical Sciences
CIOMS	The Council for International Organisations of Medical Sciences
CL	Compulsory Licence
CMIE	Centre for Monitoring Indian Economy
CMRF	Chief Minister's Relief Fund
COPRA	Consumer Protection Act
CPHC	Comprehensive Primary Healthcare
CPI	Consumer Price Indices
CRAM	Contract Research and Manufacturing
CRM	Common Review Mission
CSO	Civil Society Organisation
CSSM	Child Survival and Safe Motherhood
CT	Compute Tomography
CTRD	Centre for Tribal and Rural Development
CVI	Child Vaccine Initiative
CY	Chiranjeevi Yojana
DBFOT	Design, Build, Finance, Operate, and Transfer
DCGI	Drug Controller General of India
DEG	Deutsche Investitions-und Entwicklungsgesellschaft
DISPRUD	Delhi Society for Promotion of Rational Use of Drugs
DLHS	District-Level Household Survey
DOTS	Directly Observed Chemotherapy, Short Course
DP	Drug Policy
DPCO	Drugs Price Control Order
DPT	Diphtheria, Pertussis, and Tetanus
EHP	Essential Health Package
EMRI	Emergency Management and Referral Institute
EPI	Extended Programme on Immunisation
EWS	Economically Weaker Sections
FDC	Fixed Dose Combination
FDI	Foreign Direct Investment
FERA	Foreign Exchange Regulation Act
FICCI	Federation of Indian Chambers of Commerce and Industry
FPP	Family Planning Programme
FTA	Free Trade Agreements
FYP	Five Year Plan
GATS	General Argument on Trade in Services
GAVI	Global Alliance for Vaccines and Immunisation
GFATM	Global Fund to Fight AIDS, Tuberculosis, and Malaria

GIS	Geographical Information Systems
GMP	Good Manufacturing Practices
GNP	Gross National Product
GP	General Practitioner
GRADE	Grades of Recommendation Assessment, Development, and Evaluation
GSK	Glaxo Smith Kline
HA	Health Assistants
HFA	Health for All
Hib	Hepatitis B, H Influenza B
HLEG	High-Level Expert Group
HMIS	Health Management and Information System
HMOs	Health Maintenance Organisations
HMRI	Health Management Research Institute
HPV	Human Papilloma Virus
HRLN	Human Right Law Network
HSR	Health Sector Reforms
IANS	Indo-Asian News Service
IARC	International Agency for Research on Cancer
IAVI	International AIDS Vaccination Initiative
IBIS	Invasive Bacterial Infections Surveillance
ICD	International Classification of Disease
ICGEB	International Centre for Genetic Engineering and Biotechnology
ICMR	Indian Council of Medical Research
ICPD	International Conference on Population and Development
ICRA	Information and Credit Rating Agency
IDD	Infrastructure Development Department
IDFC	Infrastructure Development Finance Company
IDMA	Indian Drug Manufacturers' Association
IDPL	Indian Drugs and Pharmaceuticals Ltd
IFC	International Finance Corporation
IFFI	International Finance Facility for Immunisation
IFPMA	International Federation of Pharmaceutical Manufacturers' Associations
IFRI	International Forestry Resource Institute
IHH	India's Healthcare Industry
IJMR	Indian Journal of Medical Research
IMNCI	Integrated Management of Neonatal and Childhood Illnesses
IMPACT	International Medical Products Anti-Counterfeiting Taskforce
IMR	Infant Mortality Rate
INSAL	Indian Association for Study of the Liver
IOM	Institute of Medicine
IPHS	Indian Public Health Standards
IPR	Intellectual Property Rights
IPV	Injectable Polio Vaccine

IRDA	Insurance Regulatory Development Authority
ISID	International Society for Infectious Diseases
ISO	International Standards Organisation
ISQ	International Society for Quality
ITSU	Immunisation Technical Support Unit
IVCOL	Indian Vaccine Corporation Limited
JCAHO	Joint Commission on Accreditation of Healthcare Organisations
JCI	Joint Commission International
JNNURM	Jawaharlal Nehru National Urban Renewal Mission
JRM	Joint Review Mission
JSA	Jan Swasthya Abhiyan
JSSK	Janani Shishu Suraksha Karyakram
JSY	Janani Suraksha Yojana
KHSDRP	Karnataka Health Systems Development and Reforms Project
KMPG	Klynveld Peat Marwick Goerdeler
KPMCH	Kali Prasad Chowdhury Medical College and Hospital
KSHSRC	Karnataka State Health System Resource Centre
LAC	Local Audit Circle
LIC	Low-Income Countries
LIG	Low-Income Group
LMICs	Low–Middle-Income Countries
LOCOST	Low-Cost Standard Therapeutics
MARCH	Medically Aware and Responsible Citizens of Hyderabad
MCH	Maternal and Child Health
MCI	Medical Council of India
MDG	Millennium Development Goal
MLA	Member of Legislative Assembly
MLC	Member of Legislative Council
MMMHRV	Mahila Mattu Makkala Hakkugala Samrakshana Vedike
MMWR	Morbidity and Mortality Weekly Report
MNREGS	Mahatma Gandhi National Rural Employment Guarantee Scheme
MoHFW	Ministry of Health and Family Welfare
MPCE	Monthly Per Capita Expenditure
MPW	Multi-Purpose Worker
MRSA	Methicillin-Resistant Staphylococcus Aureus
MRTP	Monopolies and Restrictive Trade Practices
MSBY	Mukhyamantri Swasthya Bima Yojana
MSF	Medicines Sans Frontiers
MVI	Multi Vitamin Concentrate (Intravenous Invusion)
NABH	National Accreditation Board for Hospitals and Healthcare Providers
NABL	National Accreditation Board for Laboratories
NACP	National AIDS Control Programme
NCDC	National Centre for Disease Control
NCEUS	National Commission for Enterprises in the Unorganised Sector
NFHS	National Family Health Survey

NGO	Non-Government Organisation
NHEC	National Health Entitlements Card
NHP	National Health Policy
NHS	National Health Services
NICE	National Institute of Clinical Excellence
NIHFW	National Institute of Health and Family Welfare
NIMS	Nizam Institute of Health Sciences
NISTDS	National Institute of Science Technology and Development Studies
NITAG	National Immunisation Technical Advisory Groups
NLEM	National List of Essential Medicine
NMCC	National Manufacturing Competitiveness Council
NPPP	National Pharmaceutical Pricing Policy
NRC	NITAG Resource Centre
NREGS	National Rural Guarantee Scheme
NRHM	National Rural Health Mission
NSS	National Sample Survey
NSSO	National Sample Survey Organisation
NTAGI	National Technical Advisory Group on Immunisation
NTP	National Tuberculosis Programme
NUHM	National Urban Health Mission
NVBDCP	National Vector Borne Diseases Control Programme
O&M	Operation and Maintenance
OAE	Own Account Enterprises
OBC	Other Backward Castes
OECD	Economic Cooperation and Development
OOP	Out Of Pocket Expenses
OPD	Outpatient Department
OPEC	Organisation of Petroleum Exporting Companies
OPV	Oral Polio Vaccine
OTG	One Time Grant
PAP	Poverty Alleviation Programme
PC	Planning Commission
PDS	Public Distribution System
PE	Private Equity
PFI	Population Foundation India
PHC	Primary Healthcare
PHFI	Public Health Foundation of India
PIP	Programme Implementation Plans
PPP	Public–Private Partnership
PSU	Public Sector Undertaking
PSU	Public Sector Units
PVTGs	Particularly Vulnerable Tribal Groups
QMS	Quality Management System
R&D	Research and Development
RCH	Reproductive and Child Health

RDA	Recommended Dietary Allowances
RGSSH	Rajiv Gandhi Super Specialty Hospital
RIMS	Raichur Institute of Medical Sciences
RKS	Rogi Kalyan Samitis
RMSC	Rajasthan Medical Service Corporation
RNTCP	Revised National Tuberculosis Control Programme
RSBY	Rashtriya Swathya Bima Yojana
RTI	Reproductive Tract Infection
RTI	Right to Information
SAE	Serious Adverse Events
SAM	Severe Acute Malnutrition
SAP	Structural Adjustment Programme
SCA	Service Contract Agreement
SCCS	Self-Controlled Case Series
SDGs	Sustainable Development Goals
SHG	Self Help Group
SHRC	State Health Resource Centre, Chhattisgarh
SHSRC	State Health Resource Centre
SIHFW	State Institute of Health and Family Welfare
SIVAC	Supporting National Independent Immunisation and Vaccine Advisory Committees
SLIM	Society for Less Investigative Medicine
SME	Small and Medium Enterprise
SPHC	Selective Primary Healthcare
SSK	Swasthya Suvidha Kendras
STG	Standard Treatment Guidelines
SUD	Sudden Unexpected Death
TCC	Treatment Counselling Centres
TCS	Tata Consultancy Services
TDB	Technology Development Board
TH	Tertiary Hospital
TPA	Third-Party Administrator
TPPA	Trans-Pacific Partnership Agreement
TRIPS	Trade-Related Aspects of Intellectual Property Rights
UHC	Universal Healthcare
UHIS	Universal Health Insurance Scheme
UIP	Universal Immunisation Programme
ULB	Urban Local Bodies
UNCTAD	United Nations Conference on Trade and Development
UNFPA	United Nations Population Fund
UPSS	Usual Principal Subsidiary Status
USAID	United States Agency for International Development
VGF	Viability Gap Funding
VHNWSC	Village Health, Nutrition, Water Supply, and Sanitation Committee
VL	Voluntary Licence

VPD	Vaccine Preventable Diseases
WB	World Bank
WHA	World Health Assembly
WHO	World Health Organisation
WSP	Water and Sanitation Programme
WTO	World Trade Organisation

List of Figures

List of Tables

List of Maps

Part I
Ideas, Concepts, History, and Practice of UHC in India

Chapter 1
Universal Health Coverage: The Trojan Horse of Neoliberal Policies

Imrana Qadeer

Promises made by governments at a given point of time may not be as realistic as they sound especially, if the ambitions of planning for a given sector appear contrary to the overall trends. A careful analysis of the content and historical continuities helps to assess how realistic they are. This is an examination of the acceptance of universal healthcare by Indian policy-makers by briefly reviewing the historical contexts of (a) capitalist development and the place of welfare and technology therein; (b) the Indian context of universal healthcare; and (c) initiation of policy for achieving universal healthcare. This chapter is an attempt to highlight the trends and the challenges till 2013, the year in which the last of India's Five Year Plans, formulated since 1951, saw the light of day.

The International Context

High growth rates in capitalism came with low employment and welfare and were challenged by the socialist system despite its lower growth rates. In the 1930s, when capitalism faced its first crisis, it used the strategy of state investment into the welfare sector to tackle market stagnation and solve the problem of unemployment. Thus, welfare too became the political face of a capitalist alternative to the socialist model; a model where capitalist states regulated markets and invested in it. The politics of solidarity in Europe, cooperation within the Western block, congenial international arrangements between the United States (US) and its allies and unequal terms of trade with the former colonies gave some stability to the capitalist order under US leadership. It offered consumerism and aid to its slow-growing periphery—countries that were no more colonies but were reintegrated as primary producers and as external markets. Though it is also argued that wars and the ensuing production and arms sale

I. Qadeer (✉)
Council for Social Development, New Delhi, India

I. Qadeer et al. (eds.), *Universalising Healthcare in India*,
https://doi.org/10.1007/978-981-16-5872-3_1

were greater forces in the making of this system rather than welfare, it is accepted that the welfare sector expansion played an important role in rejuvenating the economy. The emergence of institutions like the International Monetary Fund (IMF), World Bank (WB), and General Agreement on Tariffs and Trade (GATT) undoubtedly helped to concentrate power over the 1930s to 1960s in the hands of the Western block, where most of the trans- national corporations were located (Beaud, 2004: 213–26).

The search for new markets created inter-imperialist conflicts within capitalist economies. The hegemony of the US over this search was threatened and the oil crisis added to the woes of the Western countries, which intensified the business of loans and aid and fresh wars in West Asia. Yet, it failed to contain the next global crisis. The Asian countries, despite their relative economic resilience, started getting trapped in the debt burden.

Capitalist economies failed to retain their growth rates which fell from 4.9% in the 1960s to 2.9% in the 1980s (Schmidt and Hersh 2000: 1–16). The system had no option but to revert to surplus extraction without welfare—the neoliberal model of the 1970s. Broadly speaking, neoliberalism refers to the capitalist restructuring that has occurred since the 1970s and celebrates unhindered markets as the most effective means of achieving economic growth and public welfare' (Maskovsky & Kingfisher, 2001, p. 105). It is a global hegemonic project to destroy local processes and its policies of privatisation, deregulation, liberalisation are for profit maximisation in the name of monetary efficiency. Under it the state 'rolls back' its function so that welfare, including health, is transformed from a service into a revenue generating commodity. Governmentality therefore reimagines interpretations of social and cultural relations and reassembles them to govern from a distance. The collapse of the USSR and absence of its ideological resistance helped this shift. Lowered demands reduced profitability of production leading to the growth of finance capital, which maximised profits through constantly shifting investments in global production sites, making speculation rather than production the key to profits. Information technology became the instrument of this growing phenomenon of finance capital. To control peripheral economies, lending and trade on unequal terms became instruments for extraction of profits by the international financial and political institutions. The North, especially the US, protected its own agriculture and labour to the extent possible and attempted to practise austerity, while the former socialist states were forced to face the consequences of the economic shock and the developing periphery of the capitalist system was offered Structural Adjustment Policies (SAP). In the process, many countries that constituted the periphery were forced to undermine their welfare sectors and use them for extraction of surplus. Transforming the structural contours of infrastructures for the health and education sector and reinvesting in them became a policy alternative. The strategy was to deepen the links between public and private sectors, shift state subsidies to private sector, focus on technology-based services (with promotion of hi-tech) and commoditise them, and create low cost alternatives for the poor to contain social unrest. Thus, balancing corporate interests, elite demands for personalised hi-tech services and needs of the majority were attempted. The interest in welfare markets and poverty reduction was again revived in this neoliberal model of development (Bello, 2002: 91–106).

A few interesting lessons can be drawn from this brief history. The first is that, historically, welfare has been the field of action in the two major global economic crises; in one, it was the field for investment and in the other, the focus of financial cutbacks and restructuring that revived revenue generation. Second, technology played a crucial role in both eras. The outburst of new technologies during the Industrial Revolution led to absorption of labour and expanded employment, making welfare possible by increasing paying capacity. The nature of technological inventions in sectors such as medicine (antibiotics, vaccines, chemicals for vector control, nutritional supplements), drinking water supply (filtration plants and piped water supply) and sanitation (sanitary pits and waste disposal technologies), and transport (roads, railways, bus systems), made extensive population coverage possible and economically feasible, thereby scaling up these services. The second crisis of the 1970s preceded by the electronics-based communication revolution was tackled partially by this very technology for faster movement of financial capital across the globe (Perez, 2002); it increased wealth without actually increasing production. The invention of the chip revolutionised the invasive power of medical technology, made it more individualised, costly and restrictive of employment within the sector. This character discouraged scaling up of its services that are concentrated in the medical markets for those who could afford it or in tertiary care public institutions. The old technologies were downgraded or discarded in the name of modernity and advancement, irrespective of their relevance in the context of countries of the periphery. These new technologies backed by Health Sector Reforms (HSR) helped promote loans, international trade and private insurance systems in medical services and served the interests of the corporate sector, not necessarily the public health interests of these countries.

These trends have had a detrimental effect on the welfare sectors of the countries constituting the periphery of the capitalist system. SAP meant rollback in the welfare sector including health, handing over medical care to the private sector, opening public hospitals to private investments and their commercialisation, casualisation of workers in the name of efficiency, public private partnerships and a techno-centric focus. This helped deepen the links with the global market and between public and private sectors, penetration of local markets by multinational corporations, shifts of subsidies from public to private, commoditisation of health services and change of role of the state from commanding to overseeing and stewardship (Qadeer, 2009: 228–248).

It was inevitable that these policies unfolded differently in different countries, given their historical and political contexts and political orientation. Latin America, which accepted SAP much earlier, as well as South Africa had a different trajectory of building their welfare sectors as compared to India. Their democratic systems were relatively more inclined to limit the weakening of welfare due to reforms and invested more in the health sector (Heller, 2009; World Bank, 1994: 200–210), even though hi-tech curative services dominated. In India, particularly, the influence of the guidelines offered by the World Bank was significant in shaping the financial systems and restructuring healthcare systems (World Bank, 1993). Woven into the evolutionary story of its consolidating elite—the landlords, the industrial bourgeoisie and the emerging middle classes—India's official acceptance of SAP not only further integrated the country into the periphery of the capitalist system but also set the stage for a major transformation of its welfare sector including health sector. The neoliberal challenge to expand and transform the scope of the medical market compelled governments to ignore Comprehensive Primary Healthcare (CPHC) and opting for Universal Health Coverage (UHC). Any analysis of UHC in contemporary India therefore, cannot be serious without locating it in this historical context and linking it up with the neoliberal strategies of the Indian state—now opting out of its commitments to CPHC, without openly rejecting it.

The National Context of UHC for India

The concept of universality in health services is not new to India. The British realised the importance of epidemic controls for self-protection and economic expansion and winning over people for consolidating the regime and in the latter half of their rule, started introducing services for the common man. The nationalist movement further pressed them to implement welfare policies and in 1942, the Bhore Committee (Government of India (GoI), 1946) was set up by the British to evolve a blue print of health services for the country. The Five Year Plans used some of its recommendations, the Mudalair Committee Report (GoI, 1961) reviewed the achievements, and the Government of India accepted the Alma Ata Declaration on CPHC which was supposed to be people-oriented, based on needs and affordable technology, at the core of the developmental process, and funded and provided by the state (World Health Organisation (WHO), 1978). In these efforts to achieve universality, the two core principles were free services for all and state provisioning.

While the Bhore Committee report was the blueprint till the Fifth Five Year Plan, from the Sixth and the Seventh Plan onwards, medical care was opened to non-governmental and private sectors. Significant expansion of the private sector from the 1970s onwards and increasing state subsidies for it made it an important player after the mid-1980s. The Bhore Committee lost its attraction for the state which formally accepted SAP and the first set of HSR in the early 1990s, bringing down the investment in health to 0.96%, 0.88% and 0.91% of Gross Domestic Product (GDP) over 1991–92, 1995–96 and 2003–04, respectively (Rao et al., 2005: 239–255), opening medical care to markets, introducing user fee and contractual services in public institutions and Public Private Partnership (PPP). This first phase of reforms based on receding state control did not mean retreat of the state (as is often professed), but a much more hardened state, re-engineered as the safety net for capitalism (Lang, 2002) and nicknamed as the 'steward'. Its direction became anti-poor, anti-welfare and least concerned about the prevailing hunger even among children as is evident from the inability to meet the Supreme Court's directives on hunger (Right to Food

Campaign, 2008). This transformed state, through consistent policy changes, consolidated the markets and the interests of those who had access to it. It is therefore heavily guided by class (Patnaik, 1995: 195–219).

Social and political pressures and conflicting interests within the government did bring about some limited pro-people policies and programmes such as Mahatma Gandhi National Rural Employment Guarantee Act (MGNREGA) and Right to Information Act. In services however, the trend to push for market expansion and partnerships with the private sector prevailed. The WHO through the Commission on Macro Economics and Health heralded the second phase of HSRs that proposed investing in health (WHO, 2001). This was a measure to support higher growth rates in economies in distress through commoditisation of health services and its techno-centric growth rather than to improve equity in public health. The slogan of inclusive development was used by the government's flagship programme, the National Rural Health Mission (NRHM), promising full coverage to the rural population. In reality, it reduced CPHC to Essential Primary Level Care primarily limited to reproductive health and family welfare with disease control and infrastructure maintenance acquiring the lowest priority over time (Accountability Initiative, 2015: 4). The district's secondary level institutions were given autonomy at the cost of their service links with tertiary level institutions, liberating tertiary public institutions from their referral responsibilities, to join the market. This autonomy also meant institutional growth guided by the market pressures rather than the priorities of population's epidemiological needs. Thus, the more paying services grew at the cost of a more balanced expansion of services.

The achievements of NRHM did not match the accepted United Nations (UN) millennium goals of: (i) halving 'extreme poverty' by the target year 2015, (ii) child mortality (under five) was to be reduced to 2/3, (iii) Maternal Mortality Rate (MMR) to 3/4, (iv) HIV/AIDS, tuberculosis and malaria were to be combated (though in collaboration with the pharmaceutical companies), and (v) sanitation and drinking water supply were to be improved with better technology (UN, 2014). Thus, while it distorted the structure, its performance was inadequate. A recent review indicated some success in improving drug supplies, increasing the number of functional PHCs in addition to creating Accredited Social Health Activists (ASHA). It pointed out that NRHM never received the required financial support of INR 900 per capita and functions with an allocation of only INR 270 per capita (Dhar, 2011). This is in contrast to India's defence expenditure being INR 170,913 crores for the year 2011–12, a sum which inevitably impacts inputs into welfare and leads to a health expenditure of INR 28,353.06 crores (GoI, 2016: 4; Centre for Budget and Governance Accountability (CBGA), 2012: 30) for the same period. The budget for the year 2016–17 in health and defence is over INR 33,000 and INR 246,000 crores showing the widening gap between the two (GoI, 2016).

In this milieu of contradictory pressures from donors to restructure the health sector and invest in it on one hand, and from popular movements to consider health and food security as a fundamental right on the other, the Indian state shifted its commitment from CPHC to UHC. The latter was defined by the High Level Expert Group (HLEG)—camouflaging differences between the two concepts—as follows:

Ensuring equitable access for all Indian citizens in any part of the country, regardless of income level, social status, gender, caste or religion, to affordable, accountable and appropriate, assured quality health services (promotive, preventive, curative and rehabilitative), as well as public health services addressing wider determinants of health delivered to individuals and populations, with the government being the guarantor and enabler, although not necessarily the only provider, of health and related services (Planning Commission (PC) 2011a: 3).

From the case studies though, of Brazil and South Africa that accepted reforms and were referred to earlier, it is evident that despite high investments in health, equity remained an issue while medical markets flourished. How will India face this dilemma, unravelled by the policies that unfolded after the year 2009?

Contemporary Official Strategies to Provide UHC in India

The preamble of the Draft National Health Bill was a rather lofty document promising "protection and fulfilment of rights in relation to health, and well-being, health equity and justice, including those related to all the underlying determinants of health and healthcare" (GoI, 2009: 6). It granted health as a fundamental human right that requires an overarching legal framework but the framework focused only on responsibilities of state as a steward not as provider. Explicit definitions of terms were neglected by the Bill making multiple legal interpretations possible. For example, it used terms such as essential public health system, essential health facilities and healthcare services but did not make explicit their boundaries or, which of these would be universal. The understanding of universal access was monetary—financial support for approaching a provider, public or private—affordable for the state, irrespective of actual services.

While certain key social determinants were a part of the core responsibility of the state (safe drinking water, housing, sanitation, food), neither minimum standards to be achieved for these were spelled out nor were specific mechanisms set up to ensure inter-ministerial convergence. Third, the Bill was more concerned with the private providers and did not specify the responsibility of the public sector except for its role in public health services for the marginalised. The issue of universalisation therefore remained vague and devoid of a time plan. Fourth, by putting the private and public providers in the same basket of an integrated system, the Bill ignored not only the basic contradictions of the two, but also tilted the balance in favour of profits for the private sector by ensuring payments for services by the state without articulating shared objectives or conditions and liabilities of this partnership. Fifth, the Bill proposed state and district level Public Health Boards to implement obligations, formulate rules and regulations for recruitment from the open market, develop mechanisms for PPP and empower decentralised monitoring committees, but no principles for this implementation or regulation were articulated. No institutional redressal mechanisms for non-medical services like drinking water, sanitation, etc., were mentioned, nor were schedules, by-laws and rules circulated. In other words, the Bill remained a policy document of the steward—the agency in service of—rather than a law for—the private sector.

Following the Bill, the Twelfth Five Year Plan Approach Paper, apparently oblivious of the financial cutbacks on public sector in health and the ensuing loss of its pride and prestige, lamented about the sector's lack of capacity to deliver services. Ignoring failures to contain malaria, tuberculosis, leprosy and filariasis, it proposed expansion into new areas like handling deafness, care of the elderly, oral fluorosis, mental diseases, cancer, etc. It limited prevention to education and counselling, ignoring the conditions of poverty. While it proposed participation and community-based validation for the primary level services, not a single thought was spared for the regulation of tertiary institutions of the private sector that are at the core of the business of medical tourism. Promising more resources, insurance system, training and expansion of health manpower and drugs, the approach paper accepted that publicly financed healthcare does not necessarily mean provisioning of services. It emphasised the virtues of public–private partnerships, publicly financed insurance schemes such as the Rashtriya Swasthya Bima Yojana (RSBY), of outsourcing diagnostics and of a universal healthcare system on the same lines (PC, 2011b).

In 2010, the PC set up a HLEG that laid out a plan for rebuilding universal healthcare services. While the conceptualisation of content and structures was not much different, the key difference from CPHC's underlying principles was that the state was fully responsible for ensuring access, but for provisioning it could use all the private providers as partners under contract. The main challenges thrown up by the definition were (a) resource mobilisation for strengthening of public sector and subsidies for the private providers; (b) working out the integrative processes within the public sector programmes and between public and private sectors; (c) the regulatory mechanisms of the two sectors and conditions for partnership; (d) time plan for achieving universal care; (e) prioritising the needs of those below the poverty line and those sitting on it (an equal proportion); and (f) defining the private partner's responsibility in national disease control programmes, maintaining national health statistics and monitoring mechanisms. To handle these, the HLEG upheld the principle of universality, equity and higher investments in the health sector. It was clear that the state must be "primarily and principally responsible for universal healthcare which is an entitlement to comprehensive health security" (PC, 2011a: 3). Hence, public sector services must be strengthened, improved and brought to centre stage to ensure 'access and services' to all sections of the people. They recommended that user fees in public institutions should be discontinued; participation of citizens must go beyond existing forms of community involvement in preconceived programmes of provisioning and monitoring healthcare. It was argued that UHC could succeed only if it was founded on common interests of all sections, social solidarity and cross-subsidisation across classes. Hence, it proposed a single universal method of financing through general and differential health taxation and recommended that "70% of it should go to primary healthcare" (Ibid.: 12).

Despite these positive recommendations, four basic problems are noteworthy. The recommendation to augment the services, private sector institutions and individuals could be contracted in under clearly prescribed contractual conditions may sound feasible but, given the present balance between private and public sectors and their non- existent regulatory mechanisms, it was impractical. It did not follow any analysis of either the divisions within or the nature of private sector or where best regulated linkages are feasible. Countries like Sri Lanka have successfully used their primary providers to help in primary level care while the state focused on building an efficient and well-regulated secondary and tertiary level services in the public sector offering effective, epidemiologically appropriate services. Such a system provides professional and moral authority to the state's regulatory mechanisms. Given a relatively undermined public sector in India itself needs to evolve, the licence for partnership could act as a Trojan horse for the masters of industry, waiting to transform fully, need-based tertiary care into a full-fledged medical market. An open proposition of PPP—even if conditional—at all levels without strengthening state services opens spaces for the powerful corporate sector that has been pressing the government for spaces at all levels of services to earn huge revenues (CII & McKinsey, 2002: 93–118).

The second problem area is the package of services at different levels itself which is left to the experts who till date have not found answers to the challenge of integration of vertical programmes. They themselves first need to grasp the boundaries of systems covering medical service, healthcare service and comprehensive health. They have stuck to fertility control programmes based on technology and failed to locate fertility within the same social determinants that cause ill health. Similarly, the official experts continue to project Primary Level healthcare as CPHC as, hi-tech in medical care and the norms of care set by corporate hospitals are acceptable to them. As a vision document, it was necessary for HLEG to set guidelines for developing the package using epidemiological reasoning for technological choices at different levels.

Thirdly, the recommendations totally ignore the vast presence of traditional practitioners in the country and the fact that in 14 major states, about 20–98% households reported using them in the past three months and in five of these the use was 60–98% (Priya & Shweta, 2010: 129–40). Equally disturbing is the neglect of the present system of medical education which does not sensitise doctors to the prevailing national dilemmas of universalising healthcare. Trained to judge services through international standards, doctors are encouraged to migrate to achieve those.

Fourth, while health security is inclusive of a broad range of welfare services, these are left to overall planning without confronting the extent of non-availability of food, drinking water, housing and sanitation and its impact on health. By ignoring the constraint these social determinants impose on achieving health through technology-based services, the group of experts remained confined to intra systemic techno-managerial solutions giving them priority over social and structural issues. UHC then might achieve universality of access for a limited number but not necessarily health for all.

The Steering Committee for Health constituted by the PC to guide the Twelfth Plan (PC, 2012), while considering the recommendations of HLEG, altered its own approach to public health by selectively choosing from the HLEG recommendations. It emphasised flexibility in its own approach, stewardship role of the state, importance of using the strengths of the private sector and accepted the recommendation of purchasing-in services from private providers and a multi-sectoral approach without clearly articulating it.

Low financial input and dependence on insurances, PPPs and pressure on states to contribute remained its financial strategy. It planned for a reduction in Out of Pocket Expenses (OOPE) from 71 to 51% by the end of the plan and saw UHC as Essential Health Package (EHP) of clinical services provided by in-patient and ambulatory care covering Reproductive and Child Health (RCH), emergency services, essential medicines for most of the disease burden in the country (Ibid.: 13). It also proposed pilot UHC projects for universal care in one district of each state and testing different mixes of providers (Ibid.: 25–26) enrolling households under empanelled providers, both public and private. They would be credited for the cash-free services they provide by a system of per capita capitation fee. It appears that undue urgency for UHC rather than a long-term perspective guided the Steering Committee. It had a flawed notion of public health itself separating clinical care from all other activities of the sector even though it claimed a "systemic approach" (Ibid.: 4) and at the same time wished to rely upon private providers. This managed care like model was primarily dependent on state resources and had little in common with the US experience of managed care that covered not the poor but those who could pay through Health Maintenance Organisations (HMOs) that controlled and managed medical providers (Sekhri, 2000).

Despite underlining the financial and structural problems of the public sector and saying that "strategies of provision of inputs and creation of infrastructure under NRHM have not translated into assured healthcare services for the people" (Ibid.: 6), it paid little attention to the problems it identified such as disconnect of disease control programmes with other social sectors, weak use of traditional systems, poor practice and drug regulatory system and public health management. It selectively picked up the strategy of contracting-in private providers from the HLEG and added referrals services through involving private providers. Timelines and linkages of NRHM and UHC remained vague and the age-old strategy of focusing on high fertility states and integration of vertical programmes into NRHM was restated. Significantly, the responsibility of reviving public sector infrastructure was left to the state in the name of the state's autonomy and flexibility. Training a range of personnel, developing health information systems and handing social determinants of health through a cadre of public health were mentioned, but the process and principles for accomplishing these were not. The committee essentially believed that the health sector primarily focuses on the delivery of curative services. It thereby ignored the history of evolution of public health service in India that, apart from using curative care for prevention, built promotive programmes by provisioning food and food supplements and sanitation and drinking water to vulnerable populations. Except for the proposal of State Public Health Acts and a system for providing free drugs for EHP, not much was new.

Strengthening of tertiary care was an independent task and private sector facilities were put centre stage with the logic that it caters to 60% of inpatients. The members never explored its referral linkages or asked who constituted this 60% and what were their illnesses? The potential of primary and secondary level care in reducing the heavy burden on tertiary institutions was ignored along with the fact that the majority of the poor still depend upon public sector tertiary care. Given this perspective and the space provided to the representatives of the private sector and industry and the market bias, the HLEG's relatively rational recommendations displeased the PC whose internal steering committee has prepared a road map for health sector reforms and delivery of UHC where a major role is given to the private sector and the private insurance companies. In its own assessment report to the Prime Minister, the PC is reported to have criticised the HLEG for its neglect of traditional systems. Referring to the well-established private sector, it commented that with the major share of personnel, beds and patients, the private sector has to be partnered with for healthcare. It found that, "The [HLEG] report has not taken cognizance of the existence of a functioning health system built over decades, or assessed its potential or reasons for gaps,"… "The HLEG report instead proposes creation of a new set-up for implementation of its goal… has focused exclusively on UHC (universal healthcare) and, thereby, lacks holistic prospective," The Commission's report also argued that, "The steering committee report, in contrast, has prepared a road map for health sector reforms and delivery of UHC." It added that increase in public health spending will not translate into lower OOPE on health as projected by the HLEG (Makkar, 2012: unpaged). This is a reflection of PC's vision and understanding of UHC and Primary Healthcare due to which it has failed to keep its promise to invest adequately in the health sector every year of the Eleventh Plan. The Commission members refused to interpret Universal Healthcare not as cashless clinical services to lower OOPE alone but, as a strategy for state-funded CPHC in a time-bound plan where the marginalised have a priority in services. The objection of the Ministry of Health to this overhaul by the PC did not have much effect. Those in power have their own vision of UHC where reduction of OOPE is more critical as it means higher state subsidies for the private sector.

For them HLEG's vision is not desirable but partnership with the private sector is in the name of a holistic perspective.

> Caught between the welfare approaches of the HLEG, however constrained, the report and the crass neoliberalism of the Steering Committee, the chapter on health in the Twelfth Plan (PC 2013) attempted to find a midway but could only make it less crass. For it, UHC is "some form of coverage" (Ibid.: 10) meant for equity in healthcare through assured EHP for a large percentage of people. "Inevitably, the list of assured services will have to be limited by budgetary constraints," (Ibid.: 8) while delivery is through managed care model. How will it link up to the public health programmes to form an effective preventive strategy beyond reducing pain and suffering is not clear. For example, if 75% of the tuberculosis (TB) cases are to be diagnosed and 85% treated over the next 10-15 years to reduce disease incidence then, how would public and private institutions or NRHM and UHC coordinate and cooperate in achieving this task? Lacking in such precise planning and a vision, the Twelfth Plan, like all previous such documents, leaves crucial questions unanswered.

Emphasising the necessity of strengthening public health services—NRHM/National Health Mission (NHM) and the national disease control programmes—the draft Chapter calls them 'the second step' of UHC. Unfortunately, Primary Health Centres and Community Health Centres that also provide clinical care are sidelined by the urgency to achieve UHC through managed care within two plans as it ensures absence of a level playing field for the ill functioning public sector institutions that may not be able to compete with private/corporate setups. Their strengthening should be the first step but the draft document incorporates all the Steering Committee's fragmented recommendations for public health, UHC, PPPs and state-funded insurances like the RSBY based on the argument that the existing resources of the private sector cannot be ignored. As of today, RSBY functions as a type of PPP (Bajpai & Saraya, 2012) and the challenge of integration, coordination and convergence remain ideas awaiting translation into plans. Interestingly, while public sector institutions are encouraged to mobilise their own resources through autonomous functioning, PPPs are helped from industry's corporate social responsibility funds. Meanwhile, no mention is made of the private and corporate tertiary sector's profits and its role and responsibility.

While the Eleventh Plan itself proposed a 3% investment in the health sector and the Twelfth Plan proposes 2.1%, only 0.42% of the GDP goes to drinking water and sanitation. These investments are the same as in the Eleventh Plan (CBGA, 2011: 21), reflecting the real concern for social determinants. With the huge burden of subsidies promised to the private sector, what would remain to run and strengthen public sector services and infrastructure is not clear. Even the shortages for NRHM perhaps cannot be met. The document puts heavy pressure on resource-starved states to finance their health plans and other welfare services, and on districts to take responsibility of creating PPPs, revealing the power relation between states and the centre.

The Trends and the Challenges for the Future

As we saw in the earlier sections, the nature of technology and its organisation had been at the core of the public health planning for India. The first wave of technology that came to India between 1930 and 1960–70 was such that much of it could be scaled up within available resources. In other words, within a public health perspective—by judicious choice of technology and its clinical application in an organised form—organised medical interventions could transcend individual orientation of medicine to impact the history of diseases through national disease control and eradication programmes. This was initially hampered by inadequate planning strategies that selectively picked on the Bhore Committee's recommendations and over time focused on urban-based super-specialisations rather than rural and urban basic health services. Later, the planning process was overshadowed by the needs of the growth-oriented model of development where costly and individualised technologies promised greater revenues from the emergent medical markets at home and abroad during the latter half of the twentieth century. In the West (the home of modern medicine), this shift was credited to the success of the first phase of medical technologies and also to the accompanying improvements in the living standards of the people that contributed to the control of infectious and nutritional maladies. The movement of technological evolution from mass based to hi-tech individualised care in such a milieu was uneventful as some of the basic mass-based services remained.

However, pushed by the global medical market, its premature transfer to the periphery of the capitalist system—where countries were still struggling with a huge burden of malnutrition, infectious and non-infectious diseases—created a crisis in their health sectors.

Instead of making the right technological choices from the old and the new, India chose to accommodate the hi-tech medical market for its neoliberal developmental model. India's Tenth Five Year Plan emphasised Essential Primary Healthcare and welcomed private participation in healthcare (PC, 2002: 83–91). Following in its steps, the Eleventh Five Year Plan welcomed medical tourism and hi-tech based tertiary care and went ahead to rationalise it by proposing, "the people's growing lack of trust in the public system" (PC, 2008: 68). The Steering Committee (PC, 2012) and the Twelfth Plan thus share one major vision, which is fragmentation of services into UHC, NRHM, state-led insurances and tertiary care, all based on an intermingling of public and private sectors in different ways. The PC documents are significantly silent on the role of corporate medicine and its pressure to participate in all levels of care giving (CII & McKinsey, 2002). While the UHC is ultimately seen as a network of curative services, NRHM remains an independent effort at providing an EHP, with RCH and family welfare at its core and selected vertical disease control programmes at its periphery. This has further fragmented clinical care, marginalising tertiary care within the scope of the public sector and shifting it into the hands of more powerful corporate and private sectors. The public sector tertiary care is to survive on PPP (for which the private partner can get 20% funding from the state), help from corporate social responsibility funds and self-generated resources according to the Twelfth Plan proposals! For effect, however, the six All India Institute of Medical Sciences (AIIMS) like institutes of the future are projected without any planned regional referral function.

Second, the push and the urgency for UHC is being used to rationalise a partnership between public and private sectors with an emphasis on tertiary care. While the HLEG at least envisages a conditional partnership (without specifying them), the PC documents mentioned above, treat them as equal partners in a homogeneous system without any conditionality, or even identifying the complexity of the private sector and the problems at each level. There is an assumption that given the fact that there are a number of private and public providers, there is one uniform, homogeneous system. So both public and private providers are made a part of the single healthcare system. This is a flawed vision as the centrality of profit for the private sector makes their objectives contradictory. If at all they make a system, it is parasitic where one sector thrives on the other taking advantage of its power relationship. Given the political context where industry guides national planning and has identified the health sector as a major source of revenue, where political leadership translates corporate responsibility as a means of guiding the functions of the state and as a right and duty to enter the social sector (rather than using ethical practices in business): the power balance between the two sectors is evident.

Third, these documents are insensitive to the fact that clinical medicine is a powerful instrument of prevention and when organised to achieve efficient coverage of population, can lead to control and prevention and thereby change the history of disease. They promote only insured individualised medical care under UHC with no perspective of disease control. No concern has been shown as to how the private and public providers will coordinate and collaborate to ultimately synchronise their services to achieve public health goals. Hence, mechanisms of coordination and cooperation (in addition to regulation) are not debated though the need for regulation is accepted.

Fourth, while the need for defining essential care at various levels and developing the package of its content is recognised by the HLEG, it identifies no specific areas. Both the Steering Committee and the chapter on health in the Twelfth Plan define it as RCH, emergency services and essential medicines for most of the disease burden in the country and family welfare. None of them articulate the key epidemiological principles for defining essential services. Consequently, no systematic evidence-based effort is made for defining essential care needs of different social groups living under very different conditions. Average estimates of disease burden that continue to guide the planners hide the social and economic determinants of diseases and help adopt priorities not relevant to the marginalised.

These planning documents then are trying to accommodate the hi-tech medical market in India's healthcare system. This new avatar of universal healthcare, is poised to take the health system further away from the initial dream of universal and comprehensive healthcare and it must be critiqued. Especially because, despite the Draft National Health Policy (NHP) 2015 that promised to declare health as a right and provide free primary healthcare universally, the final policy document found this an expensive proposition and opted for targeting the poor through State-led insurances and public private partnerships in a range of programmes that have further strengthened the private institutions (Draft NHP, 2015; NHP, 2017).

Universal healthcare is not just about coverage. It has to be visualised as a Rubik's cube that requires all sides to be tackled together. It is not only necessary then to reassert the positive recommendations of the HLEG but also to go beyond and spell out the steps for defining the content of CPHC and steps to strengthen public services and not be contrained by UHC. Also, it needs to be extricated from its isolation. The mistake made by the Bhore Committee of assuming that poverty and under-nutrition will be dealt with through economic planning must not be repeated. Welfare and livelihood are essential along with rebuilding the public health system within which aspects of comprehensive care left out by HLEG need to be addressed for genuinely inclusive development. For this, public health researchers must define the minimum standards of key non-health inputs which, if not achieved, act as a deterrent and a constraint for health services.

The primary task at hand is to revive the destroyed public sector in health, and ensure infrastructure and human resources necessary for CPHC in a phased manner over the next 10 years. Reviving the morale of its workers, building management systems that are responsible, accountable and transparent and can regulate, monitor, be supportive and people-friendly should be prioritised. The unfinished agenda of defining the components of EHP, reviewing existing programmes and their integration, handling the task of training appropriate personnel, provisioning of drugs, etc., needs to be completed. This basically means taking forward the work of reviewing

NRHM, expanding it, addressing its weaknesses and making it more comprehensive; reforming medical education and linking up with traditional system provider networks. This is obviously antithetical to the present trend, wherein catastrophic expenditure on illness and the urgency to reduce it, has become the logic behind linking the private sector in all possible ways with the public sector to further accelerate the shift of public subsidies for expanding India's medical market.

Regulatory bodies alone are no panacea, given the balance of power and the stewardship role of the state that is subservient to the corporate sector. Only with a well regulated, strong public sector and community-based monitoring can we hope to regulate the private sector and work with its primary and selective secondary providers. If in the future, the commitment to rebuilding the core of the public sector is met, it can begin to support the primary providers by the end of it. Otherwise it would be subsumed by schemes of PPP in the name of state-led insurances which are already corroding it. Innovative methods would be required for regulating the traditional providers as well. The corporate monopoly of the different levels of services must be arrested to contain costs. If this sector is efficient and has international standards, it must stand on its own without subsidies from the state. There is evidence to show that while it continues to draw on state resources, it has failed to respond to the needs of the disadvantaged and state regulatory mechanisms (Qadeer & Reddy, 2006: 4–20).

The public health movement in India has a major responsibility in developing its constructive criticism. It must demand articulation of minimum standards of welfare and their implementation, create blueprints for rebuilding the public sector health services, and work towards stopping of commercialisation of public institutions and giving subsidies to corporate sector partnerships so that sufficient resources could be made available for the task at hand. Analysing the results of investing in health and welfare in the present context and critiquing choices of technology therefore is a central task.

Notes

Maskovsky, J., & Kingfisher, C. (2001). Introduction: Global capitalism, neoliberal policy and poverty. Urban Anthropology and Studies of Cultural Systems and World Economic Development, 30, 105–121. [Google Scholar]

Perez, Carlota. 2002. *Technological Revolution and Financial Capital: The Dynamics of Bubbles and Golden Ages*. Cheltenham, UK: Edward Elgar.

Priya, Ritu, and A.S. Shweta A. 2010. *Status and Role of Ayush and Local Health Traditions under the National Rural Health Mission: Report of a Study*. New Delhi: National Health System Resource Centre, Ministry of Health and Family Welfare, Government of India.

Qadeer, Imrana. 2009. "Political and Economic Determinants of Health—A Case of India." In *History of Social Determinants of Health*, edited by Harold J. Cook and Sanjay Bhattacharya, 228–247. Hyderabad: Orient BlackSwan.

Qadeer, Imrana, and Sunita Reddy. 2006. "Medical Care in the Shadows of Public Private Partnership." *Social Scientist* 34 (9/10) (September–October): 4–20.

Rao, Sujatha K., S. Selvaraju, and Somil Nagpal. 2005. "Financing of Health in India." In *Financing and Delivery of Healthcare Services in India*, Section IV, Background Papers. New Delhi: National Commission on Macroeconomics and Health, Ministry of Health and Family Welfare, Government of India. August.

Schmid, Johannes Dragsbaek, and Jacques Hersh. 2000. "Introduction: Globalisation or the Coming of Age of Capitalism." In *Globalisation and Social Change*, edited by Johannes Dragsbaek Schmidt and Jacques Hersh. London: Routledge.

Sekhri Neelam K. 2000. "Managed Care: the US Experience." In *Bulletin of the World Health Organisation* 78, No. 6: 830–844.

Right to Food Campaign. 2008. "Tool for Action." Supreme Court Orders on the Right to Food. New Delhi: Right to Food Campaign.

United Nation (UN). 2014. *The Millennium Development Goals Report*. NY: United Nation. Accessed January 17, 2015. http://www.un.org/millenniumgoals/2014%20MDG%20report/MDG%202014%20English%20web.pdf.

World Bank. 1994. *World Development Report, Infrastructure for Development*. The World Bank. Oxford, NY, New Delhi: Oxford University Press.

World Bank. 1993. *World Development Report, Equity and Development Making Services Work for the Poor*. Washington: World Bank.

World Health Organisation. 1978. *Primary Healthcare: Report of the International Conference on Primary Healthcare*. Alma Ata, USSR, (September) 6–12. Geneva: WHO.

World Health Organisation. 2001. *Macroeconomics and Health: Investing in Health for Economic Development Report of the Commission on Macroeconomics and Health*. Geneva: WHO.

References

Accountability Initiative. (2015). *'NHM' Budget Brief 2015–16*, 7, No. 4. Centre for Policy Research.

Bajpai, V., & Saraya, A. (2012, April). Rashtriya Swasth Beema Yojana: A public health perspective. *The Indian Journal of Social Work, 73*(2): 265–286.

Beaud, M. (2004). *A history of capitalism*. Aakar Books.

Bello, W. (2002). *Deglobalisation: Ideas for a new world economy*. Zed Books.

Centre for Budget and Government Accountability (CBGA). (2011). *Reclaiming public provisioning priorities for the 12th five year plan*. CBGA.

Centre for Budget and Government Accountability (CBGA). (2012). *Unfulfilled promises?* CBGA.

CII and McKinsey and Company. 2002. *Healthcare in India: The road ahead. A report by CII–Mckinsey and Company with support from the Indian Heart Care Foundation*. Kriti Graphics.

Dhar, A. (2011, September 15). National rural health mission 'a minor success'. *The Hindu*, Accessed December 5, 2012. www.theHindu.com/todays-paper/tp-national/article2454690.ece

Government of India. (1946). *Report of the health survey and development committee (Bhore Committee)*. Manager of Publications.

Government of India. (1961). *Report of the health survey and planning committee* (Mudaliar Committee). Ministry of Health.

Government of India. 2009. *Draft national health bill.* Ministry of Health and Family Welfare. Accessed June 1, 2016 http://www.prsindia.org/uploads/media/Draft_National_Bill.pdf.

Government of India. (2016). *Union budget 2016–17, expenditure budget* (Vol. II), Ministry of Finance. Accessed August 12, 2016 http://www.unionbudget.nic.in/vol2.asp?pageid=4.

Heller, P. (2009). *Democratic deepening in Brazil, India and South Africa: Towards a comparative framework.* Paper prepared for Seminar: Metropolis and Inequalities, São Paulo, Brazil, March 24–26, Accessed December 7, 2012. http://www.fflch.usp.br/centrodametropole/antigo/static/uploads/seminario/Patrick_Heller.pdf.

Lang, T. (2002). The new globalisation, food and health. In B. Davey, A. Gray, & C. Seale (Eds.), *Health and Disease: A Reader,* Open University Press.

Makkar, S. (2012, February 23). Inclusive healthcare may be nixed. *Live Mint*. Accessed February 23, 2017. http://www.livemint.com/Politics/RVnaSi5wbq66IjzNe2EPqL/Universal-healthcare-plan-may-be-nixed.html.

Maskovsky, J., & Kingfisher, C. (2001). Introduction: Global capitalism, neoliberal policy and poverty. *Urban Anthropology and Studies of Cultural Systems and World Economic Development, 30*, 105–121. [Google Scholar].

Patnaik, P. (1995). A note on the political economy of the 'retreat of the state. In *Whatever happened to imperialism and other essays.* Tulika.

Planning Commission. (2002). *Tenth five year plan, 2002–2007* (Vol. 2), Planning Commission.

Planning Commission. (2008). *Eleventh five year plan, 2007–2012* (Vol. 1). Planning Commission.

Planning Commission. (2011a). *High level expert group report on universal health coverage for India.* Government of India.

Planning Commission. (2011b). *Faster sustainable and more inclusive growth: An approach to the twelfth five tear plan.* Government of India, Planning Commission.

Planning Commission. (2012). *Report of the steering committee on health for the twelfth five year plan.* Health Division, Planning Commission. Government of India.

Planning Commission. (2013). *Twelfth five year plan, 2012–17*. Planning Commission.

Qadeer, I. & Arathi, P. M. (2017, April 29). National health Policy 2017 Public policy, private care. *The Front Line.* http://www.frontline.in/cover-story/public-policy-private-care/article9604214.ece accessed on 24.1.2021

Chapter 2 Universal Healthcare and Health Assurance Through Healthcare Industry and Market Mechanisms: Evidence Versus Ideology

Indira Chakravarthi

Background

In 2013 the Planning Commission (PC) of India outlined a new strategy for health in the Twelfth Plan period, 2012–2017, for rolling out Universal Health Coverage (UHC), as part of a long-term plan that would unfold over two or three plan periods (Government of India (GoI), 2013). These plans were based on the report of the 'High Level Expert Group (HLEG) on Universal Health Coverage for India' (GoI, 2011) that it had constituted in October 2010, for developing a framework for providing accessible and affordable healthcare to all Indians. The National Health Policy (NHP) 2017 added another dimension to the goal of UHC—that of assured access termed Health Assurance (GoI, 2017). This policy lays down 'universality' as one of its principles, defining it as systems and services designed to cater to the entire population, not targeted to any sub-group and to prevent exclusion based on social or economic grounds. It states that "(t) he approach to providing assured services is free and universal access to primary healthcare services provided by a network of public primary care health facilities, supplemented by strategic purchase of secondary and tertiary care services—largely from public facilities, supplemented first by purchase from not—for profit private sector and then from the commercial private sector"(Ibid.: 8). In 2019 NITI Aayog made concrete recommendations for implementing these and moving towards UHC 2030, by consolidation of financing mechanisms and of providers, by measures such as risk-pooling and organising the private sector market (NITI Aayog, 2019). International institutions too continue to recommend engaging with the private healthcare sector for achieving UHC (UHC 2030, 2019; Clarke et al., 2019).

There is repeated reference in recent times to 'UHC', at both national and international levels, but the idea is not a new one.[1] Provision of universal health services—namely, same quality of curative and preventive services available to all as a right

I. Chakravarthi (✉)
Nehru Memorial Museum and Library, New Delhi, India

I. Qadeer et al. (eds.), *Universalising Healthcare in India*,
https://doi.org/10.1007/978-981-16-5872-3_2

irrespective of their ability to pay—through a publicly funded national health services system had been a central feature of many European nations, as also of the planning process in India since the 1950s. How it was achieved to a large extent in many countries and why this has not been achieved in India is subject for a separate discussion. These repeated announcements for achieving health for all, for universal healthcare, by themselves constitute evidence that the earlier proclamations regarding UHC have not fully materialised or, progressed beyond rhetorical pronouncements towards practice, implementation and actual strengthening of health systems. Given this, it would be prudent to be cautious about the promise of UHC once again by the current political establishment. It should not detract from the true nature and intentions underlying the developments in healthcare policy over the last two decades and the current proposals for reforms in the healthcare system for UHC.

This chapter begins with a brief look at the historical legacy and significance of UHC as a way of ensuring and implementing a genuine right to healthcare for a population, followed by a discussion on the plan and policy proposals in India for universal coverage. Given the emphasis of recent policies on engaging with the private sector, the paper next examines the developments in the private healthcare sector in the country, specifically at the corporate private sector and what is being hailed as the 'healthcare industry'. The last section presents experiences of other countries with mixed systems of healthcare providers, with corporate healthcare providers, regulation and the possibility of achieving universal healthcare in such a scenario in India.

UHC: Legacy of Social Protection and Welfarism

The concept of organised healthcare services and subsequently of universal healthcare, is an outcome of the impact, through the eighteenth-nineteenth century, of the kind of industrialisation, economic growth and development pursued in Europe and North America: the four d's of large-scale disruption, deprivation, disease, death (Szreter, 1997) and the political debates and struggles that took place then over the changes taking place, over disease causation and health (Bump, 2010; Hamlin, 1997).

The German Bismarckian system of the late nineteenth century of compulsory health insurance by employers for their low-paid workers (sickness funds) initiated the tradition of universal healthcare systems (Gaffny, 2013). Comprehensive and genuinely universal healthcare systems took shape in Britain and several other European countries in the post-Second World War period and over time have come to represent the idea of solidarity-social protection-welfarism in these states, as well as became the model for former colonies such as India. Financed through general taxes, this system provided comprehensive healthcare as a right, with medical services free at the point of service. While there were several problems, yet the,

> Poorest individuals could avail themselves of some of the most advanced medical care in the world without worry that their illness would bankrupt their family and without the stigma of charity. A true right to health care had been legislated into existence. Universal health

> care, from this perspective, represented a truly massive and historical achievement. (Gaffny, 2013:12)

(However, as discussed in a later section, the universal healthcare system is being dismantled in these countries too).

While there is no universal definition of universal healthcare, analysis of its usage and operationalisation bring out some of its underlying assumptions and principles (Bump, 2010). These are: a central role for the government in healthcare, a public commitment to collective responsibility and redistribution, public values in support of some health equity, a well-functioning health system providing financial protection and a range of services, financing of health services through general taxation, provision through an efficient health system based on a horizontal approach as against the vertical approach, to address many problems simultaneously and hence offering a wide range of healthcare services. Another important feature is that the transition to universal heatlhcare is an intensely political process, and the existing UHC systems in many countries were achieved mainly through domestic processes and re-alignments of extant political forces. International resources and assistance had not played a role in these discussions and processes (Ibid.), thus raising questions about the need for external assistance to developing countries to move towards universal healthcare, "we need to think carefully about what potential supporting roles may be played by international actors" (Ibid.: 41).

UHC in India: Policy Proposals and Measures

As mentioned before, the independent Indian state, inspired by the National Health System (NHS) of Britain, undertook a process of instituting such a system for India, to provide comprehensive primary healthcare. For various reasons, largely political and administrative, the goal envisaged in the post-independence period for the health services in India has not been fully realised. While there is substantial infrastructure, trained personnel, technology and well-equipped institutions for education and research, and adequate production capacities in the public and private healthcare sector, they are riddled with several problems (Qadeer, 2011).

With the adoption of neoliberal economic policies in the early 1990s and the accompanying health sector reforms, the original conception of universal healthcare has got transformed into UHC, to mean coverage of financial protection and provision of affordable and accessible medical care services. For the Twelfth Plan, UHC meant that each individual would have assured access to a defined essential range of medicines and treatment at an affordable price, which should be entirely free for a large proportion of the population (GoI, 2013). The HLEG defined universal healthcare as "ensuring equitable access to all Indians to affordable, accountable, appropriate healthcare services…delivered to individuals and populations, with the government being the guarantor and enabler, although not necessarily the only provider of healthcare and related services" (GoI, 2011: 3). While the HLEG recommended that general taxation should be the principal source of healthcare financing and that there should be no fees of any kind for health services, it also recommended that "(p)urchase of all healthcare services under the UHC system should be undertaken either directly by the central and state governments through their Departments of Health or by quasi-governmental autonomous agencies established especially for the purpose" (Ibid.: 13). Thus, the HLEG recommended separation of financing and provisioning, and 'purchase' of services from a fragmented system consisting of competing providers, instead of the system envisaged since the 1950s (but never effectively implemented), of a fully publicly financed, integrated health system, planning for and providing universal, comprehensive health services. According to the Twelfth Plan, the health system would "continue to have a mix of public and private service providers, and the two need to coordinate for delivery of a continuum of care" (GoI, 2013: 9). In order to make this mix work, a strong regulatory framework was essential to ensure that the UHC programme is most effective in controlling cost, reducing provider-induced demand and ensuring quality (Ibid.: 13).

The essential official proposal was as follows. Many countries were opting for coordinated care models where primary, secondary and tertiary care was delivered as an integrated framework with the participation of both the public and private sector. Given the reality of public–private providers, the Twelfth Plan document asked what are the possible ways of organising a network of public and private providers to attain UHC goals? (GoI, 2013: 13). While the PC talked of the need to strengthen public health infrastructure at all levels, it also talked of supplementing this infrastructure by private providers as well as PPPs (Ibid.: 13). According to the Plan, the UHC would take two plan periods for its realisation, but the move in terms of pilots and incremental coverage could begin in the Twelfth Plan itself (Ibid.: 13). It suggested that various options of financing and organisation should be explored by states and encouraged and financed to run one to three pilots to test out the models. Such as, "(t)he pilots could explore different models for providing universal access to an Essential Health Package (EHP)… including… a combination of public and private facility networks"(Ibid.: 15).

The NHP 2017 retained much of these strategies and proposals: assurance of universal availability of free, comprehensive primary healthcare services as an entitlement, and ensuring improved access and affordability of secondary and tertiary care services through a combination of public hospitals and strategic purchasing of services from the private health sector. This policy explicitly recognised the presence of the growing corporate sector and its contribution to employment, to medical tourism and economic growth; and recommended that the government actively intervene and influence the growth of this private health care industry and medical technologies to ensure alignment with public health goals, and enable contribution to making health care systems more effective, efficient, rational, safe, affordable and ethical (GoI, 2017). Instead of asking why the government health system has become weak and ineffective and why there is such a vast private sector, the state serves it as a 'fait accompli' and proposes to 'strengthen' the public health system for universal health coverage by accommodation and strengthening of the private sector within the health system, rather than explore other options that have been proposed over the years.[2]

Thus, in all the recent discourse and proposals, the term UHC has been used largely to camouflage discussion on financing of medical care, on how to accommodate the expanding healthcare industry. Its use now bears little resemblance, if at all any, to its original conception of healthcare as a right and as a public good to be provided as part of wider public health goals.

The biggest concern with such plans and proposals is the accommodation through all these strategies of an unregulated, increasingly commercialised private sector within the public health system and an expanded role for it in the provision of secondary and tertiary care services. This is despite lack of comprehensive information on its characteristics and workings, on efficiency and equity, quality of care, employment conditions, cost and adherence to rational, ethical practices in private sector. An effective regulatory framework to align the private healthcare sector with public health goals and to make it effective, efficient, rational, affordable and ethical is still lacking (GoI, 2017: 22). There are no rigorous evaluations yet on the terms and conditions and functioning of public–private partnerships (PPPs) in the healthcare sector (Datta, 2009; Prashanth, 2011); evaluations by government agencies of PPPs in Karnataka and researchers have highlighted several failures, such as noncompliance with rules, misuse of funds, lack of accountability, poor quality of care, lack of availability of qualified human resources, leading to several of them being ended (Belagere, 2020; PHRN et al., 2017; Karpagam et al., 2013). However, such evidences on the private sector continue to be ignored in policy making.

Private Healthcare Services in India

Healthcare as 'Big Business Opportunity', Engine of Growth

Since the 1990s, the provision of health services has become increasingly commercialised, and projected as a revenue/profit generating activity (Chakravarthi et al., 2017; Lefebvre, 2010). By 2016–17 the hospital industry in India was estimated to be worth Rs 4 trillion (US$ 61.79 billion) and was expected to almost double to Rs 8.6 trillion (US$132.84 billion) by 2022 (India Brand Equity Foundation (IBEF), 2019). Healthcare delivery, which includes hospitals, nursing homes and diagnostics centres, and pharmaceuticals, constitutes 65% of the overall market (IBEF, 2016). Healthcare in India was reported to be one of the largest service sectors, contributing about 4% of Gross Domestic Product (GDP) (Chakraborty, 2016), and expected to grow to around 6.1% of GDP and employ about 8 million people (Federation of Indian Chambers of Commerce and Industry (FICCI), 2014).

Increasingly over the past decade, there is strong advocacy and promotion by the industry of the idea that "Health care infrastructure should not just be viewed as a social good but also as a viable economic venture with productivity" (FICCI, 2008:

11). The Confederation of Indian Industry (CII) projects the healthcare sector as one with immense importance for the national economy, due to its rising contribution to Gross Domestic Product (GDP) and the potential to be an engine of growth for the nation as it can create 70–80 million jobs in the next 10 years (Bakshi et al., 2010). Since 2002, CII has been regularly organising India Health Summit to promote private investment in the healthcare sector and lobby for concessions and favourable policies[3,4]. One of the demands of FICCI Health Services Division is that the government should attract private healthcare investment to supplement the public funding deficit in healthcare allocations, by giving various fiscal and non-fiscal incentives. Some of the proposals suggested by this FICCI are:

1. The role of private healthcare providers in creating affordable, accessible, and quality healthcare infrastructure should be recognised through sensitisation of the decision-makers by providing appropriate information through dialogue.
2. PPP projects for building health infrastructure should be facilitated through healthy dialogue between the public and the private sector, and extensive stakeholder consultation by involving the civil society organisations, NGOs and the government to leverage each other's strengths.
3. The private sector should be encouraged and incentivised to make the required amount of investment particularly in Tier 2 and Tier 3, cities and in those states lagging behind in the development of the health sector.
4. The non-viable concept of free treatment by the private sector in lieu of incentives should be replaced with third party payment by the government or insurance system (FICCI, 2008).

PPPs are being viewed as having the potential to create an enormous market with a reliable, multi-year revenue stream for private investors (CII, 2011). In short, the industry views the scenario thus:

> The first wave of healthcare provision in India was the government run healthcare network. The influx of the private players defined the second wave. Now a discerning and interconnected nation demands a new incarnation: Healthcare 3.0, which will transform the ground rules of healthcare. Healthcare 3.0 will ordain that revenues are linked to patient satisfaction. Seamless public-private partnerships will be the backbone of the new dispensation, emerging as fundamental to growth. (Bakshi et al., 2010: v)

'Targeting New Segments'—Setting Up Clinics and Hospitals Outside Metropolises and Big Cities

According to the Centre for Monitoring Indian Economy (CMIE) projects entailing investments of 231.9 billion INR, were likely to be completed during 2015–17. Among these, projects worth 72.4 billion INR were likely to be commissioned by the end of the 2015, 76.7 billion INR in 2015–16 and 82.8 billion in 2016–17 (CMIE, 2015).While there were a few projects by the government among these, the bulk of the investments were from the private sector. Apollo Hospitals was implementing ten projects across several states, expected to be completed during the 2014–16 period, entailing an investment of 12.9 billion INR. Fortis Healthcare also set up two hospitals in Karnataka (investment of 350 million INR in one of these) and one in Telangana at an investment of 2.1 billion INR (D'Souza, 2014). The share of Foreign Direct Investment (FDI) equity inflow too had increased from 13% during 2000–2005 to around 25.5% in 2013, though was subject to year to year fluctuations (Hooda, 2015). A significant number of multinational players had increased their presence through partnerships and investments in joint venture projects. Corporate hospitals are also expanding into Tier 2 and Tier 3 cities, as well across north and east India, beyond Kolkata to cities such as Asansol, Siliguri in Assam, Bhubaneshwar in Odisha.

The lack of hospitals and medical facilities outside metropolitan cities and urban centres, and the availability of government health insurance programmes such as Rashtriya Swasthya Bima Yojana (RSBY), Arogyasri, etc., is being exploited by corporate hospitals such as Apollo, to set up what has been termed Apollo Reach Hospitals. As part of the plans to expand and penetrate different, underserved markets, Apollo Reach hospitals are being set up since 2008 in Tier 2 and Tier 3 cities, with 100–200 beds, in the name of taking high-quality healthcare closer to the masses so that patients in these locations do not have to travel to Tier 1 cities for comprehensive medical treatments (Apollo Hospitals, 2011). For Apollo Hospitals, the leading corporate healthcare company in India, indicators such as revenue from operations, profit before tax, profit after tax and earnings per share have all steadily increased over the past five years. For instance, profits after tax increased since 2011, from INR 1839 million to 3168 million in 2014 to 3399 million in 2015 (Apollo Hospitals, 2015).

Healthcare companies and corporate hospitals in India now have marketing and business development departments, with the marketing division becoming increasingly active. While the code of medical ethics by the Medical Council of India (MCI) prohibits doctors from advertising or marketing to solicit patients, there are no such restrictions on corporate hospitals. There has been a substantial increase in marketing and advertising expenses of the top hospital chains like Apollo Hospitals and Max Healthcare over the last five years (Kanchan, 2015).

Infusion of Private Equity

The hospital and diagnostic centres attracted FDI worth 3.21 billion US$ between April 2000 and September 2015, according to the data released by the Department of Industrial Policy and Promotion (DIPP); FDI into the hospitals and diagnostics sector increased from US$ 6.93 million in 2001–02 to US$ 684.58 million in 2013–14, though subject to year to year fluctuations (IBEF, 2016). In Rupee terms, FDI equity inflow to hospitals and diagnostic centres increased to INR 3995 crore in 2013–14 from as low as 31 crore INR in 2001–02 (Hooda, 2015). Among others, Max Healthcare Institute Ltd., Fortis Hospital Ltd., Apollo Hospitals Enterprises Ltd., Colombia Asia Hospital Pvt. Ltd., DM Healthcare Pvt. Ltd., Kanishka Healthcare Ltd., Narayana Health (earlier Narayana Hrudayalaya Pvt. Ltd.) attracted the highest

FDI equity inflow (about more than the 100 million US $) in the hospital sector between March 2000 and October 2014. In addition to these, Seven Hills Healthcare Ltd., Nova Medical Centres Pvt. Ltd., Vasan Healthcare Pvt. Ltd., Escorts Heart Super Speciality and Research, International Hospital Limited, Quality Care India Ltd. and Thyrocare Technologies Ltd. also attracted high FDI inflows. Most of the FDI inflow to these major corporations located in five metropolitan cities, namely New Delhi, Chennai, Bangalore, Hyderabad and Mumbai are routed via Mauritius, Singapore and the USA (Ibid.).

Healthcare has become an attractive new sector for investment by venture capital and global private equity funds, such as TPG Capital and Sequoia USA, Temasek and Quadria Singapore, and IHH Berhad of Malaysia (Chakravarthi et al., 2017). According to business reports there has been an increase of Private Equity (PE) funding in healthcare. The healthcare industry is reported to be 'flush' with PE funds (Dutta, 2008). Private equity investments into the private healthcare provider sector were reported to be 552 million $ in 2014, slightly lower than the 786.2 million in 2013, according to Thomson Reuter's data (Reuters, 2015). The investment of PE funds was reported to be taking place not just for established hospital chains in urban areas but also for hospitals in tier II and tier III cities, rural and semi-urban areas, diagnostic centres and medical equipment.

Acumen Fund (a US-based social venture capital fund) and Hindustan Latex Ltd (HLL, a government enterprise) have formed a joint venture called Life Spring Hospitals, which was creating a chain of small hospitals (20–25 beds), to provide maternal and child healthcare services for the low-income group in urban areas. As of 2012, Life Spring had 12 hospitals in Hyderabad, and aimed to set up 200 hospitals across cities such as Delhi, Mumbai and Bangalore over the following five years.[5] ICICI Venture, through I-Ven Medicare in mid-2007, had invested in not so-renowned names in healthcare such as 36 million US$ in Sahyadri Hospital, Pune; 24 million in Vikram Hospital, Mysore; 16.25 million in Medica Synergy, Kolkata and 10.25 million in RG Stone, New Delhi. Apollo Hospitals has had PE investments from companies such as Schroders (Dutta, 2008). PE firms were also reported to be investing in independent diagnostic centres. Such as: Industrial Credit and Investment Corporation of India (ICICI) Venture had invested 35 crore INR in Metropolis Health Services in 2006. Venture Capital firm Sequoia Capital India had invested 10 million $ in Dr Lal Path Labs (FICCI, 2008). Some other such investments include Deutsche Investitions- und- Entwicklungsgesellschaft (DEG) investing $12.21 million in Ivy Hospitals, International Finance Corporation (IFC) and Standard Chartered investing over $46 million in Fortis Healthcare, and Multiples Alternate Asset Management investing $33.15 million in Vikram Hospitals, among others (Team VCC, 2013).

Role of Development Finance Institutions

Since 2006, there has been an increase in funding by bilateral and multilateral development finance institutions to private healthcare providers in the form of equity investments and loans: from around just US$ 0.4 bn to US$ 1.9 bn in the period 2007 to 2015, and an estimated US$ 1.7 bn was committed over 2016 and 2017 alone (Hunter & Marriott, 2018).

The International Finance Corporation (IFC), a member of the World Bank (WB) group, is the largest global development institution focused exclusively on the private sector in developing countries.[6] IFC's Venture Capital Division provides equity financing to early and growth- stage companies including information technology, healthcare, education, and agribusiness. At the IFC's International Private Health Conference in May 2011, it was stated by one IFC functionary that, "Health care has become a major global industry, growing faster than GDP in most countries… as the world recovers from the international financial crisis, the expansion of the private health sector continues rapidly across emerging markets" (IFC, 2011 unpaged). According to the Principal Investment Officer, IFC-South Asia, India is a very important market for the IFC and the World Bank Group, particularly in the healthcare sector. IFC had a strong investment portfolio in the Indian healthcare sector, with commitments of over US$ 450 million, representing over 30% of its global health investment portfolio (Babu, 2014). As of May 2009, it had invested about US$ 200 million in the private healthcare sector in India (IFC, 2009), including several large hospital chains such as Apollo and Max for their expansion and in smaller facilities such as EYE-Q, NephroPlus and Ivy Hospitals, as detailed in Chakravarthi et al., 2017. Commonwealth Development Corporation (CDC) of UK has similarly provided capital to healthcare businesses in India[7]: in 2013 CDC with (Dubai-based Abraaj group) made a direct equity investment of 17.5 million US $ in Rainbow Hospitals, an Andhra Pradesh-based paediatric and maternity healthcare business, for expansion to Chennai, Pune, Kurnool and Vizag, to set up tertiary paediatric centres (Team VCC, 2013). In 2015 it invested INR 300 crore for around 10–15% stake in Narayana Health, to fund its expansion in Kolkata, Bhubaneshwar, Lucknow and Bangalore (PTI, 2015).

Discussion

Currently, in India, we see that the provision of medical care has become a highly sought after sector by capitalist institutions, with a growing network of corporations supplying medical care for profit (McKinlay, 1978). The 2017 National Health Policy reported that the government had invested heavily in building a positive economic climate for the healthcare industry and there was now a robust healthcare industry with double digit growth, generating revenues and employment (GoI, 2017). The healthcare sector (medical care sector) is getting rapidly transformed from a heterogeneous one comprising small hospitals and nursing homes owned by individual doctors. A crucial feature of the private sector in India is the consolidation of the healthcare industry, and the spread of for-profit hospitals, a process which is being facilitated through policy measures, organised advocacy by the healthcare industry, as well as by powerful institutions such as the IFC and development partners such as the Department for International Development (DFID). We witness rapid developments in the private medical care sector, such as the expansion of the corporate sector to smaller cities and towns, forming referral networks, setting up of smaller facilities for specialised, single-specialty care such as maternity care- eye care-cardiac care-dialysis-diagnostics, etc., setting up primary care clinics for out-patient needs and consultations, attracting doctors towards such arrangements, getting into PPPs and expanding insurance schemes.

Analysing the phenomenon of entry of financial and industrial capital in medicine and healthcare in the US in the 1970s, McKinlay pointed out that the industrial and financial capital institutions in medical care impose the same logic (profitability through expansion) in this field that they have been doing in other sectors of the economy since around the turn of the twentieth century (Ibid.). Their presence has ramifications at all levels. There is an urgent need to comprehend the behaviour and power of corporations that have the resources to raise finance, to hire marketing expertise to package and sell services, to create and sell new demands and to influence/restructure medical practice and the nature of services sold/offered, the pricing of services and the kind of technologies used. There arise several concerns about the private finance capital investments in healthcare. When the capital market provides funds to the healthcare companies it expects a return just as in any other area of enterprise. In his discussion on the role of capital markets in the healthcare system in the US, Silvers says: "The capital market is dominated by an economic perspective, which leaves little room for broader measures of welfare. Those who lend money want it back" (Silvers, 2001: 1022–23). So, all institutions with outstanding debt must meet their financial obligations first if they are to continue, notwithstanding concerns about patient welfare being a priority. Furthermore, access to equity capital comes with a price tag, such as expected returns of 40% or more, shared control or shared ownership (Venkatesan, 1997 cited in Grazier & Metzler, 2006).

The healthcare industry, specifically the hospital sector within this healthcare industry, is adopting a moralistic stance and talks of working towards universal, affordable and high quality healthcare to the millions of Indians who are deprived of such services. This, the industry persons say, is possible through 'innovative' business and market mechanisms, and are making plans along these lines for expansion, penetrating new markets, targeting new segments, training and attracting medical professionals, etc. However, the actual goals of the industry are clearly those of commerce, profits and expansions, and bear no relation to these stated goals of service provision. They are in reality a total antithesis to the vision and provision of healthcare as public good and a public service, to be provided through a comprehensive, universal, healthcare system.

What are the implications for a mixed health system of the presence of this expanding for-profit private sector and the influx of finance capital into healthcare? The government's plans and proposals need to be placed in the context of the growing presence and influence of the corporate and finance capital in medical care, as well as the larger ideological shift that has occurred since the 1980s against provision of welfare services by the state.

Is this the way towards a health system for 'universal healthcare' or towards the entrenchment of the 'healthcare industry'? Is it possible to align the activities of such an industry to meet the objectives of comprehensive, universal and equitable healthcare?

Experiences from other countries shed some light on the impossibility of achieving universal care through such measures. There is not much evidence that such a mixed system is better, more equitable or efficient. On the contrary, there is plenty of evidence of the adverse and pernicious effects of corporate investment, of private capital, as well as of having a system of public funding, private provisioning and of introducing competition and managed care. One such case is that of the UK NHS.

Impact of Market-Oriented Reforms on Expenditure, Quality and Comprehensiveness

Macro-economic measures aimed at curbing public expenditure on health were introduced in the mid-1970s in the UK. Extensive documentation and analysis of the UK experience of reform of NHS, through a range of market prescriptions, point to the erosion of universality, comprehensiveness and equity, and to the enormous transaction costs and waste associated with market-based mechanisms in healthcare (Pollock, 2005). It was observed that: costs were driven up, not down; bureaucracy continued to expand, instead of decreasing, inequities of all kinds were aggravated, not reduced and new inequities were created; more services that had been free were to be charged for, or would simply disappear from the NHS, to be provided only by the private sector, for those able to afford them. Comprehensiveness and universality became things of the past…Healthcare moved increasingly rapidly away from being a right, back towards being a commodity—as it had been before 1948 (Ibid.: 35). Comprehensiveness has clearly been abandoned, whether explicitly, as with most long- term residential care and routine optical care, or implicitly, as with dentistry, which is available at NHS terms only to children…Universality has gone in as much as the services provided both by GPs and hospitals vary increasingly from place to place…The emphasis is now on 'decentralisation' and 'choice', but there are no mechanisms for providing democratic local control…(Ibid.: 83).

The management reforms of the 1980s and the introduction of the internal market in the early 1990s saw the NHS's administrative costs rise from 6 to 12%. Making and monitoring hundreds of thousands of contracts, billing for every treatment (to achieve payment by results), and paying for accounting, auditing, legal services and advertising—not to mention shareholders' profits—are bound to swallow a large part of the new money. As a result of outsourcing of non clinical work in the NHS, turnover of support staff rose, cleaning standards fell, while the poor quality of hospital meals became notorious… managing the outsourcing contracts and monitoring their performance often consumed more administrative time than had previously been needed to manage the services in-house…the main effect of outsourcing, however, was to replace the professional culture that had previously prevailed in NHS hospitals with a business culture focused less and less on medical values and more on accounts (Ibid.: 40–41).

Another consequence of the market was that it had become virtually impossible to track NHS expenditure, and the lack of transparency was set to worsen (Ibid.: 227). At a deeper level still are the implications of the so-called mixed economy of healthcare. Quite apart from some £4 billion a year of tax revenues going to the private long-term care industry, more and more of the NHS budget itself now ends up in the accounts of private companies providing everything. (Ibid.: 84). Finally, the independent regulator was to regulate the medical markets that are sought to be created through these reforms. The mandate of the regulator had nothing about comprehensiveness, universality and equity (Ibid.: 85, 234).

Other than these problems associated with markets and the difficulties and barriers in regulating them, the major casualty of the introduction of markets has been loss of the population focus in the health system, which is what public health is all about to begin with.

Adverse Impacts of Corporate Presence

In India, sections of the medical profession are now expressing concern about the increasingly unethical and irrational medical practices, arising from the practices adopted by corporate and other big private hospitals to increase their revenues. It has been pointed out that big private hospitals adopt measures such as offering 'commissions' to doctors in solo outpatient clinics and to those who practise in smaller hospitals (public or private), which do not have all the facilities, to refer their patients to these big hospitals. This system is widely known as 'cut practice' and the doctor becomes effectively an agent, whose commission gets related to the number of patients he/she sends to the big hospital (Berger, 2014; Kanchan, 2015). There are also accounts of targets being given to doctors for conducting a certain number of procedures or surgeries in the hospital or keep patients longer than necessary in the hospital to increase hospital revenues (Gadre & Shukla, 2016). Such mechanisms are making it difficult for rational and ethical medical practice. In 2014, cardiologists at the prestigious All India Institute of Medical Sciences (AIIMS), Delhi, decided to launch an initiative called the Society for Less Investigative Medicine (SLIM), to tackle the increasing practice of advising excessive medical investigations. There are also accounts of doctors suffering from 'dual loyalties', towards their corporate employers and towards their patients; sometimes the two come into conflict and often interests of the patient are undermined (Jesani, 2014). These revelations and accounts raise serious concerns about how the government intends and plans to curb these irrational, unethical practices and align the activities of the corporate and other private hospitals with public health goals.

In Australia it was found that corporate investment clearly undermined the capacity of the state to intervene in the healthcare sector and there was lack of political and bureaucratic control over the planning of appropriate hospital services. Among the problems of introducing competition in this sector was the lack of information sharing between hospitals, such as of disease infection rates and about financial performance on grounds of 'commercial sensitivity'. Such inhibition of information sharing decreased the capacity of the state to monitor, regulate and control (White & Collyer, 1998). In Malaysia, it was observed that "the profit motive does not appear to have resulted in vigorous competition and improvements in the quality of services. Nor had competitive pricing resulted in lower costs to consumers" (Barraclough, 1997: 653). Further, many doctors and nursing staff had left the public sector for the better pay, work conditions and prospects in the private sector. Yet another issue was that existing charitable hospitals were finding it more difficult to cross-subsidise their poor patients due to the need to be competitive with commercial hospitals. In the context of similar developments in the US, it was observed that with the coming of the corporation has come, "the pursuit of market logic above all" (White, 2007: 396). This review of studies of the market mechanisms in medical care in the US over more than a decade (1993–2005) indicated that some of the features of the market—particularly how investors allocated capital—had been incompatible with the pursuit of a more efficient and equitable healthcare system (White, 2007). Competition had little ability to rationalise (re-organise) healthcare systems; costs were driven more by market power over prices than by management of utilisation; competitive or financial threats compelled a very large portion of all providers (including non-profit providers) to merge with larger entities, with resulting loss of local managerial control. Other reviews showed that the economic benefits promised by for-profits had not been demonstrated. Rise in investor-owned hospitals had increased rather than lowered costs of healthcare.

Bravemann and Bennett (1995) in their analysis of the problems in the US of the healthcare system and how to reform it, draw attention to the presence and impact of for-profit corporatisation on every aspect of healthcare, on the pressures to achieve efficiency at the cost of quality and equity. They observe that, "(t)he health-care industry now provides a deep feeding trough for the insatiable appetites of for-profit corporations" (Bravemann & Bennett, 1995: 266). They point out that even if multiple payers (insurance companies) were replaced by a single- payer the problems would not go away, managed competition would persist among multiple providers, for-profit providers would compete among themselves for re-imbursement from the single payer. A single payer would eliminate the wastage associated with insurance companies, but profiteering by providers and suppliers would remain; even with single-payer reform, extensive mechanisms for managed care would be necessary to control profiteering and waste. In conclusion they say,

> Perhaps it's time to do battle with the real monsters and dare to question publicly the role of rapacious profit-making in health-care as well as the practice of unregulated fee-for-service medicine and the treatment of health care as a consumer commodity like any other. Achieving universal coverage with high-quality services that are distributed equitably and sustained by public funding will necessarily involve some limits on physician autonomy and patient choice as well as on profiteering. (Ibid.: 267)

Another review of many studies of the US healthcare system arrived at the following indicting conclusions:

> The US has four decades of experience with the combination of public funding and private healthcare management and delivery, closely analogous to reforms recently enacted or proposed in many other nations. Extensive research…shows that for-profit health institutions provide inferior care at inflated prices. The US experience also demonstrates that market mechanisms nurture unscrupulous medical businesses and undermine medical institutions unable or unwilling to tailor care to profitability. The commercialization of care in the US has driven up costs by diverting money to profits and by fuelling a vast increase in management and financial bureaucracy, which now consumes 31% of total health spending…The poor performance of the US healthcare is directly attributable to reliance on market mechanisms and for-profit firms, and should warn other nations from this path. (Himmelstein & Woolhandler, 2008: 407)

Experience of USA with Private Capital Financing

In the context of the US it has been found that the capital market has had a major role in restructuring the healthcare sector (Silvers, 2001). Firstly, the capital market provides the funds it does to the health sector and expects a return just the same as in any other area of enterprise. Reliance on private investment sources in the United States has fundamentally shaped the focus of the industry in a manner dramatically different from the systems found in other countries where governments supply capital. For all the disclaimers about the importance of patients, service and community, the fact is that all institutions with outstanding debt must meet their financial obligations first if they are to continue. As the level of outside financing has grown, other differences blur and traditional concern for the public or even attending physicians may come second after profitability (Ibid.: 1027–1028).The resulting market discipline extends to both for-profit firms and non-profit organisations in several ways. The implications for access, quality and cost coming from the role of private capital in the health sector are very uneven depending on location, health status, and insurance coverage. The important question that emerged was, whether the requirements of private capital can be made compatible with larger needs of society to provide service to marginal populations? In other words, will the government be able to set payment levels and subsidies so as to allow privately financed providers to meet these needs while staying solvent and avoiding suboptimal decisions in the pursuit of paying customers? (Ibid.: 1028).

Conclusion

UHC and Health Assurance in Times of for-Profit Healthcare: Evidence Versus Ideology

Thus, there is a wealth of information on the distortions produced by for-profits healthcare providers, on how the presence of markets and competition in healthcare systems has not achieved objectives such as universality, efficiency, cost-control and a regulated private sector. If such overwhelming evidence is to be ignored, and governments and policy-makers insist on imposing market prescriptions for universal access, then is it anything other than neoliberal ideology at work for the benefit of a few?

As it is well known, health sector reforms are not unique to India. The restructuring of economies worldwide since the late 1980s have had significant implications for healthcare: there has been restructuring of health services in the name of efficiency. Shaoul's analysis of the health sector reforms in the UK show how the chief characteristic of all these economic, financial and organisational 'reform' measures, is that they are 'the techniques used by the private sector to generate profit out of the production of commodities for distribution to the providers of finance' (Shaoul, 2003: 152). The reforms comprised a series of measures under the umbrella of 'new managerialism'. The underlying assumption was that the tools of private sector management could improve the output, enhance profits, and contain the 'problem' of rising cost of healthcare. The emphasis on financial management as a proactive tool to manage public healthcare was to achieve these objectives, not simply to record income and expenditure. This approach was accompanied by emphasis on the three es—economy, efficiency and effectiveness —and the growth of performance measures which attempted to capture and compare the performance of public sector providers. It represented a change in the way that public health was managed in two significant respects: from planning on the basis of perceived needs, to managing by financial numbers; and from decision- making and control by the service professionals to decision-making and control by managers. As rightly pointed out by Shaoul, through these measures a transformation of social relations is being affected. Firstly, the relations of production in health are being realigned so that they match those of the private sector. Second, services funded by the public through taxation are being organised by the state to serve more directly the financial interests of the private corporations, not the public, via outsourcing, partnership arrangements, and insurance. Third, the public is being reconstituted as the 'customer' for the goods and services so produced (Ibid.).

While these measures may appear and are presented as a form of decentralisation that permits local decision-making, their real function is to create the structures and mechanisms for the private sector to more easily control, own and direct public services and public policy. Such services can then get integrated into the wider international economy as they are taken over by the transnational corporations, through provisions such as General Agreement on Trade in Services (GATS). These trends in the financing and organization of healthcare, specifically, the active attempts by state and non-state actors to accelerate and deepen financialisation[8], create new markets and opportunities for accumulation in the name of 'development', have been situated within a trajectory of capital formation (Hunter & Murray, 2019: 2); they describe the transformation of healthcare into saleable and tradeable assets for global investors and extraction of revenue from situations of vulnerability, with little concern for the consequences for equity in healthcare.

In other words, in reality, the social welfare functions of the state are being integrated into the world economy, not for the benefit of the population at large as they are made out to be, but for the benefit of capital. Terms such as 'universal healthcare,' 'healthcare as a right,' 'equity,' 'choice', etc. are merely being used to give the so-called 'human face', rather a mask to conceal what is essentially becoming an unhealthy, unjust accumulation of profits in the name of providing healthcare.

Notes

1. The terms Universal Healthcare, Universal Health Coverage and Universal Access to Healthcare are often used interchangeably. For some UHC means that basic medical services should be available at low or no cost; for others it means everyone should have health insurance. Health activists point out that UHC is not simply a question of extending the existing healthcare system to cover the entire population, but of transforming it to a new system in which health services are a right and not as a commodity, and is part of comprehensive welfare services. It functions with the principle and objective of providing good quality health services to the entire population, regardless of income level, social status or place of residence. Since the First World War UHC has been propounded by international institutions as a goal for health systems of developing countries: first by the Rockefeller Foundation (1920s), then by the League of Nations (1930s), in the WHO Alma Ata Declaration of "Health for All" in 1978, in contemporary times by the World Bank and WHO.
2. As pointed out by Banerji, 'considerable thought has been given to re- orienting this health service system and over the years several commissions, committees and study groups have pondered over it. Almost all of them have emphasised the need for radical change.' (Banerji, 1985: 42).
3. https://www.cii.in/sectors.aspx?enc=prvePUj2bdMtgTmvPwvisYH+5EnGjyGXO9hLECvTuNu2yMtqEr4D408mSsgiIyM/, last viewed 25.01.2021.
4. https://www.mycii.in/image/eventimages/eventmainimages/E000038024_CII%20Brochure.pdf, last viewed 25.01.2021.
5. https://acumen.org/investment/lifespring/?sector=health&region=india; and http://www.lifecarehll.com/page/render/reference/LifespringLowering_Cost_And_Raising_Access_To_Maternal_Care_In_India, last viewed 25.01.2021.
6. IFC promotes private sector investment through direct and indirect investment, extending loans, informing government policy, as well by providing support and technical assistance for private sector growth through its institutions.

7. https://www.cdcgroup.com/en/our-approach/where-and-what-we-invest-in/sectors/health/, viewed last 25.01.2021.
8. Financialization in its broadest sense is the 'increasing role of financial motives, financial markets, financial actors and financial institutions in the operation of the domestic and international economies' (discussed in Hunter & Murray, 2019).

References

Apollo Hospitals. (2011). *Vision 20.6: A blueprint for smarter healthcare: Annual report 2010–2011*. Apollo Hospitals Enterprise Limited.

Apollo Hospitals. (2015). *Annual report 2014–2015*. Apollo Hospitals Enterprise Limited.

Babu, G. (2014). *IFC eyes strong opportunities in India's healthcare sector*. Business Standard, November 8, 2014. Accessed May 25, 2016. http://www.business-standard.com/article/companies/ifc-eyes-strong-opportunities-in-india-s-healthcare-sector-114110701321_1.html

Bakshi, A., Prathipati, S., Shriram, S., & Vaidya, M. (2010). Gearing up for healthcare 3.0. In Background Paper for CII Seventh India Health Summit. Dec 2–3, 2010. McKinsey and Company.

Banerji, D. (1985). *Health and family planning services in India: An epidemiological, socio-cultural and political analysis and a perspective*. Lok Paksh.

Barraclough, S. (1997). The growth of corporate private hospitals in Malaysia: Policy contradictions in health system pluralism. *International Journal of Health Services, 27*(4), 643–659.

Belagere, C. (2020). Public private partnerships in healthcare not a good idea: Experts. *The New Indian Express*. 3rd January. https://www.newindianexpress.com/nation/2020/jan/03/public-private-partnership-in-healthcare-not-good-idea-experts-2084375.html

Berger, D. (2014, May 4). Corruption ruins the doctor-patient relationship in India. *British Medical Journal, 348*, g3169.

Bravemann, P., & Bennett, T. (1995). Let's take on the real dragon: Profiteering in healthcare. *Journal of Public Health Policy, 16*(3), 261–268.

Bump, J. B. (2010, October 19). *The long road to universal health coverage: A century of lessons for development strategy*. PATH.

Chakraborty, S. (2016). *India's services sector grew 10% a year in 2015–16: CII report*. Business Standard, April 21, 2016. Accessed March 15, 2017. http://www.business-standard.com/article/economy-policy/india-s-services-sector-grew-10-a-year-in-2015–16-cii-report-116042001082_1.html

Chakravarthi, I., Roy, B., Mukhopadhyay, I., & Barria, S. (2017). "Investing in health": Healthcare industry in India. *Economic and Political Weekly, 52*(45), 50–56.

Clarke, D., Doerr, S., Hunter, M., Schmets, G., Soucat, A., & Paviza, A. (2019). The private sector and universal health coverage. *Bulletin of the World Health Organization, 97*, 434–435.

CMIE (Center for Monitoring Indian Economy). (2015). Health services industry on an expansion spree: Projects worth Rs.231.9 billion to be commissioned by March 2017. Industry Outlook 20th January. CMIE Mumbai. Downloaded on February 21, 2016 from http://www.cmie.com/kommon/bin/sr.php?kall=wclrdhtm&nvdt=20150120104104593&nvpc=099000000000&nvtype=ANALYSIS+%26+OUTLOOK. Accessed March 5, 2016.

Confederation of Indian Industry (CII). (2011, November 2011). Addressing the unfinished agenda: Universal healthcare. Healthcare Background Paper.

Datta, A. (2009, August 15). Public private partnerships in India: A case for reform? *Economic and Political Weekly, 44*(33), 73–78.

D'Souza, M. (2014). Health services industry to witness capacity addition of 34,674 beds by March 2016: Incremental capacity to come at a cost of Rs.209.1 billion. Industry Outlook.

November 28, 2014. CMIE Mumbai. Accessed February 21, 2016. http://www.cmie.com/kommon/bin/sr.php?kall=wclrdhtm&nvdt=20141128114644883&nvpc=099000000000&nvtype=ANALYSIS+%26+OUTLOOK&ver=pf

Dutta, R. (2008, June). It's raining funds. *Express Healthcare.*

Federation of Indian Chambers of Commerce and Industry (FICCI). (2008). *Fostering quality healthcare for all. FICCI Heal 2008—Recommendations for the road ahead.* FICCI Health Services Division.

FICCI. (2014). Sectoral investment landscape across India: An overview. knowledge Paper for Twelfth Pravasi Bharatiya Divas, January 7–9, 2014. New Delhi India. Accessed March 15, 2017. http://ficci.in/spdocument/20362/Knowledge-Paper-Book.pdf.

Gadre, A., & Shukla, A. (2016). *Dissenting diagnosis: Voices of conscience from the medical profession.* Delhi Random House. Chapters 1, 2, and 4.

Gaffny A. (2013). Austerity and the unravelling of European healthcare. *Dissent, 60*(2) (Spring), 10–15.

Government of India. (2017). National Health Policy 2017. Ministry of Health and Family Welfare.

Government of India. (2011). High level expert group on universal health coverage for India. Planning Commission.

Government of India. (2013). Health. In *Twelfth Five Year Plan (2012–2017) Social Sectors* (Vol. III). Sage.

Grazier, K. L., & Metzler, B. (2006, January 4). Healthcare entrepreneurship: Financing innovation. *Journal of Health and Human Services Administration, 28*(4), 485–503.

Hamlin, C. (1997). *Public health and social justice in the age of Chadwick: Britain, 1800–1854.* Cambridge University Press.

Himmelstein, D., & Woolhandler, S. (2008). Privatisation in a publicly funded healthcare system: The U.S. experience. *International Journal of Health Services, 38*(3), 407–419.

Hooda, S. K. (2015, April). Foreign investment in hospital sector in India: Trends, pattern and issues. ISID Working Paper, No. 181. Institute for Studies in Industrial Development.

Hunter, B. M., & A. Marriott, (2018). Development finance institutions and the (In)coherence of their investments in private healthcare companies. In B. Tomlinson, E. R. Palo-mares, & L. A. Pano (Eds.), *The reality of aid* (pp. 33–44). IBON International.

Hunter, B. M., & Murray, S. F. (2019). Deconstructing the financialization of healthcare. *Development and Change, 50*(5), 1263–1287.

India Brand Equity Foundation. (2019, July). *Healthcare.*

India Brand Equity Foundation. (2016, January). *Healthcare.* http://www.ibef.org/industry/healthcare-india.aspx, accessed May 25, 2016.

IFC. (2009). IFC and India's Apollo Hospitals join forces to bring affordable healthcare to smaller cities in India. Accessed December 3, 2012. http://www.ifc.org/wps/wcm/connect/ada2c7004970bfe099b9db336b93d75f/Apollopercent2BHospitals.pdf?MOD=AJPERES.

IFC. (2011). IFC International Health Conference 2011: Private healthcare is growing rapidly in emerging market countries, says IFC. Accessed January 17, 2016. http://www1.ifc.org/wps/wcm/connect/industry_ext_content/ifc_external_corporate_site/industries/health+and+education/news/events_presentations/event_2011internationalconference.

Jesani, A. (2014). Professional codes, dual loyalties and the spotlight on corruption. *Indian Journal of Medical Ethics, 11*(3), 134–136.

Kanchan, M. (2015, July 25). Business of hospitals. *Economic and Political Weekly, 50*(30), 25–27.

Karpagam, S., Roy, B., Seethappa, V. K., & Qadeer, I. (2013). Evidence-based Planning—A myth or reality: Use of evidence by the planning commission on public-private partnership. *Social Change, 43*(2), 213–226.

Lefebvre, B. (2010). *Hospital chains in India: The coming of age? Asie Visions 23.* Institut Francais des relations Internationales (Ifri) Centre Asie.

McKinlay, J. B. (1978, October). On the medical-industrial complex. *Monthly Review, 30*(5), 38–42.

NITI Aayog. (2019, November). Health system for a new India: Building blocks. NITI Aayog.

Pollock, A. (2005). *NHS plc: The privatisation of our healthcare.* Verso.

Prashanth, N. S. (2011, October). Public private partnerships and health policies. *Economic and Political Weekly, 46*(42):13–15.

PTI. (2015, January 14). Britain's CDC invests $48 Million in Narayana Hrudayalaya. *Economic Times.*

Public Health Resource Network (PHRN), Jan Swasthya Abhiyan, and Oxfam. (2017). Public private partnerships in healthcare outsourcing of Haemodialysis services in Delhi: A case study. PHRN and Oxfam.

Qadeer, I. (2011). *Public health in India: Critical reflections.* Danish Books.

Reuters. (2015, August 28). Malaysia's IHH buys global hospitals for $ 195 Million. *The Economic Times.*

Shaoul, J. (2003). Global capital and healthcare reform: The experience of the UK. In K. Sen (Ed.), Restructuring health services: Changing contexts and comparative perspectives. Zed Books and European Commission.

Silvers, J. B. (2001, October). The role of capital markets in restructuring of healthcare. *Journal of Health Politics, Policy and Law, 26*(5), 1019–1030.

Szreter, S. (1997, December). Economic growth, disruption, deprivation, disease, and death: On the importance of the politics of public health for development. *Population and Development Review, 23*(4), 693–728.

Team VCC. (2013). CDC and Abraaj Group Invest $17.5M in Rainbow Hospitals August 13. Accessed May 25, 2016. http://www.vccircle.com/news/healthcare-services/2013/08/13/cdc-and-abraaj-group-invest-175m-rainbow-hospitals

UHC2030. (2019) Private sector contributions towards universal health coverage UHC2030. Private Sector Constituency Statement.

White, J. (2007, September). Markets and medical care: The United States, 1993–2005. *The Milbank Quarterly, 85*(3), 395–448.

White, K., & Collyer, F. (1998). Healthcare markets in Australia: Ownership of the private hospital sector. *International Journal of Health Services, 28*(3), 487–510.

Chapter 3
National Health Policy 2017: Securing Interests of Profits

Indranil Mukhopadhyay

The ability of the nation state to take independent policy course gets undermined under neo-liberalism. Any policy measure that contradicts the interests of the big corporate is a virtual non-starter under the current context. Even if the national governments are under tremendous pressure from the masses to take up something radical, the affiliates of finance capital would twist the discourse in such a way that either such efforts are undermined or at least the corporate interests are properly served. Developments in Greece, series of bailouts and subsequent austerity measures in US depict the power of finance capital to arm twist nation states to push through its agenda. Thus it is not at all astonishing that the current discourses on 'Universal Health Coverage' would reflect the interests of market forces and use state as a means to achieve its interest. In this paper, we would like to highlight some of the important concerns on approach of the Twelfth Plan chapter on Health and the Draft National Health Policy 2015 (NHP 2015 henceforth) and National Health Policy 2017 (NHP 2017 henceforth), and open a debate on the service delivery mechanism envisioned there and attempt to unravel the plot of further expansion of market.

The Current Policy Context: The Consensus and Few Contentions

Health system in India is among the most privatized in the world wherein the share of private spending on health is among the highest. Of the total spending on health 68% comes from people's pocket, while government share is 29% (NHSRC, 2016). Such regressive form of financing leads to indebtedness; pushes people towards poverty, untreated ailments and preventable deaths. In recent years global debates on health financing is centred around eradication of 'financial hardship' through 'Universal

I. Mukhopadhyay (✉)
School of Government and Public Policy, O.P. Jindal University, Sonipat, India

I. Qadeer et al. (eds.), *Universalising Healthcare in India*,
https://doi.org/10.1007/978-981-16-5872-3_3

Health Coverage' (UHC), essentially financed through government resources. The Sustainable Development Goals also calls for reduction of financial hardship as a central goal of UHC.

UHC and health for all mean entirely different things. While health for all prerequisites a progressive socialization of health care, gradual undoing of commoditization of health care, primary health care approach integrated under the notion of social determinants; universal coverage merely means that a financing system is developed to cover majority of people against out of pocket expenses. Under UHC, governments are being seen as a major purchaser of health services (and not the only provider) and different forms of purchasing mechanisms are proposed including tax financed health insurance, mandatory social insurance and managed care models.

The idea of UHC is doing the rounds in India for almost a decade now. It was first floated through the National Health Bill (MoHFW, 2009), by the Central government in late 2009 which was shelved subsequently without much deliberation. Lancet published a special volume on universal coverage of health in India in early 2011 (Lancet India Group, 2011) and Planning Commission (PC) set up the High Level Expert Group on Health (GoI, 2011). All these reports have pointed out towards alarming levels of out of pocket expenditure and suggested that UHC should be an immediate priority. Lancet 'call for action' lays bare what all is on the cards (Lancet India Group, 2011 p. 763). It propsoed to setup an 'Integrated National Health System' including public and private health providers. According to them, '…comprehensive health insurance that is financed through a combination of public, employer, and private sources'(ibid.).would be rolled out Apart from financing and regulating, the roles of government as envisioned in the volume are to ensure provisioning in rural and underserved communities and preventive and promotive work.

The High Level Expert Group (HLEG) report made a departure from the global discourse in suggesting that enhanced public spending on health to 2.5% of the Gross Domestic Produce (GDP) should be largely devoted towards strengthening public systems. It also recommended against insurance mechanisms and called for bringing different government insurance programmes under the same umbrella. It rejected insurance sighting the evidence that bulk of out of pocket expenses was in out-patient services and on drugs and diagnostics. Instead the HLEG suggested that a national health package would be provided as a guarantee to all citizens and services would be jointly provided by the public sector and the private sector. It suggested two models to engage private sector, one is a 'coordinated care model' based on public provisioning complemented by contracted in private sector; the other is more like a 'managed care model' where private and public facilities would be part of a network to provide health services to empanelled citizens. The final health chapter of 12th Five Year Plan (FYP) has proposed various UHC models which would be piloted in different districts and states would be provided incentive funds for the proposed National Health Mission (NHM) to take up the pilots.

With change in government at the Centre, there are some crucial developments, with potential to alter the way health care has been delivered and financed in India.

The Planning Commission has been replaced by the *Niti Aayog*, thus ending six-decade long practice of devolving Plan funds to states. On the other hand, the Fourteenth Finance Commission had promised to devolve greater share of tax revenue to states. In the health policy scenario, we have had the draft NHP 2015, with its own contradictions and sliver-linings. Subsequently, the NHP 2017 came into being, with further aggressive attempt to handover public resources in the interest of profit. In fact there is a reversal from the limited but concrete gains made by National Rural Health Mission (NRHM) due to cutbacks in public spending perhaps due to an inevitable paralysis because of the ideological rift between the Niti Ayog and the Ministry of Health and Family Welfare (Sethi, 2015)

National Health Policy 2017: Healthcare an Avenue for Quick Returns Over Investments?

When NDA came to power, health policy circle was abuzz with rumours about major policy pronouncements from the Prime Minister on the Independence Day. Given the overwhelming mandate it was expected that the current dispensation would provide some concrete direction to health policy. Draft National Health Policy, circulated at the end of 2014 for public comment, promised health assurance of some nature. It is stated that Primary level health care would be universalized, largely delivered through public services. However, secondary and tertiary level care would remain targeted and would be provided free only for poor and vulnerable populations, through strategic purchasing from the private sector—clearly making avenues for profiteering and potential fragmentation of health care services. NHP is unique in various ways- in terms of its total surrender to neo-liberal dictum, in its attempt to visualise health care industry as a vehicle of economic growth and in the conceptualisation of regulation as an impediment in fostering growth of 'health care industry'.

Earlier the 12th Five Year Plan gave a call to expand and strengthen public sector—a laudable proposition no doubt—but also pitched for creating conditions for further expansion of market in health care. Emphasis was given to increase district level capacities to provide different range of services at various levels including primary, secondary and tertiary. It also called for rapid expansion of medical and paramedical education to fill huge human resource gaps with conversion of district and sub-divisional hospitals as centres of training and education. Almost at the same breath the 12th Plan wanted to 'find a workable way of encouraging cooperation between the public and private sector in achieving health goals'—essentially hinting towards public-private partnerships (PPPs) and contracting-in (Planning Commission, 2012 Vol III, p. 9). The PC and later NHP 2015 had hinted that transformation towards such managed care model would require a longer time horizon and as an interim strategy proposed greater coordination between public and private sector to provide 'continuum of care'.

We can clearly identify the multiple strategies of marketization of health care suggested under the 12th Five Year Plan. The range include contracting in private providers in urban areas, more organised forms of PPPs and developing managed care models by including private providers along with public facilities within the managed network. Such large scale attempts of privatization were being justified to enhance patient choice, increase efficiency of resource use based on the assumption that private sector is more efficient and offers good quality care compared to public sector in delivery of health care services. It was being argued that the inherent problems of private provisioning would be overcome by combining incentives and effective regulation of both public and private sector.

The NHP 2017 takes forward the privatization agenda further by proposing 'strategic purchasing' of care from private and public sector alike through insurance like mechanisms.

The consequences of using public resources to finance a private sector led model of provisioning are well known- induced demand for unnecessary provisioning of services, drive towards more technology intensive interventions and over-emphasis on diagnostics and; above all high cost of care. One of the reasons why private sector needs to indulge in such unethical practices is the failure to achieve economies of scale for the investments made on capital intensive equipment and diagnostics. In order to create product discrimination and provide 'state of the art' technologies, there is always a tendency to over supply some of the high end services like Compute Tomography (CT) scans, magnetic resonance imaging (MRI) etc. It is often the case that if one follows standard treatment protocols, given the patient load, usage would be less and hence returns would be less compared to investments made to procure such services. One of the ways to achieve economies of scale is to plan on epidemiological basis and develop systemic ways of cooperation between providers for sharing the load and ensure continuum of care. Public owned and managed district health systems with clear referral links are the main feasible approach by which many nations have achieved this goal. But if the reliance is only on demand side financing of private providers, then this possibility is lost.

Making Resources Available to States and Enhancing Capacity to Spend: The 'Cloud-Rain Conundrum'

It is quite often argued that there is no dearth of money in public sector however states do not have the capacity to absorb funds. It is quite usual to write the epitaph of public sector to build the argument that direct provisioning is not an efficient option and insurance kind of mechanisms are more effective ways of ensuring health security and access. The question of fund absorption and quality of care are not isolated from overall spending. The relationship between spending and quality is like rain and cloud. A cloudy sky is necessary to have rain but it is not sufficient. It does not always rain if the sky is clouded and it never rains if the sky is not clouded.

Though mere increase in the magnitude of spending may not be sufficient to increase the quality of spending, it is important to recognise that spending is an absolute necessity to improve quality.

Public Spending on health in India is among the lowest in the world when compared in terms of share in GDP and per capita spending. There were only seven countries in the world (Myanmar, Guiana, Lao PDR, Pakistan, Azerbaijan, Cote d'Ivore, Singapore) which spent lesser proportion of GDP on health in 2010 (WHO, 2013). Some developing countries like Brazil, Chile, Costa Rica, Cuba, Colombia, Thailand, Malaysia and South Africa, have made significant efforts in recent history towards provisioning of universal access to health, spend much higher proportions of GDP on health (Table 3.1). Governments in neighbouring countries like Sri Lanka, China, and Nepal could mobilise more resources towards health than what was done in India. Per capita public investment on health, is almost at the same level with the average of the low income countries (LICs) and much lower than the low middle income countries (LMICs). Countries like Brazil, Thailand, and South Africa which have recently made attempts to universalize health care, have stepped up public spending on health to 3–5% of GDP over the period of a decade or so. Lack of public

Table 3.1 International comparison of Government expenditure on health (2004–2014)

		Out of pocket expenditure (OOPS) as % of total health expenditure (THE)		General government health expenditure per Capita in Int$ (purchasing power parity)		General government health expenditure (GGHE) as % of gross domestic product (GDP)	
Regions	Countries	2004	2014	2004	2014	2004	2014
BRICS	South Africa	11	6	292	554	3.2	4.2
	Brazil	33	25	344	607	3.3	3.8
	Russia	33	46	316	958	3.1	3.7
	China	54	32	79	408	1.8	3.1
	India	68	62	26	32	1.0	1.2
Asian							
Neighbours	Bangladesh	58	67	17	25	1.0	0.8
	Bhutan	28	25	120	206	3.2	2.6
	Pakistan	61	56	24	45	0.7	0.9
	Myanmar	85	51	5	48	<	1.0
	Nepal	55	48	23	55	1.6	2.3
	Sri Lanka	44	42	96	207	2.0	2.0
	Thailand	26	12	206	467	2.3	3.2
	Malaysia ara>	34	35	317	574	2.1	2.3

Source World Health Organisation (2010)
*Derived from WHS

spending has resulted in heavy dependence on household out of pocket expenses (OOP) leading to inequity in access, untreated morbidity, unavoidable deaths and various forms of financial hardship while seeking care including impoverishment, health care spending shooting above the affordable limits (call catastrophic expense) and indebtedness (Garg & Karan, 2009; Ghosh, 2011; NCMH, 2005; Selvaraj & Karan, 2009).

As of now, states spend more than two third of total public spending on health. Given constitutional responsibilities, any major expansion in public spending on health has to happen through States. Given the unsatisfactory situation of State finances, whereby States are being asked to cut expenditure to meet fiscal deficit targets- major reallocation in favour of health looks unlikely if the entire onus is left to the states.

The need of the hour is that both Union and state governments need to step up their expenditure significantly. However, since the NDA government came to power in 2014 we see systematic cuts in Union government allocations towards health, this despite the repeated commitment under NHP to augment public investment. National Health Mission budget allocation and expenditure has gone down during the Modi era (Mukhopadhyay & Sinha, 2019; Sundararaman et al., 2016).

Introduction of NRHM had brought in additional funds, albeit limited, for health sector; recent trends are quite disturbing. It is being observed that contrary to popular perceptions. states are absorbing more central funds following the introduction of the flagship NRHM. During 2008–09 and 2012–13, expenditure by states increased by seven percent, after adjusting for rise in prices while Union Government expenditure remains stagnant (Fig. 3.1). States like Tamil Nadu, Himachal Pradesh and Rajasthan have demonstrated that a rejuvenation of the public health system is possible and cost effective as well. The Centre's spending on health as a percentage of GDP is the

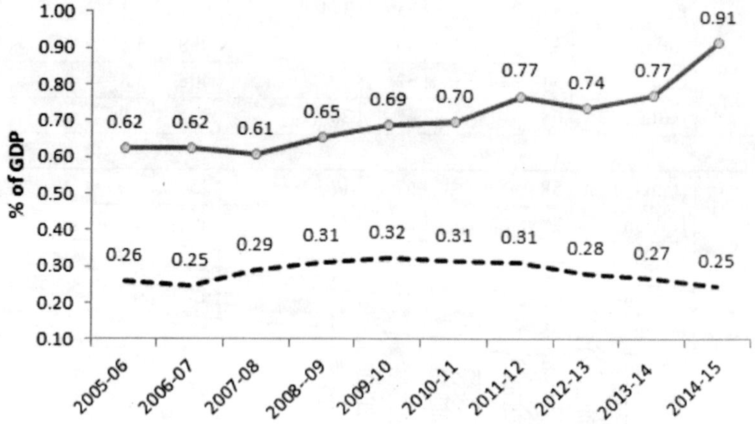

Fig. 3.1 Union and state government expenditure on health (adjusted for inflation): widening divide. *Note* 2013–14: state figure is RE, union is actual expenditure; 2014–15: State is BE, union is RE. *Source* Authors calculation based on budget data. (RBI, 2016; Government of India, 2016)

lowest in the last four decades (Fig. 3.2), even lower than the early 1990s. Utilization of NRHM funds increased to more than cent percent after 2010–11 in some cases (Fig. 3.3).

It is true that during the initial years of the Mission considerable portion of funds remained under-utilised especially in the High Focus States[1] (Indranil & Trisha, 2009). Further increment in public spending was scuttled arguing that states are not capable of spending funds that are being provided to them and hence the increase in investment is futile. Recent trends show that fund absorptive capacity is gradually increasing in the high focus states and higher percent of NRHM funds are getting invested towards creating systems (Mukhopadhyay, 2012a).

Several expert groups (HLEG), Parliamentary Standing Committees have advocated for enhancement of public investment in health to 2.5–3% of GDP. The NDA government seemed to concur, announcing its National Health Assurance Mission.

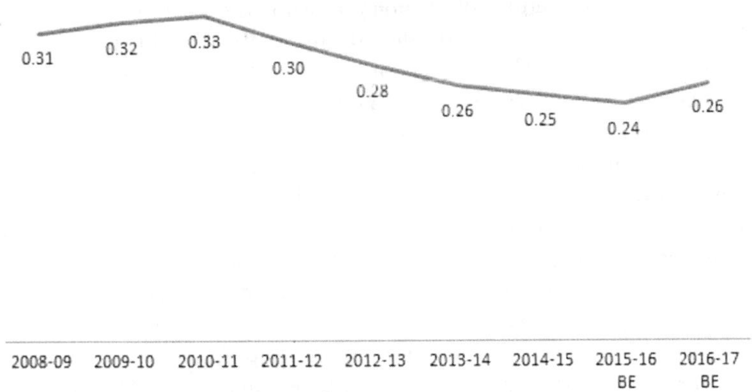

Fig. 3.2 Centre's spending on health as % of GDP: on a slippery slope. *Source* same as Fig. 3.1

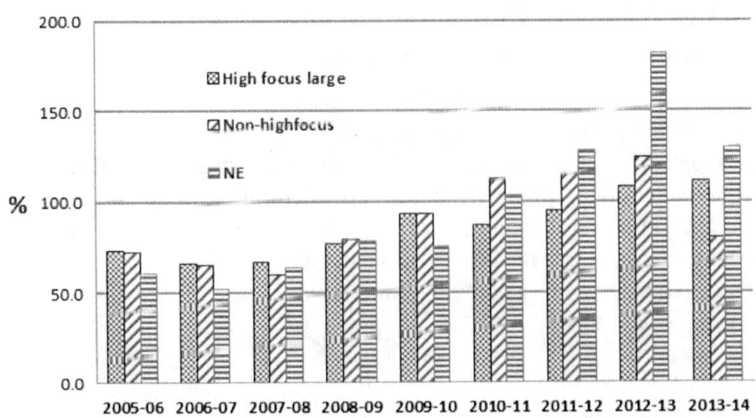

Fig. 3.3 Utilisation of NRHM/NHM funds by states. *Source* MIS, NRHM various years

But the budget cuts are a major dampener. Finance Commission transfers and further restructuring of resource sharing, with additional taxation rights devolved to states are essential to meet the commitments of public spending. Under 14th Finance Commission, the Union Government is claiming to increase the share of states in total taxes. Meanwhile, many Central Sponsored Schemes are being withdrawn and the system of central assistance to state plan is being dismantled. The net effect on health sector is quite debilitating. Within NRHM, fund flow arrangements have undergone several changes over the last few years, creating situation of confusion and stalemate. The reduced Government spending on health has a perilous effect on the quality of health services delivered through government facilities. Implementation of the NHM has been halted across states. Salaries of doctors and nurses are due; mothers are being denied financial assistance after delivery. There is an unwritten embargo against any new intervention under the NHM. Integrated Child Development Scheme (ICDS), one of the oldest programs to improve nutrition is facing its severest crunch.

As per the recommendations of the 6th Common Review Mission (CRM) of the NRHM, Government expenditure on the NRHM in the 12th Plan period must be increased to at least the scale that was originally envisaged in the Framework of Implementation document (2005–2012). Over the last few years, states have begun taking steps to improve poor fund absorption and increase efficiency of fund utilization, and this is an important first step. Future reform measures must focus on institutional innovations and appropriate changes in rules and regulations to enable better use of investments. However we also caution that unless there is sufficient and corresponding increase in investment, the focused reforms alone will not make the critical difference for improving health care and health outcomes (NRHM, 2013). Though health is a State subject, they need to be financially empowered to invest more in health. But that cannot be at the cost of withdrawal of efforts from the Centre. The central Government needs to enhance its own spending to match State efforts.

Private Provisioning: Consolidation of Capital and Destruction of Petty-Production

As discussed earlier, the NHP has proposed multiple strategies to engage with the private sector. The idea is to push through a thorough restructuring of health system in the country by giving private sector a permanent place in government financed provisioning. Though it is being argued that the current strategy is innovative and designed to provide people the best care as early as possible in the given context, the fact is that such a system is a continuation of neo-liberal policies followed over the last two decades in India.

Increasing domination of private sector in service delivery (Table 3.2) led to high dependence of people on their own means to manage health care expenses, leading to indebtedness and poverty; prolonged deprivation of a large section of population from any access to modern health care system and uncontrolled escalation of

Table 3.2 Share (percent) of private sector in total hospitalized episodes and short duration ailments

Year	Hospitalisation		Short duration ailments	
	Rural	Urban	Rural	Urban
1986–87 (42nd round)	39.97	39.56	74.29	72.79
1995–96 (52nd round)	54.71	56.93	80.29	81.65
2004–05 (60th round)	58.39	61.76	77.72	80.83
2014 (71st round)	58.1	68	71.7	78.8

Source Based on NSSO estimates, 42nd, 52nd, 60th and 71st round

costs of care (Garg & Karan, 2009; Ghosh, 2011; Mahal et al., 2002; Selvaraj & Karan, 2009; Indian state has not only ignored the agonies of people, it has adopted a whole range of 'health sector reforms' like gradual withdrawal from providing health services, introducing user fees, cut backs in public spending on health, privatisation and commercialisation of existing facilities and services, provision of subsidised land and other incentives to systematically help private sector grow (Baru & Nundy, 2008; Dev & Mooij, 2002; Ravindran, 2010; Sen, 2001; Sita Prabhu, 1994; Tulasidhar, 1993). Though these reforms were pushed in the name of preventing so called 'error of wrong inclusion', i.e. free up public subsidy from the undeserving rich and redistribute among poor; it ended up with enormous 'error of wrong inclusion' by pushing out the deserving poor who had to suffer not only the economic costs but also the corresponding social costs. One should see the current design as an ambitious step forward in the process of enhancing market penetration. During the early 1980s, private sector in India largely comprised of individual practitioners, both qualified and unqualified, essentially providing primary level, outpatient care of extremely variable quality across urban and rural areas in the country (Baru, 2003; Jesani & Anantharaman, 1990). The growth of secondary and tertiary hospitals was relatively new phenomenon, limited to metro cities and few affluent rural pockets of the country. Like every other sector of the economy, growth of organised and advanced capitalist forms of production requires state support in different forms. The case of health sector is no different.

In the 1980s, when medical care was gradually opened up to private sector and PPPs were made part of national strategy (MoHFW, 1983), the objective was to help market grow. Introduction of neo liberal reforms in the 1990s accelerated the process. Continuous cutbacks in expenditure halted the process of expansion of government health services and reduced quality of care (Dev & Mooij, 2002; Tulasidhar, 1993). A large and relatively affluent section of the middle class moved out of the government health services and formed the market base for organised private sector (Baru, 1998, 2003). This was supplemented by various forms of input subsidies including land, import subsidies on machinery and equipment and tax concessions. Large government investments made in medical education allowed private sector to access subsidised, cheap but good quality doctors. Freeze in government recruitments left little choice to the medical graduates but to join private sector or fly abroad. PPPs were expanded to channelize government revenues to provide further impetus to private sector growth. Adherence to selective primary level care approach pushed citizens further away from public sector for wide range services including chronic care especially related to non-communicable diseases (Rao et al., 2005; Qadeer, 2002; Sen, 2012).

Then, the relevant question is, why the same international agencies which advocated vehemently in favour of cutback in public spending and introduction of user fees are today talking about increased public spending on health and abolition of user fees. In order to understand the question better we need to study the structure of private health sector today. Over the years, the corporate health sector though very few in absolute numbers, has really penetrated in the big cities. These arc large establishments with huge bed strengths. Apart from these, there are small establishments in the form of nursing homes providing wide range of secondary care services. But the large majority are still the individual practitioners. While there is no comprehensive data for the entire private sector, some recent data sources can provide some partial picture. Survey of unorganised enterprises conducted by the National Sample Survey Organisation (NSSO) covers enterprises operating in service sector including health sector (MoSPI, 2003, 2009). There are two rounds of surveys which provide data for the years 2000–01 and 2006–07. The data on corporate health sector is collected by Centre for Monitoring of Indian Economy (CMIE). Together the two data sources give picture of individual practitioners, small nursing homes, diagnostic facilities and the corporate sector hospitals and diagnostic chains. Two important things come up if one analyzes these two data sets.

According to the NSSO survey, in 2001–02, all these practitioners and facilities put together were approximately 1.3 million unorganized enterprises[2] providing health services in the country, excluding public facilities. Four out of every five enterprises (1.1 million) were Own Account Enterprises[3] (OAEs) and the rest were (0.23 million) establishments[4] (Fig. 3.4). OAEs are individual or household run business providing health services without hiring a worker on a fairly regular basis. An overwhelming majority (Eighty percent) of the OAEs are located at the villages where as most

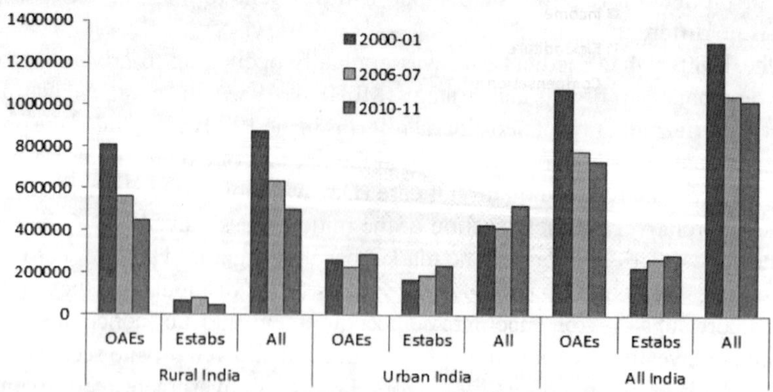

Fig. 3.4 Un-organised health enterprises in India (in '000 s). *Source* Unit records, NSSO 57th round and 63rd round

of the establishments are in the urban areas. As per the 2006–07 survey, number of unorganised enterprises has declined to 1.05 million. This decline is mainly on account of a decline in OAEs (0.78 million), whereas number of establishments has increased (0.27 million). Thus between 2000–01 and 2006–07 more than 40,000 new establishments have come up, largely in the urban areas. Simultaneously, OAEs have gone down by almost 0.3 million. These clearly point out that rapid transformation towards organised forms of production is taking place in urban areas of the country. Disappearance of general practitioners from Delhi is a reflection of such tendencies. Further insights are required on the process through which these practitioners are being included in the medico industrial complex. Though the NHP recognises this heterogeneity of structure within private sector, it fails to device an appropriate strategy to suit the current health system realities.

At the same time corporate sector has rapidly expanded over the last two decades. In 2001 there were some 35 corporations listed with Centre for Monitoring of Indian Economy (Fig. 3.5). By 2006, the number jumped to 93. In 2001 total income was only INR 8510 millions. This increased INR 35,300 million in 2007. This meant an annual average increase of 18% in real terms (adjusted for inflation). This is more than double the real GDP growth rate during this period. Private Investments did not grow at the same rate till 2005, though we observe sudden jump in 2006 and 2007 (CMIE, 2013). Meanwhile, news reports on merger and amalgamations suggest that consolidation of the corporate sector itself is going on rapidly.

Compensation to employees did not increase too much. Out of the total income earned only a sixth went to the employees. One of the pathways through which capitalism increases income is by squeezing wages. Figure 3.5 clearly depicts such tendency in health sector. It is expected that a lot of squeeze in wages would happen on the paramedical and nursing staff, while hefty payments are made to the specialist doctors. Mass exoduses of experienced specialists from All India Institute of Medical

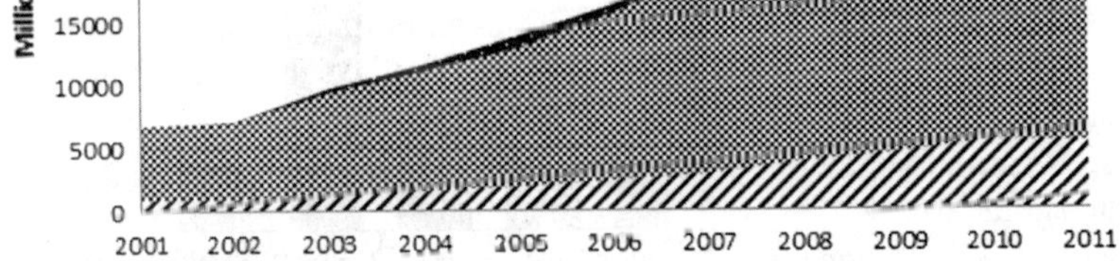

Fig. 3.5 Income, investments and compensation to employees in corporate health sector (constant prices). *Source* CMIE, PROWESS data source

Science who are being lured by astronomical salaries clearly substantiate such developments (PTI, 2012). Exploitation of semi-skilled labour on one hand and sharing part of the profit with the upper echelon of the professionals on the other helps hospitals manage hefty income. At the same time there is a gender and caste dimension to the problem. Unlike the medical professionals in the country who are mainly upper caste men, most of paramedical staffs and nursing staffs come from diverse deprived sections of the society and also largely women. The so called claim to efficiency of the private sector is based on cost minimization which often leads to deterioration of quality and at the same time exploitation of women and deprived sections of the society.

Capitalist development in health is far from being complete. The rate at which individual practitioners are being replaced with organised capital is quite overwhelming. Transition towards managed care models would definitely accelerate the process. Given the assurance from government about cashless services, a lot of people would tend to enrol themselves with the better looking secondary and tertiary care institutions where ever they are available. In order to incentivize the growth process further, the government of India has included health sector in Viability Gap Funding scheme under which 20% of expenses would be borne by the government if hospitals and medical colleges are setup in non-metros. This, coupled with the market guarantee mechanisms provided under 'managed care' model, can create conditions for further expansion of private sector.

Is Regulation the Panacea?

Consequences of private sector led growth on people are well- documented. Evidences of RSBY suggest that cashless insurance mechanisms fail to reduce out of pocket expenses (Sakthivel & Karan, 2012). A number of studies show that with such Government Funded Health Insurance (GFHI) schemes, health care is becoming more expensive rather than cheap with people having to pay large amounts of money out of pocket, often for unnecessary procedures. It has to be noted that more than two thirds of out-of-pocket expenditure on health is incurred on account of outpatient care (67%). The evidence from these schemes shows that care is seldom 'free', particularly when it is sought at private hospitals. Out of every 100 cases of hospitalisation under various GFHIs, only 3 get free care. Further, people, even when they are insured, spend more money when they are admitted in a private hospital than what they would have spent seeking care in public hospitals'. More than 60% of those seek care in private hospitals under GFHIs face catastrophic expenses at the 10% threshold.

One of the key arguments in favour of the GFHIs is that it brings in better access to health care as it opens up possibilities of accessing free care in private sector, particularly where government hospitals do not function or don't exist. However, as we have observed earlier, reality in India is that private hospitals have either grown where public hospitals already exist or in metro cities, state capitals and other big cities where there is greater purchasing power. There are hardly any private hospitals in rural areas and remote parts of the country.

Furthermore, these schemes have favoured the betteroff sections of the society, while the official promise has been to improve access for the poor and marginalised. For instance, only 10.6% of the people belonging to the poorest sections in rural areas and 8.6% in urban areas are covered under all the GHFIs. Whereas coverage among the richest sections are 17.7% and 15% in rural and urban areas respectively. If we leave out the hospitalisations related to child birth, hospitalisation rate among women remain lower (4.1%) compared to overall hospitalisation rate of 5.4%. Women also face financial hardship as 18% of those seeking care resort to borrowing—the main source of financing high cost of care under GFHIs.

Uncontrolled greed for profit by private sector has also burdened women disproportionately. Numerous incidents of unethical practices, over charging, unnecessary care and in extreme situation deaths due to medical negligence and denial of care have been reported. Thousands of women have been subjected to unnecessary procedures like hysterectomies under these GFHIs (Economic Times, 2019). Complete absence of regulation of private sector has remained a major challenge in assuring fair prices as well as adequate quality care in private sector. Ignoring all the evidence, the current government has launched another GFHI scheme-Pradhan Mantri Jan Arogya Yojna (PMJAY). The scheme offers health insurance coverage up to Rs. 5 lakh per family for 10 crore families across the country, with the promise of free hospitalization care for the poor and marginal sections of the society. This scheme is basically an expansion of the Rashtriya Swasthya Bima Yojana (RSBY) and numerous government funded health insurance (GFHI) schemes run by state governments.

Experience of Organisation for Economic Co-operation and Development (OECD) countries shows that the cost of care is increasing faster than growth of GDP and every day a larger share of resources is being invested to finance health care while entitlements are getting gradually curbed (Fig. 3.6).

There is an effort to deliberately underestimate problems of private sector and hush up the real issues under the garb of regulation. Global experience suggests that most of the developing countries do not have the capacity to regulate private health sector and especially corporate hospitals. In India, there is very limited experience in terms of regulating private sector. Until recently, there were no efforts to enumerate total private health enterprises at the national level. Thus the question of regulation has been limited to the field of manufacturing, sale, quality and prescription of drugs and pharmaceuticals (the Pharmacy Act, the Drugs and Cosmetics Act and Dangerous Drugs Act); Medical and clinical practice related (COPRA, the Indian Medical Council Act, and the Human Organ Transplant Act); registration and inspection of facilities and the Nurses, Midwives and Health Visitors Act) (Mukhopadhyay, 2012b). Apart from these, there were state level legislations in some states for registering private sector. Though these legislations are there on paper there is hardly any initiative from the state governments to even register private clinical establishments, not to speak about regulating them.

As a result these institutions remain highly unregulated. Very recently the Clinical Establishment (Registration and Regulation) Bill, 2010 has been passed in the

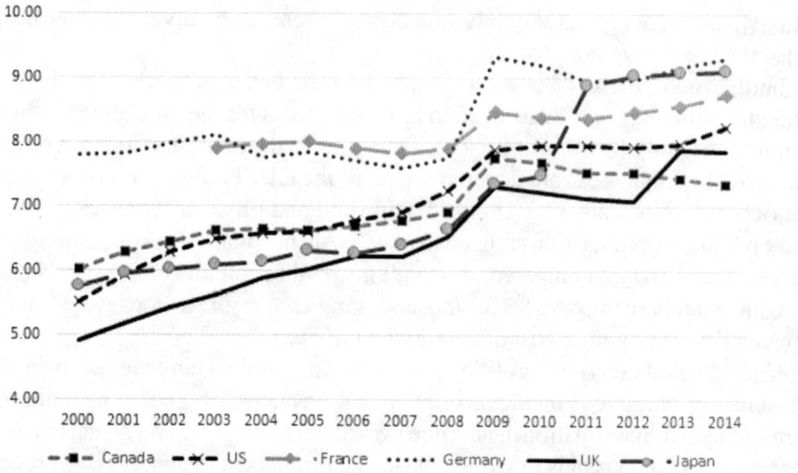

Fig. 3.6 Government health expenditure on health as percent of GDP: some OECD countries. *Source* WHO, National Health Accounts

Rajya Sabha. The Bill makes it mandatory to register all health establishments, with or without beds, both public and privately owned, barring establishment under the jurisdiction of armed forces. The Bill is absolutely silent about the regulation of prices in the private sector. One of the major maladies of accessing private sector is high and differential prices charged by private facilities. It is important in this context that there are restrictions on prices that the private sector can charge. Its failure to propose any regulation on prices is a reflection of the dominance of private hospital lobby over the Government.

The NHP 2017 views the existing version of Clinical Establishment Act as an outdated act, stated to be 'intrusive' and there is no mention of need to ensure key components of regulation such as patient rights, regulation of rates, standard treatment guidelines, multi-stakeholder bodies to oversee regulation, etc. In the watered down accreditation, a non-binding voluntary mechanism is proposed as a 'first step' instead.

Conclusions

The noble objectives of the NHP 2017 to ensure equity, to ensure continuum of care and to facilitate rational use of technology would necessarily fall apart because of contradictory design-a design based on privatization that is being pushed by the given global order and the class composition of the present national Government. The prerequisite of strong public sector in ensuring greater access has been demonstrated in all kind of contexts, from the most developed countries like UK, Sweden, middle income countries like Costa Rica and Chile or developing countries like Cuba, Sri

Lanka, Thailand, and Brazil etc. Like all other Plans, the 12 FYP and subsequently the NHP 2017 has retained the rhetoric of strengthening public sector and at the same time paved the way for its further monopolization by the private sector. These tendencies if not halted will overpower the entire agenda of system strengthening through NHM.

This may require bringing qualified general practitioners from various systems of medicine into the public fold before they get completely integrated into the medico industrial complex. Experience of initial decades of NHS of Britain shows that the General Practitioners (GPs) can provide cheaper services, can be regulated, rational treatments can be ensured through them and most importantly indirectly curb the growth of tertiary hospital sector. The political context under which such radical transformations had happened in UK was vastly different from the neo-liberal regime that we are living in. The strength of progressive political and civil society movements would be tested at such a juncture. Whether it can really push the agenda towards rebuilding public provisioning based on Primary Health Care approach or allows the vested interests to make use of public money to further the interest of profit and greater downfall of public sector is to be seen in the days to come. Small ray of hope is seen in the provisioning of free drugs in public sector. An entitlement which was unobtrusively dropped during the era of liberalization may now bring patients back to public facilities and create demand for better services. However, the battle to rebuild public sector in a Primary Health Care approach cannot be fought in isolation and in current context of neo-liberalism possibilities of rejuvenating government health services are really bleak. Under the present regime, where exploitation of labour is taking place in most advanced and pervasive form, state still plays its role in generating demand. But only in a manner which doesn't interfere in the process of production or price setting. That is why artificial means of demand generation like cash transfer, voucher schemes, insurance and other market guarantee schemes are promoted; which allow market to operate freely and make plunder over peoples' money. That is why health care, food and nutrition, water services are packaged and epitaph of universal and comprehensive public provisioning is written in unprecedented hurry.

Notes

1. There are ten High Focus States: Uttar Pradesh, Bihar, Orissa, Madhya Pradesh, Rajasthan, Chhattisgarh, Jharkhand, Uttarakhand, Himachal Pradesh and Assam.
2. Unorganised Enterprise: The unorganized sector comprised the following types of enterprises: (i) All the enterprises except units registered under Section 2m(i) and 2m(ii) of the Factories Act, 1948 and Bidi and Cigar Workers (condition of employment) Act, 1966. (ii) All enterprises except those run by Government (Central, State, local bodies)/Public Sector Enterprises.
3. Own-account Enterprise: An Own-Account Enterprise (OAE) is defined as a unit which is engaged in the provision of health service on a fairly regular basis but without employing any hired worker.

4. Establishment: An enterprise, on the other hand, is defined as a unit that employs at least one hired worker on a fairly regular basis. A hired employee is one who is a paid or unpaid apprentices, paid household member/servant/resident worker in an enterprise.

References

Baru, R. (1998). *Private health care in India: Social characteristics and trends*. SAGE Publications.

Baru, R. (2003, January). Privatisation of health services: A South Asian perspective. *Economic and Political Weekly, 38*(42), 4433–4437.

Baru, R., & Nundy, M. (2008, January). Blurring of boundaries: Public–private partnerships in health services in India. *Economic and Political Weekly, 43*(4), 62–71.

Centre for Monitoring Indian Economy Pvt. Ltd. (2013). *Prowess database*.

Dev, S. M., & Mooij, J. (2002, March). Social Sector Expenditures in the 1990s: Analysis of central and state budgets. *Economic and Political Weekly, 37*(9), 853–866.

Economic Times. (2019). Hysterectomy tops Ayushman claims; red flags raised; July 22, 2019; https://economictimes.indiatimes.com/news/politics-and-nation/hysterectomy-tops-ayushman-claims-red-flags-raised/articleshow/70323579.cms?from=mdr

Garg, C. C., & Karan, A. K. (2009). Reducing out-of-pocket expenditures to reduce poverty: A disaggregated analysis at rural-urban and state level in India. *Health Policy and Planning, 24*(2), 116–128. Accepted November 11, 2008.

Ghosh, S. (2011). Catastrophic payments and impoverishment due to out-of-pocket health spending. *Economic and Political Weekly, 46* (47).

Government of India. (2011). *High level expert group report on universal health coverage in India* (submitted to Planning Commission). Planning Commission of India.

Government of India. (2016). Union budget: Expenditure budget of various years; www.indiabudget.nic.in.

Indranil, & Trisha, A. (2009). *Safe-motherhood, public provisioning and health financing in India* (report). Centre for Budget and Governance Accountability.

Jesani, A., & Anantharaman, S. (1990). *Private sector and privatisation of health care services: A review paper*. ICSSR-ICMR Joint Panel on Health, Foundation for Research in Community Health.

Lancet India Group for Universal Health Care. (2011, January 12). India towards universal health coverage. *Lancet, 377*.

Mahal, A., Singh, J., Afridi, F., Lamba, V., Selvaraju, V., & Gumber, A. (2002). *Who benefits from public sector health spending in India?* National Council for Applied Economic Research.

Ministry of Health and Family Welfare (MoHFW), GoI. (1983). *National health policy*. Ministry of Health and Family Welfare.

Ministry of Health and Family Welfare (MoHFW), GoI. (2009). *National health bill*. Ministry of Health and Family Welfare, Government of India.

MOSPI. (2003). *Unorganised service sector in India: 2001–02, NSS 57th round*. National Sample Survey Organisation, Ministry of Statistics and Programme Implementation.

MoSPI. (2009). Service sector in India (2006–07) Operational characteristics of enterprises. NSS 63 Round. Report No. 528 (63/2.345/1). National Sample Survey Organisation, Ministry of Statistics and Program Implementation; February 2009. New Delhi MoSPI 2006. *Morbidity, health care and condition of the aged*. National Sample Survey Organisation, Ministry of Statistics and Program Implementation, NSSO 60th round (Jan-June 2004).

Mukhopadhyay, I., & Sinha, D. (2019). Painting a picture of Ill-health. In Azad, Chakraborty, S., Raman, S., & Sinha, D. (Eds.), *"Quantum leap in the wrong direction"*, Orient Black Swan, Feb 2019; ISBN-10: 9352876180

Mukhopadhayay, I. (2012a). Health System Strengthening and the Importance of Public Investment: A Study of NRHM in Bihar. *BMC Proceedings, 6*(Supplement 5), O11.

Mukhopadhayay, I. (2012b). *Public health care expenditure in India: A study of Kerala, Tamil Nadu and West Bengal* (Unpublished Ph.D. thesis). Submitted to the Centre for Social Medicine and Community Health (CSMCH), Jawaharlal Nehru University.

National Health Systems Resource Centre. (2016). *National health accounts estimates for India (2013–14).* Ministry of Health and Family Welfare, Government of India.

National Commission on Macroeconomics and Health. (2005). *Report of National Commission on Macroeconomics and Health.* Ministry of Health and Family Welfare, Government of India.

National Rural Health Mission. (2013). *Report of the 6th common review mission.* National Rural Health Mission Ministry of Health and Family Welfare, Government of India. http://nrhm.gov.in/monitoring/common-review-mission/6th-common-review-mission-crm.html

Planning Commission. (2012). *XII Five Year Plan: Social sector* (Vol. II). Government of India.

Press Trust of India. (PTI). 2012. *AIIMS faces Exodus of doctors*, PTI, 26.

Qadeer, I. (2002). Primary health care: From adjustment to reform. In K. Seeta Prabhu & R. Sudarshan (Eds.), *Reforming India's social sector, poverty, nutrition, health and education.* Social Science Press.

Rao, S., Nundy, M., & Dua, A. (2005). Delivery of health services in private sector (background papers). *Financing and Delivery of Healthcare Services in India.*

Ravindran, S. (2010). Health Sector Development Projects of the World Bank. In M. Kelley & D. D'Souza (Eds.), *World Bank in India: Undermining Sovereignty, distorting development*. Orient Black Swan.

Reserve Bank of India. (2016). State budget: State finances: A study of budget, RBI, various years.

Sakthivel, S., & Karan, A. (2012, May). Why publicly financed health insurance schemes are ineffective in providing financial risk protection. *Economic and Political Weekly, 47*(11), pp.60–68.

Selvaraj, S., & Karan, A. K. (2009). Deepening health insecurity in India: Evidence national sample surveys since 1980s. *Economic and Political Weekly, 44*(40).

Sen, K. (2001). Health reforms and developing countries: A critique. In I. Qadeer, K. Sen, & K. R. Nayar (Eds.), *Public health and poverty of reforms: A South Asian perspective.* Sage.

Sen, G. (2012, February). Universal health coverage in India. *Economic and Political Weekly, 47*(08), 25.

Sethi, N. (2015, August 25). NITI Aayog against free health care, bats for more private sector role. *Business Standard.*

Sita Prabhu, K. (1994, April 16–23). The budget and 'structural adjustment with a human face'. *Economic and Political Weekly, 29*(16/17), 1011–1013

Sundararaman, T., Mukhopadhyay, I., Muraleedharan, V. R. (2016). No respite for public health. *Economic & Political Weekly, 16*, 39–42. ISSN: 0012-9976; ISSN (Online)-2349-8846.

Tulasidhar, V. B. (1993, November). Expenditure compression and health sector outlays. *Economic and Political Weekly, 28*(45), 2473–2477.

WHO. (2010). *World health statistics.* WHO.

WHO. (2013). *Global health expenditure database.* WHO.

Chapter 4
Interrogating the Proposed Universal Healthcare in India Through a 'Quality' Lens

Prachinkumar Ghodajkar

Introduction

Rising health inequalities, catastrophic healthcare costs pushing people below the poverty line, along with glaring gaps between economic growth rates and health status of people have raised many questions about the post-liberalisation health sector reforms in India. Having one of the lowest rates of public spending on health has become a source of discomfort for the country in the face of failure to achieve the targets set for Millennium Development Goals (MDGs). Other developing countries with similar health expenditure patterns, of about 5% of Gross Domestic Product (GDP) (public and private together), have achieved much better health indices as compared to India. This turns the focus on to the problems of the existing healthcare delivery mechanisms and models. The quality of services delivered through available health services is another important concern and India shows a very dismal performance. The Global Burden of Disease 2016 data was used to compute Health Access Quality Index (HAQ) Index. India stands at the 145th position, among 195 countries ranked, much behind neighbouring counties like China (48th), Sri Lanka (71st) and Bangladesh (133rd) Bhutan (134th) (GBD 2016 Healthcare Access and Quality Collaborators, 2018).

The discussion around universal healthcare offers an opportunity to rethink the model of healthcare delivery and debate the core issues of good quality services. Perceived 'quality' constitutes one of the important reasons for increasing utilisation of healthcare services from the private sector. The impression of poor 'quality' of services in government hospitals is increasingly becoming the rationale for the introduction of market mechanisms and privatisation of different services through mechanisms such as public-private partnerships. The underlying assumption is that quality of services provided in private hospitals is good. Along with the logic of 'quality', the other reason influencing the principles and philosophy of proposed

P. Ghodajkar (✉)
Centre of Social Medicine and Community Health, Jawaharlal Nehru University, New Delhi, India

I. Qadeer et al. (eds.), *Universalising Healthcare in India*,
https://doi.org/10.1007/978-981-16-5872-3_4

models of health service delivery for universal healthcare is that the resources of the existing large private sector should be used in a 'meaningful' way to provide services.

The revealed preferences of people (in the form of large-scale use of the private sector), along with quality criteria like patient satisfaction, are increasingly being used to justify the continuation and augmentation of the private sector in a significant way. The High Level Expert Group on Universal Healthcare in India (HLEG), appointed in 2009 by the erstwhile Planning Commission (PC), and Report of Steering Committee on health for the Twelfth Five Year Plan (2012) recommendations now make provisions for this through public money. The convenient assumption among the dominant players in policy making, the economists, is that the revealed preferences are a reflection of what people really want (Adam Smith's 'rational man'). However, as Thomas Rice and Lynn Unruh argue, preferences are neither static, nor inborn nor given. Preferences are influenced by past experiences, expectations, peers, community pressures and expectation, marketing and media. They further argue that people often do not get the information that they need to maximise their preferences. Often even when information is available they might not use it to their maximum benefit (Rice & Unruh, 2009). The information asymmetry in the health sector accentuates this problem and the intermediate player, the doctor makes many choices on behalf of or for the patient. This makes health services different from the rest of the service industries.

The literature on quality of healthcare shows different streams of thought; some with prime focus on quality of care delivered to 'a patient', while others delve into quality of the 'health service system' providing care services to a population. Both are interdependent but involve different perspectives for addressing quality improvement initiatives. The history of the discourse on quality shows that the shift towards purchasing, rather than funding, health services has resulted in increased attention on ways of measuring hospital performance and quality of hospital care (Draper & Hill, 1996). Increased governmental and societal focus on health service quality demands nuanced understanding of different concepts of healthcare and quality of care. A different definition or conceptual understanding may lead to different policy paths, strategies and active measures (Priya, 2005).

Evans et al. note that, In 1980 Donabedian defined quality of care as 'that kind of care which is expected to maximize an inclusive measure of patient welfare, after one has taken account of the balance of expected gains and losses that attend the process of care in all its parts.' Ten years later the Institute of Medicine (IOM, USA) defined quality of care as 'the degree to which health services for individuals and population increase the likelihood of desired outcomes and are consistent with current professional knowledge.' The IOM narrowed the goal from improving total patients welfare to improving health outcomes, but also moved the focus from patients to individuals and population, thus allowing quality of care to incorporate promotion and prevention and not just cure and rehabilitation. It also added two qualifiers: 'desired health outcomes', to emphasize the need to consider the perspective of recipient of the service, and consistent with current professional knowledge to define standards of the service (Evans et al., 2001: 442).

The IOM also differed from Donabedian on the issue of treatment of resource constraints. Donabedian's initial definition was absolutist, reflecting what was maximally feasible for the patient given the current medical knowledge. Subsequently he allowed for an individualised or socially optimal definition, incorporating the concept of value so that the quality was the maximum possible for the inputs available. The IOM returned to the original definition of quality by Donabedian and explicitly rejected the inclusion of resource constraints in the definition, on the grounds that it should not fluctuate just because resources are constrained and unavailable (Evans et al., 2001: 443).

Neoliberal economic policies are known to have a negative impact on the welfare and income of vulnerable groups. In the present era of 'reforms', the claims of providing universal access to healthcare and efforts of improving quality of healthcare, therefore, raise the question: What quality criteria of health services and which models of health service delivery will contribute to health of the population, especially the vulnerable groups?

Conceptual Underpinnings of 'Quality' in Healthcare

Much of the literature on quality has been derived from management studies meant for the industrial sector (Anadaleeb, 2001). We have an intuitive understanding of the meaning of quality, yet when one sets out to study and to apply concepts of quality, it becomes very elusive. One of the reasons for this difficulty is that quality is multifaceted. It is also important to understand the concept of quality before attempting to implement quality improvement initiatives in our daily work. Many such efforts fail, or degenerate because of the failure to understand the multi-dimensional nature of quality. It is important to accept that quality is best defined and applied in the context of a specific time, space and activity (Hock, 2005).

The definition of quality takes on a new meaning, depending on the approach taken to attain quality. Garvin suggests five main approaches to attain quality (Garvin, 1988).[1] Different stakeholders (users, clinicians and payers) have different definitions and views onquality of care. For example, the management cares more about efficiency and profits over costs, while the users care more about whether the health system could provide patient-centred services according to individual needs (Yang, 2007). Thus the question arises: who judges quality?

In a complex healthcare sector, with hegemony and power of medical professionals over knowledge on the one side, and patients whose knowledge is limited on the other side, one can encounter situations where wants (felt needs) and needs (clinically assessed) may be divergent. In a situation where an insurance company is paying for the services, the purchaser (insurers) and user (patients) may have dissimilar needs and concerns, which will lead to conflicting definitions of quality. A service or a product of high quality therefore is one that best meets the needs of the majority of users, most of the time.

When assessing quality in healthcare, one must look beyond the actual delivery of services and incorporate those factors that facilitate delivery and the inherent consequences. These have come to be known as the structure, process, and outcome of care and the quality of care should be analysed through these three aspects (Donabedian, 1966). Under special circumstances, the significance of each aspect could be different. If the purpose of measurement is to improve the operation of the health service system then process is a better index, whereas if the purpose is to assess the contribution of the health services system to individuals or even society as a whole the focus should be on the outcome index (Yang, 2007).

Not only is the technical domain consisting of infrastructure, knowledge and skill of a provider important; the interpersonal relationship between patient and care giver is also equally critical. Donabedian's deliberations brought the patient's perspective into consideration for the first time while assessing quality. Quality in healthcare has several dimensions, which he later developed into what is known as 'seven pillars of quality'.[2] Pursuit of each of the several attributes of quality can be mutually reinforcing, but the pursuit of one attribute may also be in conflict with another so a balance has to be achieved. He suggests that while assessing quality a healthcare professional must take into account preferences of both, patient as well as society. When there is a disagreement between these two sets of preferences the healthcare provider faces the challenge of reconciling the differences (Donabedian, 1990).

Levels of Quality in Healthcare Services

Roemer and Montoya-Aguilar (1988) have analysed the concept of quality of healthcare at two levels. First, at a more general level, where resources or inputs, processes and outcomes of healthcare are involved, quality becomes an attribute of the system as a whole. While appraising the quality of healthcare system from an individual's perspective it is natural to take into account the results of such care. However, in quality assessment from the point of view of the population, what matters most are changes in survival, morbidity, disability, etc. Thus, according to these authors "quality signifies proper performance (according to standards) of interventions that are known to be safe, that are affordable by the society in question, and that have the ability to produce an impact on mortality, morbidity, disability, and malnutrition" (Roemer & Montoya-Aguilar, 1988: 54).

Yang Hui suggests different definitions of quality at different levels, viz. one at an individual level and another at a population level, which is discussed below (Yang, 2007).

Definition of Quality of Care at an Individual Level

While defining quality one should focus on the core of the concept of quality of care. High quality service means conditions where one has the ability to see the doctors and get care and treatment for the disease or illness (Ibid.). Thus the construct of quality of care at an individual level has two parts: whether individuals have access to the structure and process of health services, and whether such services are effective. To interpret this, technical terms like accessibility[3] and effectiveness[4] have been used (Ibid.).

Definition of Quality Healthcare at a Population Level

Population healthcare might be a contradiction to individual healthcare. From a government's point of view, the outcomes of population health are most important. The definition of quality of individual healthcare cannot be imposed directly on to the quality of population healthcare, as social background factors affecting the quality of service have to be accounted for. Assessing quality of care at a population level brings forth three other factors: equity, efficiency and cost.

Then the quality of healthcare at a population level is: 'The ability to obtain affordable services on the basis of efficiency[5] and equity[6]' (Ibid.). The balance between equity and efficiency is a permanent theme for healthcare quality, but this does not mean that efficiency and equity are mutually exclusive. The key concern is how to integrate the factors of economic and clinical motives with the social motives.

Thus, according to Yang Hui, the quality of individual healthcare is 'the ability to obtain effective health services according to needs and aiming at maximising the health benefits'; the quality of population healthcare is 'the capacity to obtain effective services through efficient and equal means to optimise population health benefits' (Ibid.).

Challenges to Assessment of Quality in Healthcare

Healthcare services are different from other service industries. Quality in health services needs spelling out of product attributes, whereas other industries get along by simply meeting customer requirements. This is because health services both in their production and consumption are far more complex than other kinds of industries. The standard industrial quality management approaches cannot deal with this complexity. Each episode of individual patient-health service interaction consists of unique, intangible, highly variable and contentious process that cannot be compared with the market. Unlike many products and services, healthcare has intrinsic moral and ethical dimensions in its production as well as delivery (Walsh, 1999).

The principles of universality, equity, and comprehen-siveness are integral if public health perspective is used for conceptualising quality. This perspective makes it necessary to ensure that quality services are available, accessible and responsive to the felt need of different sections of the population. Baru and Kurian (2008) while highlighting the importance of a public health perspective divide the different aspects of quality as tangible and intangible dimensions,[7] which are interdependent and interlinked. The intangible dimensions make quality measurement and comparison a difficult task.

Much of thc discussion on quality involves different kinds and types of 'standards'. The standards used to assess quality of care come from the dimensions of care under study and values that one uses to judge them. The standards can be either selective or inclusive depending on the selection of dimension of care for assessment. Selection and defining the boundaries of dimension of care selected for setting up standards, the number of dimensions selected, and exhaustiveness with which performance in each dimension is explored affects the quality assessment. Judgments of quality are incomplete when only a few dimensions are used and decisions about each dimension are made on the basis of partial evidence. Some dimensions, such as preventive care or the psychological and social management of health and illness, are often excluded from the definition of quality and the standards and criteria that make it operational. The dimensions selected and the value judgments attached to them constitute the operationalised definition of quality in each study (Donabedian, 1966). Donabedian's work contributed the argument that quality cannot be judged by healthcare professionals alone but must include the patient's views and preferences as well as those of society in general because 'standards' used in quality assessment are heavily influenced or rather come from three sources, namely,

- the science of healthcare that determines efficacy
- the individual values and expectations that determine acceptability
- social values and expectations that determine legitimacy (Sale, 2005).

Social Determinants of Quality of Healthcare

Considerable progress has been made over the past decades in health status as well as of the health services provided in the country as compared to what was there at the time of independence. However there are wide differences in health status as well as for accessibility to health services for different social groups. There are also rural/urban differences. The improvement in the quality of services is also not uniformly distributed for rural and urban population. There are wide differences in the quality of services provided for different social groups. "Placed squarely in the realm of human interaction, the way providers perceive the care needed and the care they provide, and the way clients perceive the care they need and are given, depend on complex, socially and culturally constructed needs and expectations, begging the question who defines quality?" (Hartigan, 2001: 7). Quality is thus a relative concept that is influenced by complex social determinants. Disparities in the quality of care provided can be observed according to gender, class, race, ethnicity and religion, across most of the dimensions of the healthcare process (effectiveness, safety, timeliness and patient centredness) and across most of the four patient perspectives (staying healthy, getting better, living with chronic illness, and coping with the end of life). The review work done by Fiscella (2003) brings out the above mentioned disparities in different medical, surgical and counselling treatment for different types of diseases.

The causes for disparities in provision of healthcare and its quality can be broadly classified into two: recipient side factors and provider side factors. Recipient side factors can be analysed both at the individual and at community level, whereas provider side factors can be analysed at individual provider, institution and healthcare system level. For instance, people from the poorer sections may delay treatment seeking while the healthcare providers would also give them lower priority, later and less attention as against middle class patients.

Tracing 'Quality' in Healthcare Services Development in the Indian Context

Historically, various Health Committee recommendations have touched upon quality issues of specific health programmes and on dimensions which impact upon quality of the public health service system as a whole. Institution level quality of services has also been addressed to some extent. However, there has been no regulation or quality assessment of the private healthcare sector till the recent past.

The Bhore Committee (Government of India (GoI), 1946) recommendations for health services development represent the most comprehensive system design. At the time of independence, by accepting the Bhore Committee recommendations the state took the responsibility of providing comprehensive healthcare to all irrespective of their ability to pay. The health services planned and recommended in it represented a comprehensive health service system to be developed within the resource availability of the country by giving priority to health services. The design of the health service system and organisational set up recommended was internally consistent with requirements of health service delivery and was externally consistent by addressing the social determinants of health. Much of the components of what constitutes 'quality' in healthcare at healthcare system level are directly or indirectly addressed in this report. The recommendations and principles of health service delivery are relevant even today. The recommendation of developing a comprehensive multi-tier health services system becomes an important prerequisite for providing quality health services and constitutes the structural aspect of quality as suggested by Donabedian (1990).

After a decade of adopting the Bhore Committee recommendations a review of implementation of those recommendations was given in the Mudaliar Committee (Ministry of Health and Family Welfare (MoHFW), 1962) report. It recommended stopping the expansion of services and improving the services delivered through existing institutions. It represents an important shift, where expansion of services and improving coverage of service was considered less important as compared to increasing performance of already existing institutions. The Jungalwalla Committee (Directorate General of Health Services (DGHS), 1967) recognised the multiplicity in health services delivery and recommended integration of health services for optimising resources and improving the health service delivery. The Mukerji Committee (GoI, 1966–69) recommendations correspond to identification of basic health services that need to be delivered on a priority basis.

The Kartar Singh Committee (MoHFW, 1973) recommendations constituted creation of intensive and twilight zones, based on distance around sub-centres in order to rationalise and optimise the work load for the then deficient number of Auxiliary Nurse Midwives (ANMs) available. It also brought into the picture a new cadre of health workers, the Multi-Purpose Worker (MPW), by doing away with multiple individual programme health workers. This was an important development in optimisation of existing health resources and providing better quality services to the community. The Shrivastava Committee (GoI, 1975) recommended having an additional doctor at the Primary Health Centre (PHC). Recognising the importance of referral services in the multi-tier health services system, it recommended a referral service complex. Importance of better monitoring, supervision and assistance to the MPW was recognised, and was to be provided with a new cadre of Health Assistants (HA). The issue of access to basic health services for vast sections of rural population was addressed by bringing in Village Health Guides, which also served the purpose of involving and empowering the community in the healthcare process to some extent, within the then resource availability of the country. Thus many of the issues of quality addressing structural, procedural and resource optimisation factors were addressed through these recommendations. The Alma Ata Declaration (WHO, 1978) on primary healthcare articulated principles and basic elements of primary healthcare, and defined essential services to be provided. This constituted minimum services that are to be ensured, and also served as a starting point for building up comprehensive services. The Declaration brought forth very important ideas on health service delivery and development. The primary healthcare approach was about community ownership and participation, sustainability, i.e. the ability of the community to run such services in the long run, rationality and appropriate technology, accessibility, comprehensiveness, inter-sectoral coordination, etc. and all these are attributes of the 'means' for the 'end' of providing 'health for all'. Therefore, much of the discussion in Comprehensive Primary Healthcare (CPHC) is about the 'means' and ways, principles and philosophy of providing the predetermined goal of health for all. India was signatory to the Alma Ata Declaration, but chose to follow a completely different trajectory of Selective Primary Healthcare with UNICEF in the form of strategies like GOBI-FFF.[8] Despite recognition of failures of vertical programmes the new strategy of GOBI-FFF complemented the further growth of disease-specific, techno-centricvertical national health programmes.

The National Health Policy 1982 and that of 2002 laid down policy guidelines for health services. These two policy reports represent apolicy shift in health services delivery. During Health Sector Reforms (HSRs) in the 1990s, Public Private Partnerships (PPPs) were recommended in the name of improving health services and making services more efficient. This led to the promotion of the private sector and downplaying of the general health services in the public system. HSRs along with its different policies such as PPPs brought about an important shift in the notion of quality from systemic to institutional level. It represents the neglect of the state-run health service system and increased attention being given to the stand alone private and public institutes providing health services. This era brought into focus quality assessment and accreditation of hospitals and healthcare institutes through different mechanisms propounded by different accreditation organisations, discussed in the subsequent section.

Meanwhile there were other attempts at improving health services delivery which can be considered as important for quality of health services. It included rational drug therapeutics or Standard Treatment Guidelines (STGs) developed by the Delhi Society for Promotion of Rational Use of Drugs (DISPRUD). Following Delhi, a few other states developed STGs. Different national health programmes have had standard operating procedures and treatment protocols developed for the conditions covered under those specific national health programmes. Syndromic approaches for diagnosing and treating different sexually transmitted diseases STDs/reproductive tract infections (RTIs) have also been developed. Other examples include the Integrated Management of Neonatal and Childhood Illnesses (IMNCI) for neonatal and childhood illnesses. The National Institute of Health and Family Welfare (NIHFW) has developed many management training modules for different health functionaries like district health officers. Most of these endeavours represent attempts at improving process-related dimensions of quality.

There were no separate internal systems for quality improvement other than the departmental supervisory structure. Efforts to assess the quality of health services or improve their quality were largely undertaken through the external committees set up from time to time for review of health services development and functioning, and their recommendations provided the guidelines and pathways for further development. Often, they were set up when a particular change was already envisaged.

Though largely systematic (applicable for larger systems), many of the recommendations made by different committees at different points of time and other guidelines made by different institutions/organisations and committees are also applicable for improving thequality of care at the level of institutes of healthcare delivery, e.g. Medical Council of India (MCI) guidelines for medical colleges. Different programmes like Family Planning Programme, Maternal and Child Health (MCH) Programme, Child Survival and Safe Motherhood (CSSM) Programme, Reproductive and Child Health (RCH) Programme, National Tuberculosis Programme (NTP), Revised National Tuberculosis Control Programme (RNTCP), National AIDS Control Programme (NACP), National Vector Borne Diseases Control Programme (NVBDCP) etc. have had their own monitoring and evaluation mechanisms or quality assurance mechanisms in the recent past.

Contemporary Currents of 'Quality' in Indian Health Services

With some new ideas and strategies, the National Rural Health Mission (NRHM) is addressing many of the recommendations made by different committees over a period of time. It is a positive step in terms of addressing the issue of 'quality' of healthcare. While addressing the quality dimensions of larger health service systems in terms of comprehensiveness of services, integrated service delivery, access to services, finance, design and planning, NRHM has undertaken measures to improve the quality of the services that are being delivered through each facility, from the lowest upto the district hospital level. The systemic issues are addressed by intervening in input and process factors of health service delivery, as well as through demand generation by demand side financing. It also uses outcome data of health services to assess their performance. It has developed dedicated mechanisms to address the quality dimensions of health service delivery at institutional level through its Quality Management System (QMS), though it has a long way to go. NRHM addresses the concerns of the quality of the system as a whole, as well as the quality of the services through institutions of healthcare delivery.

The attempts to improve quality of the health service system getreflected in various strategies such as increased financial allocation, provision for Accredited Social Health Activists (ASHAs) at community level, provisions of increased manpower, community involvement, decentralised planning through some of the initiatives like Programme Implementation Plans (PIPs), removal of bottlenecks in financing, flexibility for expenditure, RogiKalyanSamitis at institutional level (RKS—Patient Welfare Committees), strengthening procurement and supplies, research, constant monitoring and evaluation Joint Review Mission (JRM), Common Review Mission (CRM), concurrent evaluation, Health Management and Information System (HMIS), Janani SurakshaYojana (JSY),[9] equity and special programmes for vulnerable groups.[10] However, some of the policies like public private partnership and medical insurance, deployed to fill in the gaps like availability of specialists in government hospitals, have resulted in strengthening private hospitals through public money. There have been no concrete and large-scale attempts to employ the required specialists and filling these vacant posts through regular employment. Another concern is that of casualisation of labour, through contract-based temporary employment of many health workers as well as of medical and paramedical workers. How far these interventions have contributed in improving the health status of the population and in improving the quality of services provided is yet to be seen.

Special/Specific 'Quality' Related Policy Measures for Public Institutions

The Bureau of Indian Standards (BIS) developed Indian standards for healthcare organisations, viz. hospitals and laboratories.[11] The process of development of these standards started after the Alma Ata Declaration in 1978, wherein the Indian government was a signatory to the undertaking of 'Health for All' by 2000. The first set of recommendations—'Indian standards recommendations for basic requirements of general hospital buildings', 'Classification and matrix for various categories of hospitals' and 'Basic requirements for hospital planning Part-1 up to 30 bedded hospitals'—were released in the years 1984, 1988 and 1988 respectively. However, despite their relevance, none of these standards have been followed completely even in public hospitals till today.

Indian Public Health Standards (IPHS) was one of the important initiatives taken under the flagship programme of NRHM. IPHS were developed in an attempt to improve functioning and quality of health services at all levels of institutions, from sub-centre to district hospitals and hospitals up to 750 beds with or without medical colleges. While sharing many similarities with the standards developed by BIS, the IPHS added standard treatment guidelines and protocols/standard operating procedures for different conditions under different national health programmes. Under NRHM efforts have been made to fulfil these standards at all levels in select institutes.

Quality Management System (QMS) and International Standards Organisation (ISO) certification: QMS (with some limitations) is the first system to assess quality by directly addressing systemic and service delivery issues at the level of institutes of healthcare delivery in the public system. QMS was a systematic initiative taken under NRHM toencourage and assist different healthcare organisations to develop quality management systems to improve the quality of health services at facility level. Regular monitoring and evaluation is also done to ensure that QMS is in place and functions effectively as a continuous improvement process. QMS aims at fulfilling the standards laid down by IPHS through systematic efforts (MoHFW, 2011). However, it lacks a systems approach when one considers the effect and relationship with other levels of health service delivery in a multi-tier system. Other important aspects like access and coverage of healthcare delivery are not considered effectively as a part of the framework of QMS.

For AYUSH services (Ayurveda, Yoga and Naturopathy, Unani Siddha and Homoeopathy), there is no quality assessment and improvement mechanism except supervision within the departments, which too remains non-functional owing to various reasons such as vacancies, etc. (GoI, 2010).

Special/Specific 'Quality' Related Initiatives and Interventions in Private Institutions.

The National Accreditation Board for Hospitals and Healthcare Providers India (NABH) has accredited around 120 hospitals till date, and around 450 more are in the process of accreditation. Most of these hospitals are large, multi-specialty or super-specialty private hospitals. Some of the government hospitals have also been accredited by the NABH. 'Standards for Hospitals' developed by NABH have been accredited by the International Society for Quality in Healthcare (ISQua). The approval of ISQua has been used as a claim for authentication that NABH standards are in consonance with the global benchmarks set by ISQua. The National Accreditation Board for Laboratories (NABL), another board under Quality Council of India (QCI) along with NABH, is doing quality assessment and accreditation of laboratories and investigation facilities.

The Joint Commission International (JCI) and Joint Commission on Accreditation of Healthcare Organisations (JCAHO) are USA-based organisations, performing quality assessment and accreditation of healthcare organisations. Some of the private and corporate hospitals in India have been accredited by JCAHO.

Emerging Discourse for Health Services Strengthening: Implications for Quality HLEG and Steering Committee Recommendations

The proposed Universal Health Coverage (UHC) by the HLEG (GoI, 2011) strongly advances the logic of ensuring end-users' access to healthcare services. However, ends do not justify the means. The HLEG report claims allegiance to the principle of primary healthcare. But the primary healthcare approach was about community ownership and participation (community being seen not just as passive recipient of services, or just the ones making grievances at some grievance redressal cell), sustainability, i.e. the ability of the community to run such services in the long run, rationality and appropriate technology, accessibility, comprehensiveness, intersectoral coordination, etc.—all these are prescribed attributes of the 'means' for the 'end' of providing 'health for all'. Much of the discussion around CPHC is about the means and the ways, the principles and philosophy of providing the predetermined goal of health for all. The HLEG report seems to focus only on the end goal of health for all while making a significant departure from the principles of the 'means' and the spirit of CPHC expressed at Alma Ata.

Even though the HLEG recommendations take a stand against an insurance-based system, the theme of recommendations is 'public funding' and 'guarantee of financial provision'. The actual service provision is left to either the public or 'contracted-in' private sector. In the current policy ethos, the assumption that there will be encouragement of service provision through contracted-in private providers and will result in further strengthening of the private sector through public money is not entirely misplaced. This is despite the established fundamental problems with the health services being delivered based on market principles (Light, 2000; Rice, 1997).

Monitoring each instance of patient interaction with proposed every 'contracted-in' private provider would require a mammoth bureaucracy equipped with the facility to make assessments and intervene in the complex and highly-technical healthcare delivery systems with the given information asymmetry which is favourable to doctors. At the very least, this would require specialists/doctors who have the prerequisite skills to monitor service provisioning by contracted in private providers. The proposed recommendations will have to further face the challenge of the complete lack of regulatory frameworks, monitoring and evaluation mechanisms and absence of culture of medical audits in government as well as private sector health services. In the context of the existing situation of the lack of human resources, trained doctors, paramedical workers and managerial staff in the health sector, the task of monitoring of service delivery through proposed contracted-in private providers seems an unrealistic task.

Medical audits, systems of monitoring and evaluation, guidelines and audits for appropriate and rational usage of medical technology, quality management/assessment/assurance and accreditation systems are in their infancy in the government sector and are alien to most of the private sector as well. In such circumstances, would it be possible to control unnecessary investigations and treatment administration from the contracted-in private sector? There is a similar question mark on assuring implementation of rational treatment protocols and standard operating procedures through such private hospitals given the profit- seeking principle of their operations, as can be seen from the epidemic of hysterectomies among insured patients under the RashtriyaSwasthyaBimaYojana (RSBY) in Bihar and Chhattisgarh and in the Arogyashree Scheme of Andhra Pradesh (Editorial, 2012; Shukla et al., 2012).

The proposition in HLEG recommendations to get IPHS or ISO standards implemented for those hospitals getting contracted-in raises a plethora of questions. In what percentage of private hospitals are standards related to buildings, infrastructure, and organisation of service delivery, human resources, and Government of India stipulated wages being currently followed? How many of them will be prepared to enrol in UHC? (In fact, HLEG recommends the standards will also be applicable for non-UHC private providers.) The profits in many of the private hospitals at district and sub-district level are driven by unethical practices and by compromising on many infrastructural, material and human-power standards (less human resources, less qualifications, more work hours along with unsatisfactory salaries). Another source of earning is through commissions/cut practice by referring patients, and through sale of medicines, drugs and other medical consumables. If they were to follow those standards then it would require additional investments. There will be expectation of returns on the investments. So the assumption in the proposed UHC recommendations that highly powerful and unregulated private hospitals will part with easy profit-making avenues and opt for price regulation and follow government-stipulated rates of treatment seems untenable given the ground reality.

The IPHS are for sub-centres (SCs), PHCs, Community HealthCentres (CHCs) and for hospitals with 30–50 beds, 50–100 beds and more. These standards are said to be used for quality improvement and accreditation of hospitals delivering the proposed National Health Package. Before commenting on the composition and nature of standards used in IPHS, it is important to remember that these are standards for public institutions. There are no standards laid down for private hospitals. IPHS for hospitals with thirty beds and above can be considered as useful for similar types of private hospitals. However, there are no standards for private hospitals with bed strength belowthirty, and this constitutes the bulk of private providers. Standards used for sub-centres, PHCs and CHCs cannot be used for small private hospitals as the mandate, composition, objective and circumstances of service delivery are different.

The standards for thirty-bedded hospitals and above are also for a specific composition of services with a particular kind of specialist mix and balance. Will the prescribed standards be relevant and acceptable to private sector hospitals having thirty or more beds? The specialisation and composition in terms of skill mix availability in such private hospitals is very different in different settings. This sector may comprise a small segment of the private sector but there can be no doubt about its significance and power. The biggest section of the private sector would include individual general practitioners, specialists running their own hospitals, doctor couples with different specialisations running nursing homes or hospitals and then there are private hospitals, nursing homes or polyclinics owned or run by groups of different types of specialists. The mix of specialisation in such private hospitals is based on social, physical, geographical, economical and other considerations and not primarily on epidemiological and public health considerations. Is it at all feasible to develop standards which will be applicable for such varied types of hospitals and permutations and combinations of skill mix? More importantly, will they be applicable and acceptable to the private sector? It is important to address this question as this constitutes the bulk of the total private sector.

The area requirement for 30-bedded hospitals as per IPHS is around 15–20,000 ft^2. What will be its implications in terms of availability of such land and prices? Along with other material requirements there are huge human resource requirements of trained manpower which is not available in many of the district and sub-district towns. Implementation of standards related to area, building and human resource standards, along with their working hours and minimum wages would increase the costs of running the hospital phenomenally as compared to what it is now. Will this be acceptable to the private sector? If such standards are necessary, will the government allow private hospitals to ignore it even if they are not part of the proposed UHC? Even if it is a dream come true situation and all these hospitals implement the prescribed standards by investing enormous resources, the likelihood of these financial investments being recovered from the patient is far too obvious to be ignored.

There is also the question of whether the proposed price regulation will be acceptable to the private sector, and for how long. Capital costs, concurrent costs as well as the cost of trained human resources withstandard salaries in the context of proposed price control and regulation would be seen as threatening the economic viability of private hospitals unless there is sufficient business turnover. This scenario, in turn, raises more questions about who will ensure the desired business turnover to private providers and how. Increasing the business turnover of such individual or couple-owned hospitals raises the risk of defeating the purpose of providing quality services, as there is a limit to the workload a single doctor can handle while assuring the provision of rational and quality services.

In this context, it is relevant to recall that the government could not enforce even the much watered-down Clinical Establishments Act 2010. This Act has been challenged by the Indian Medical Association (IMA). These are the real life power dynamics in which the proposed recommendations of HLEG will have to be negotiated. Needless to say, such circumstances challenge the larger goal and modalities in providing universal access to rational and quality healthcare services. The recommendation to introduce three new categories in the public health cadre, namely, all India public health services cadre, health systems management cadre and hospital managers cadre (GoI, 2011) is riddled with ambiguity and overlap in their roles and responsibilities (unclear responsibilities of public health cadre). Most importantly, it would be interesting to see how the power dynamics within these proposed different cadres of health professionals will unfold. Health services are presently dominated by the clinical specialist and super specialist. The proposed recommendations call for a change in this power dynamics by replacing it with new professionals. In a highly technical and complex field like health, and in the context of the given power dynamics where specialist doctors dominate the health sector, it would have been logical to develop these cadres and define their roles, responsibilities and power dynamics through appropriate operations research.

HLEG proposes that District Health Managers will manage thegovernment-run health service system as well as purchase of services from contracted-in private providers (Ibid.). Quality assurance, performance management (that involves recruiting and deciding career trajectories), purchasing health services, etc., accords a disproportion- ately powerful position to the health system management cadre. These managers will be in a position to cater to management needs like supply chain maintenance, financial calculations, etc., but the technical component of care delivery and rationality of care are tasks that are way out of the league of district health system managers unless they are trained medical doctors. Further, even if this cadre comprisesmedically trained doctors, there is no certainty about their understanding, perspective and expertise in handling AYUSH treatment systems.

Quality assessment and quality assurance cannot be left to health system managers alone. Quality in healthcare is unique conceptually and would need a different approach for assessment and improvement. The management-trained professionals will not be in a position to assess the clinical services provided by medical and paramedical professionals. In addition to developing inbuilt mechanisms of regular medical audits, death audits, clinical audits and their use for quality assessment, overall quality assessment should be done through a team consisting of clinicians from different disciplines, paramedical workers, experts in management and administration, epidemiologists, public health specialists, economists, representatives of Civil Society Organisations (CSOs), patients, relatives or attendants of the patients, community representatives, etc.

The HLEG recommendations acknowledge the difference between hospital services and hospitality services and allow for extra charges for providing services not covered under the proposed National Health Package and for hospitality services (Ibid.). Allowing a dual system with the public and private systems providing hospitality and luxury services will, in the long run, have its implications for UHC as well as for public health systems. Supply creates its own demand. Over time a five star hospital with luxury hospitality services will have changed the perceptions about what constitutes hospital and health services. Will such a luxury hospital providing hospitality services act as a role model for what constitutes hospital services? Will it increase pressure over time on government-run health services? Will these hospitality services become part of 'quality' assessment and the accreditation process? Will presence or absence of it affect the process of empanelling private hospitals in UHC or any other private insurance scheme?

Are hospitality services limited to tertiary level/multispecialtycorporate hospitals alone? Single specialty individually or couple- owned and run nursing homes at district and sub-district level also provide hospitality services. The most important task is to define and distinguish between what constitutes hospitality service and what constitutes necessary hospital service. Will talking to the patient courteously and spending some time explaining the condition of illness and line of treatment constitute hospitality service or necessary service? Will access to safe drinking water, hygienic food, sanitation facilities, and arrangements for attendants accompanying the patient constitute hospitality or necessary hospital service? Does prompt or timely treatment constitute hospitality service or necessary service? It is a difficult task to define the boundaries of what constitutes necessary service and hospitality service; it is not static and will vary in different socio-political and cultural contexts.

The whole idea of defining the National Health Package of HLEG and Essential Health Package (EHP) of the Steering Committee (Ibid.; GoI, 2012)—needs to be reconsidered. It is impractical to define boundaries for diseases given the fact of co-morbidities and complications associated with even simple illnesses. Universal access to comprehensive services for all illnesses needs to be guaranteed. A more holistic approach, i.e. the entire human body being treated, is in sharp contradiction with the present endeavours to define the boundaries for health and progression of disease based on National Health Package or EHP. This kind of planning is not only impractical but also unethical. Furthermore, a payment for treatment of diseases up to certain boundaries (as pre-decided in packages) within the arrangements of PPPs leaves significant scope for financial irregularities. The HLEG as well as Steering Committee recommendations vis-à-vis public private partnership, where health services will be delivered on market principles as well as the idea of a health package are antithetical to the idea of 'quality' in terms of universal access to comprehensive services. Many of the dimensions of quality as discussed above such as efficacy, effectiveness, efficiency, optimality, acceptability, legitimacy, equity, intangible dimensions like reliability, responsiveness, assurance, relevance, empathy provided by care gives, issues like time taken, queues, organisation of services, administrative procedures, services being comprehensive, ethical, safe and patient centredness have not even been alluded to or adequately addressed in the recommendations of HLEG as well as the Steering Committee. The technical domain of quality which will deal with the rationality of the treatment process has been recommended to be developed in both set of recommendations. However, the Steering Committee recommendations do not make any provision for that. The quality of clinical process and inter-personal dimension of quality are untouched in both sets of recommendations.

Mechanisms for addressing the issue of quality at the systemic and at individual service delivery level are thought about in HLEG recommendations but need further deliberations. Though Steering Committee recommendations project responsiveness to service as an important principle (along with its elements like choice, communication, confidentiality, dignity, amenities, prompt attention and autonomy), there are no concrete suggestions and pathways on to how to achieve this. Steering Committee recommendations do not have any specific systemic recommendation which addresses the issue of quality directly. The Steering Committee proposes that the existing NRHM governance mechanisms be continued and accommodates some other suggestions like developing a public health cadre, while maintaining total silence on a health system management cadre and on other institutional arrangements like the National Health Regulatory and Development Authority (NHRDA), along with its important subsidiary institutional mechanisms suggested by the HLEG report. It recommends continuation of existing public private partnerships and has nothing new to offer to the UHC except the Bachelor of Rural Healthcare cadre that is already being offered in some states. Creating competition between public and private sector services, as in the pilots recommended to be conducted in one district of each state, may theoretically be seen as one way of forcing quality improvement in both. However, there are serious doubts about whether it will work on the ground.

It can be seen from both the Committee recommendations that just to accommodate the idea of PPPs, a plethora of other institutional arrangements have to be developed and used, such as the National Health Entitlements Card (NHEC), packages like EHP/National Health Package, the cut offs like 70% spending on OPD services and 30% on indoor services, empanelment mechanisms, prescription audits, huge monitoring bureaucracy, bureaucracy to settle financial mechanisms with proposed private partners, private Jan Aushadhi stores, performance and health outcomes assessment of the families registered under each of the healthcare providers, etc. This official thrust favouring private sector was in conflict with the popularly projected welfare framework in the twelfth Plan and to some extent in a Draft National Health Policy (NHP) finalized in 2017.

National Health Policies (NHP): Draft 2015 and NHP 2017

The draft National Health Policy (dNHP) of 2015 was modified and finalized after two years as National Health policy 2017. The dNHP with many missed opportunities and limitations had made a way for making health care as a basic right of the people (MoHFW, 2014). This was done after due deliberation on the limitations and contextual reality of health sector; and the hope and impetus it offered to act on improving health services. However NHP 2017 while invoking similar deliberation puts off the promise of health care as basic right (GOI, 2017). This raises doubt on state's commitment to health of its citizens and promise of universal health care.

While invoking the phrase Comprehensive Primary Health Care (CPHC), NHP 2017 deploys a very reductionist meaning and understanding of the phrase. The CPHC as used in Alma Ata declaration was a philosophical/theoretical approach of providing health care where it had suggested a three tier system of health care, integrated at each level like Primary, Secondary and Tertiary level care. All these three levels were parts and means of providing comprehensive health care in PHC declaration of Alma Ata. However, the NHP 2017 while invoking these three levels of health care has treated them with different principles and approach.

NHP 2017 aims to provide comprehensive services at primary level of care by expanding package of services for more illnesses. It elaborates the package as '*Assuring availability of free, comprehensive primary health care services, for all aspects of reproductive, maternal, child and adolescent health and for the most prevalent communicable, non-communicable and occupational diseases in the population*' it further extends it to include *geriatric health care, palliative care and rehabilitative care services.*

It needs to be mentioned here that, comprehensiveness is not just about the horizantal spectrum of conditions covered but was also about each disease condition being managed in its entirety from its simple manifestation to severe and complicated manifestation. The NHP doesn't assure comprehensive services for all disease conditions and their varied manifestations. Unlike the dNHP 2015, this defined package of CPHC is not even free and assured to all citizens in NHP 2017. This becomes abundantly clear in policy recommendations for urban area, '*for achieving the objective of having fully functional primary healthcare facilities- especially in urban areas to reach under-serviced populations and on a fee basis for middle class populations, Government would collaborate with the private sector for operationalizing such health and wellness centres to provide a larger package of comprehensive primary health care across the country*'. On one side the policy recognizes that health care expenditure is one of the important causes of impoverishment and on other side excludes urban middle class even from free primary level care. This shows the grave limitations of universality of coverage of even primary level of care and precarious nature of equity in services delivered.

The expanded package of CPHC services provided through primary level of care would be assured service only to eligible families having health cards. These health cards could be used to govern eligibility and utilization of assured services. The recommendation of instituting gate-keeping mechanism in utilizing higher level of services complements well with the health card paving a way for targeting of population to be covered and disease conditions to be covered. The NHP 2017 aims to provide this comprehensive package of services from current sub- centres and PHCs which will be upgraded to 'Health and Wellness Centres' which will be run either by AYUSH graduates or BSc in rural health services or nurses. Therefore the nature and extent of these services, their comprehensiveness and their potential to achieve many of the targets that it has set for itself by 2025 remains doubtful.

It is prosed to upgrade the secondary level services, 'the policy also aims that ten categories of what are currently specialist skills be available within the district. Additionally four or at least five of these specialist skill categories be available at sub-district levels'. However the secondary and tertiary services are neither assured nor free for all. NHP opens the possibility of these institutions being run with market principles. The key policy shift advocated for organizational structure, 'in secondary and tertiary care—from an input oriented to an output based strategic purchasing' opens the possibility of these levels of institutions being reduced to organizations governing strategic purchase of services from private sector. The fear of these institutions either becoming institutions governing strategic purchase from private sector or institutions providing services based on market principles stems from the stated objective in policy of, 'Ensuring improved access and affordability, of quality secondary and tertiary care services through a combination of public hospitals and well measured strategic purchasing of services in health care deficit areas, from private care providers, especially the not-for profit providers'. Thus the objective is to make secondary and tertiary services affordable. This would mean these secondary and tertiary services are not assured for all and health cards serving as gate keepers.

The policy choice of purchase of services from private sector necessitates other institutional mechanism for it to be functional. The NHP recognizes it and recommends 'multistakeholder institutional mechanisms to be created at Centre and State levels—in the forms of trusts or registered societies with institutional autonomy'. These agencies are to be tasked with ensuring that purchasing is strategic. The quantum and complexities of health conditions and services for them to be purchased from institutions at the level of secondary and tertiary level would demand huge bureaucratic structure. The Policy also recommends setting up of 'a separate, empowered medical tribunal for speedy resolution to address disputes/complaints regarding standards of care, prices of services, negligence and unfair practices'. These institutional mechanisms would mean additional administrative cost taking sizable proportion of health budget. This additional administrative cost raises a doubt on how strategic is the policy of strategic purchase of secondary and tertiary services.

The promise of good quality health care services is highlighted in the goals, principles, objectives, policy thrust and regulatory framework of NHP. The Policy has proposed establishing National Healthcare Standards Organization and to develop evidence based standard guidelines of care applicable both to public and private sector. It recommends, 'creating a robust independent mechanism to ensure adherence to standard treatment protocols by public and non-government hospitals'. It is assumed that strategic purchase would be used to implement these standards in private hospitals. The need of developing evidence based standard guidelines of care was mentioned even in the Clinical Establishment Act 2010 but, the guidelines are still illusive. It remains to be seen when these institutions would see the light of the day. A decade long experience of implementing even this simpler Act has not been very impressive in its acceptance and in bringing out significant change in quality of care provided.

Health budget allocations till the year 2020, in the context of most of the targets set in the Policy for the year 2025, don't inspire much confidence that this Policy is of any consequence towards achieving universal health care. The rising proportional allocation to insurance based health schemes, financial protection schemes and now, the provision of strategic purchase for secondary and tertiary level of care hint at the direction in which health care systems are heading, raising doubts over the recommendation of, '*comprehensive facility development and obligations with regard to human resources, especially specialists needs, are to be prioritized*'. In the absence adequate expert human resources and upgraded health amenities the recommendation of '*free drugs, free diagnostics and free emergency care services in all public hospitals*' could mean getting away with providing only a few free medicines and diagnostic services along with first aid emergency services to all. The existing health care financing mechanisms through insurance based schemes like RSBY, PMJAY and provision of strategic purchase carry a potential danger of perpetuating these very institutions of expanding health coverage further. They would take away resource better used in strengthening public services. The short term arrangement carry the risk of slowly becoming permanent features of the health system.

The Way Forward

For the year 2013, the USA had a per capita total health expenditure of about 9146 $ (47.1% of this was government expenditure and 52.9% was private expenditure) (World Bank, 2016). Despite such a high per capita health expenditure of around 13–15% of their population is uninsured and does not have access to healthcare. The proportion would be even higher for those who do not have comprehensive health insurance coverage. The insurance-based model of health service delivery of USA (private insurance and public insurance for select groups) relies mainly on provisioning of health services from the private sector. For the year 2013, the UK had a per capita total health expenditure of about 3598 $ (84% of this was government and 16% was private expenditure) (Ibid.). With this expenditure (almost half as compared to the USA), UK has managed to provide better universal access to integrated medical care. The UK manages this because they have a model of health service delivery which predominantly involves public funding and public provision of services. However, this model of health services is under stress after health sector reforms were introduced in the National Health System (NHS) in the 1990s. Health sector reforms involving budgetary cuts and introduction of market mechanisms have started affecting NHS. The waiting lines for treatment and surgeries in NHS have become a source of concern.

India has a total health expenditure of about just 61 $ (32.2% of this was government and 67.8% was private health expenditure) (Ibid.). With such a low expenditure base, we cannot think of providing integrated medical care universally in the near future. A vision of insurance-based model of 'assuring' health services will not make services accessible to all even in the distant future. However, the budgetary allocations of RSBY and other insurance schemes from different states are showing a consistent rise over time. This is creating a new set of problems where much of the meagre public funding is getting diverted for strengthening private services. RSBY and other publicly funded health insurance schemes have not fulfilled their goal of reducing out-of-pocket expenditures. Rather, these schemes have contributed to irrational and unethical medical practices as seen in the reported instances of epidemics of unnecessary hysterectomies.

The foremost issue would be to define and lay down the concept of 'quality' in healthcare for UHC, along with its different dimensions and determinants. The objectives and implications of that particular definition and quality improvement efforts should be deliberated upon as there is a risk of quality assessments and accreditation systems being used for closing down public facilities and favouring corporate hospitals as against the primary and secondary level private services. This has a direct impact on making services more inaccessible. While increasing access to services at all levels, medical rationality and ethical practice have also to be built into the quality criteria. Within the public system itself, there is a need for both the general systemic strengthening measures and a specific mechanism for facility-based quality improvement. Existing mechanisms as implemented under NRHM should be reviewed and wide discussions need to be held to design quality improvement systems in each state.

The existing health service system is a result of three decades of neglect and two decades of active dismantling. In such a situation, the sudden attention to the issue of providing universal healthcare nationally as well as globally needs to be understood in a wider perspective. Many countries are opting for arrangements of healthcare insurance following the US model of health service system. However, the US model is proved to have failed in providing universal access to healthcare despite spending a substantial amount of money (around 17% of their GDP). Health service systems of countries like UK and Australia have much more to offer, principally as well as for designing a system for providing UHC. The farcical emergency situation created to provide universal healthcare needs to be countered, as it can be used to push in unscientific and irrational models under the disguise of UHC. It should be acknowledged that it would need realistic time frames for materialising health services system designs developed on the principles of public health and epidemiological rationale and evolved through wider public discussion.

The discussions around different models of UHC should take into account the experience of the countries that are providing universal access to healthcare or medical care. Rising healthcare costs have become a source of concern for many developed countries and questions are being raised over the sustainability of this continual increase in the health budgets. Rising healthcare costs have been seen as one of the important causes of economic crisis that some developed countries are facing. Health service systems in most of the developed countries rely on modern bio-medicine and are doctor-centred. Iatrogenesis is becoming an important cause of mortality; it is one of top ten causes of death in the US (Priya, 2013). This costly healthcare system based on modern bio-medicine also does not seem to have answers to many important contemporary health problems like non-communicable, chronic diseases. Increasing research evidence shows food, physical activity and stress as important causes of many non-communicable diseases. This highlights the fact that individual and communities are not just passive recipients of medical services but have an important role in healthcare.

Attempts to expand health services and build models of UHC should learn from the experience of the developed countries. Not replacing it but going beyond modern biomedicine is the need of the hour given its limitations in dealing with important health problems of current times, exorbitant costs and sustainability issues. Engaging with alternate systems of medicine like AYUSH in a very profound and systematic manner is necessary. Learning from people about their health cultures and helping communities to improve their health by aiding their efforts should be an approach towards health service system development. Community resources and practices in the form of home remedies and traditional healers, along with trained professionals and healthcare providers from all systems of medicine should be used as valuable resources while building health service delivery systems. Health service systems involving pluralist systems of medicine (democratic pluralism) should be developed by using principles of public health and epidemiological rationale (Priya, 2012). Wider public discussions are needed to evolve context-specific, self-reliant, sustainable and rational models of health service delivery. Community participation is needed at different levels, viz. assessing health status, identifying priorities, planning health services, delivering health services and monitoring and evaluation of health services. This would mean revisiting principles laid down in the Alma-Ata Declaration and sincere engagement with the politics of knowledge while involving different systems of medicine.

Notes

1. Transcendent: This philosophical approach defines quality as something absolute and universal. Quality is perceived as something experiential that cannot be resolved into measurable dimensions. Unfortunately this definition is probably the least practical.
   Product-based: Almost diametrically opposite to the transcendental approach, the product-based approach is only concerned about the most tangible aspects of quality. Quality is seen as being only what is measurable in a product. Differences in quality are represented by differences in ingredients, components and attributes. This approach is very attractive as it appears to be objective and precise.
   User-based: This customer centred approach defines quality from the individual user's perspective. High quality means greater satisfaction of the needs and wants of the user. This approach is appealing to the service providers and advocates of quality management. The International Organisation for Standardisation ISO 9000 states 'the standardised definition of quality refers to all those features of a product (or service) which are required by the customer'.
   Manufacturing-based: This approach sees quality from the perspective of the supplier or service provider. Designs or specifications that are assumed to represent high quality are laid down. Conformance means quality and deviation means reduction in quality. This approach is attractive to policy makers, engineers and designers as it simplifies matters into specifications and control of deviation.
   Value-based: Central to this approach is the concept of 'value for money'. Quality is defined in terms of conformance to costs and prices. With the rise of consumerism and the ease of obtaining information, price comparison is a

major factor to be considered when comparing quality of products and services (Garvin, 1988).

2. 1. Efficacy: The ability of care at its best to improve health.
   2. Effectiveness: The degree to which attainable health improvements are realised.
   3. Efficiency: The ability to obtain the greatest health improvement at the lowest cost.
   4. Optimality: The most advantageous balancing of costs and benefits.
   5. Acceptability: Conformity to patient preferences regarding accessibility, the patient-practitioner relation, the amenities, the effects of care, and the cost of care.
   6. Legitimacy: Concerning all of the above.
   7. Equity: Fairness in the distribution of care and its effects on health (Donabedian, 1990).
3. Accessibility: The first half of the definition of healthcare quality emphasises whether individuals have access to the structure and process of health services. The very basic dimension of healthcare structure is geographical/physical accessibility. Affordability of services is also an important aspect of accessibility as expensive care services and difficulty in seeing a doctor are barriers to access. Organisational access is one of the 'soft' components of accessibility besides the physical factors, and consists of regulations, institutional and human factors. Availability is interpreted in terms of the degree of individual satisfaction with the facilities (structure) and services (process) provided by the healthcare system, such as availability of women doctors, experts, or multi-specialty consultations (Yang, 2007).
4. Effectiveness: The second part of health services quality, effectiveness, is the outcome of services provided to meet the needs and the degree of closeness to the anticipated outcome when an individual accesses such services. Effectiveness is determined by two factors: clinical care and inter-personal care. The nature of both inter-personal services as well as clinical services is critical for the effectiveness of health services, and it is incorrect to emphasise only one aspect. The measurement methods of these two types of quality are quite different. The methods used to measure customer-centred service and communications between doctors and patients are more time-consuming, less evolved and expensive than searching hospital clinical databases via computers for assessing effectiveness of clinical services (Yang, 2007).
5. Efficiency is the ratio of returns to the cost, i.e. to maximise outcomes by the most efficient use of services. Efficiency could be divided into allocation efficiency (focus on the measures to maximise returns) and technical efficiency (focus on technical capacity). As for individuals, technical efficiency is more important, which allows individual users to maximise their expected outcomes. However, such maximisation is neither continuous nor affordable for population health services.

   Therefore, allocation efficiency should be emphasised for population health, effectively distributing resources into the areas where health could be possibly obtained. Resource allocation is determined by a society's choice, which could be justified by need and equity. Resource allocation is also an interactive process as well as an outcome in itself (Yang, 2007).

6. Equity is a relevant factor to accessibility with regard to population level healthcare processes and outcomes, and it is the degree to which all the individuals can obtain necessary services within the population. The definition of accessibility must emphasise prompt access to services according to patient/customers' needs.
7. Tangible dimensions include location of health services and their availability, accessibility, affordability to the population being served. In addition, it looks at the availability of infrastructure, medicines, manpower, transport facilities, financial resources available, distance and cost of healthcare.
   Intangible dimensions include: Functional quality: manner of services delivery, i.e. issues like time taken, queues, organisation of services, administrative procedures involved.
   Technical quality: Consists of effectiveness, comprehensiveness and rationality of care.
   Interactive quality: Includes aspects like reliability, responsiveness, assurance and empathy provided by caregiver.
   Corporate quality: Deals with the image of the organisation Accessibility: social access to organisations and personnel providing healthcare. It refers to socio-economic and cultural access (issues like caste, class, gender, which impinge upon utilisation of services) to health institutions (Baru & Kurian, 2008).
8. GOBI-FFF stands for Growth monitoring, Oral rehydration, Breastfeeding, Immunisation-Family planning, Female literacy, Food supplementation.
9. It increases access to and the demand for services as well as service utilisation through demand side financing.
10. It improves the brand value of the system in the community and improves utilisation of services and improves the health status of the vulnerable groups of the community thus serving the objective of health service.
11. These standards are laid down for 30 and 100-bedded hospitals. Standards for more than 100-bedded hospitals with or without medical colleges are not yet released. These standards are related to infrastructure and space requirements, material, equipment and other consumables required for effective functioning of the hospitals. The services to be provided along with human resource requirements have also been specified. These standards are very detailed and have meticulously elaborated on most of the dimensions required for effective functioning of these hospitals. These standards do not elaborate on STGs, rational drug therapeutics or standard operating procedures and suggest developing these with expert opinions.

References

Anadaleeb, S. S. (2001). Service quality perceptions of patient satisfaction: Study of hospitals in developing countries. *Social Science and Medicine, 52*(9), 1359–1370.

Baru, R., & Kurian, C.M. (2008). Towards an expanded conceptualisation of quality in public health. In R. Priya & S. Mehta (Eds.), *Dialogue on AIDS: Perspectives for the Indian context*. Vasudhaiva Kuttumbakkam Publications.

Directorate General of Health Services, Government of India. (1967). *Report of the committee on integration of health services*. Directorate General of Health Services.

Donabedian, A. (1990). The seven pillars of quality. *Archives of Pathology and Laboratory Medicine, 114*(11), 1115–1118.

Donabedian, A. (1966). Evaluating the quality of medical care. *Milbank Memorial Fund Quarterly, 44*(3),166–206.

Draper, M., & Hill, S. (1996). Feasibility of national benchmarking of patient satisfaction with Australian hospitals. *International Journal for Quality in Healthcare, 8*(5), 457–466.

Editorial. (2012). A 'twisted' health scheme: State health insurance schemes are being abused to profit private care providers. *Economic and Political Weekly, 47*(38), 8.

Evans, D. B., Edeger, T. T., Lauer, J., Frenk, J., & Murray, C. J. (2001). Measuring quality: From the system to the provider. *International Journal for Quality in Healthcare, 13*(6), 439–445.

Fiscella, K. (2003). *Assessing healthcare quality for minority and other disparity populations*. Agency for Healthcare Research and Quality, US Department of Health and Human Services.

Garvin, D. A. (1988). *Managing quality: The strategic and competitive edge*. Free Press.

GBD 2016 Healthcare Access and Quality Collaborators. (2018). Measuring performance on the healthcare access and quality index for 195 countries and territories and selected subnational locations: A systematic analysis from the global burden of disease study 2016. *Lancet, 391*, 2236–2271.

Government of India. (1946). *Report of the health survey and development committee* (Vol. IV). Manager of Publications.

Government of India. (1975). *Health services and medical education: A programme for immediate action—Report of the group on medical education and support manpower*. Allied Publishers Pvt. Ltd.

Government of India. (1966–69). *Mukerji committee report on basic health services*. Government of India.

Government of India. (2011). *High level expert group report on universal health coverage for India*. Planning Commission of India.

Government of India. (2012). *Report of the steering committee on health for the twelfth five year plan (incorporating reports of working groups and deliberations in steering committee meetings)*. Planning Commission of India.

Government of India. (2017). *National health policy 2017*. Ministry of Health and Family welfare. Government of India.

Hartigan, P. (2001). The importance of gender in defining and improving quality of care: Some conceptual issues. *Health Policy and Planning, 16*(Supplement 1), 7–12.

Hock, L. K. (2005). Evolving concepts of quality: The need for a contextual approach to defining quality. *Clinical Quality, 31*(3), 1–5.

Light, D. W. (2000). The sociological character of healthcare markets. In G L. Albrecht et al. (Eds.), *The hand book of social studies in health and medicine*. Sage Publications.

Ministry of Health and Family Welfare, Government of India. (1962). *Health survey and planning committee*. Ministry of Health and Family Welfare.

Ministry of Health and Family Welfare, Government of India. (1973). *Report of the committee on multipurpose workers under health and family planning programme*. Ministry of Health and Family Welfare.

Ministry of Health and Family Welfare, Government of India. (2010). *Status and role of AYUSH and local health traditions under the national rural health mission.* Ministry of Health and Family Welfare.

Ministry of Health and Family Welfare, Government of India. (2011). *Quality management in public health facilities: An implementation handbook.* Ministry of Health and Family Welfare.

Ministry of Health and Family Welfare, Government of India. (2014). *National health policy 2015 (draft).* Ministry of Health and Family Welfare.

Priya, R. (2013). Aren't technological choices central to designing health systems? *Indian Journal of Public Health, 57*(4), 212–218.

Priya, R. (2005). Public health services in India: A historical perspective. In L. V. Gangolli, R. Duggal, & A. Shukla (Eds.), *Review of healthcare in India.* Cehat.

Priya, R. (2012). AYUSH and public health: Democratic pluralism and the quality of health services. In V. Sujatha & L. Abraham (Eds.), *Medical pluralism in contemporary India.* Orient BlackSwan.

Rice, T. (1997). Can market forces give us the healthcare system we want? *Journal of Heath Politics Policy and Law, 22*, 383–426.

Rice, T., & Unruh, L. (2009). *The economics of health reconsidered.* (3rd ed.). Health Administration Press.

Roemer, M. I., & Montoya-Aguilar, C. (1988). *Quality assessment and assurance in primary healthcare.* WHO.

Sale, D. (2005). *Understanding clinical governance and quality assurance: Making it happen.* Palgrave Macmillan.

Shukla, R., Shatrugna, V., & Srivatsan, R. (2012, December 3). Aarogyasri healthcare model: Advantage private sector. *Economic and Political Weekly, 46*(49), 38–42.

Walsh, M., et al. (1999). Towards critical quality. In H. T. O. Devis (Ed.), *Managing quality: Strategic issues in healthcare management* (pp. 41–53). Ashgate Publishing Ltd.

World Bank. (2016). *Health, nutrition and population data and statistics: Thematic data.* Accessed March 23, 2016. http://datatopics.worldbank.org/hnp/ThematicData.

World Health Organisation. (1978). Primary healthcare. A Joint Report by The Director General of World Health Organisation and The Executive Director of the United Nations Children's Fund. In *Report of the International Conference on Primary Healthcare Alma-Ata, USSR*, Sept 6–12, 1978. WHO.

Yang, H. (2007). Building a conceptual framework for quality of care. *Chinese Health Quality Management, 14*(1), 1–9.

Chapter 5
Growth of Private Medical Colleges in Maharashtra and Its Implications for Universal Healthcare

Archana Diwate

Historically, the health planning exercise in India is conceived of an infrastructure for services, as well as attention to the training of required personnel, as reflected in the reports of the Bhore and the Mudaliar (Government of India (GoI), 1946; GoI, 1961) Committees and the Five Year Plans. In addition, there have been efforts when specific issues regarding manpower were addressed, as in the Multi Purpose Workers' Committee (Ministry of Health and Family Planning (MoHFP), 1973) and the Srivastva Committees of GoI (MoHFP, 1975). Despite these exercises, planning was pervaded by an urban bias, a specialist orientation in medical education, and a slowing down of the growth of infrastructure in rural areas. Over time, though the training of paramedics got neglected, a significant increase occurred in the number of medical colleges. This increase was primarily in the private sector after the 1970s. These developments during the late 1960s have been linked to the economic slowdown that brought economic growth rates to 3.3% by the year 1970 (Chandrasekhar & Ghosh, 2002: 6), and lowered investments in the health sector. It has been argued that, constrained by its social base, the ruling regime was slow to deal with persistent inequalities in society. It was unable to introduce adequate land reforms, and the nature of industrial growth failed to expand employment and consumer markets to the extent needed, despite state support (Chandrasekhar & Ghosh, 2002). A section of the organised labour class and the rich peasantry were partially accommodated by the ruling alliance (Mathew, 2002: 94), thus expanding social opportunities for certain classes. When the state could no more support the prevailing direction of development, instead of cutting on its undesirable investments, to protect the dominant classes it opted for external borrowing. As a consequence the state had to accept structural reforms that included health sector reforms, which inevitably pressed for privatisation of the welfare services (Chandrasekhar & Ghosh, 2002). These explanations largely relate to the economic and political aspects, barely touching upon the sociological dimensions of shifts in the health sector. Over the last three decades,

A. Diwate (✉)
SATHI, Pune, India

I. Qadeer et al. (eds.), *Universalising Healthcare in India*,
https://doi.org/10.1007/978-981-16-5872-3_5

specifically after 1990, the southern and western states have seen a marked increase in the number of private medical colleges over government medical colleges. While shrinking state investment and the accompanying push for privatisation explain the rise of private medical colleges, the questions we ask are: what are the socio-political dimensions that would explain the exact processes behind this trend and what are its implications? In other words, why should one be concerned about the growth of these private medical colleges?

Since the 1970s a class of rich peasants or capitalist farmers started investing their surpluses into various enterprises and, over generations, accessed higher education and gained social mobility. They contributed to the commercialisation of the economy and social services while retaining their rural roots (Omvedt, 1981; Rutten, 1986; Upadhya, 1988). Growth of private health services was a part of this process (Baru, 1987). Given their high capitation fees, only children from families of affluent professionals, bureaucrats, big businessmen, rich peasants or politicians could access private medical colleges (Ananthakrishnan, 2010; Diwan et al., 2013; Qadeer & Nayar, 2005). In fact, "students in private medical schools were more likely to have a physican parent than those in the public sector" (Diwan et al., 2013: 4). It was also observed that students from public medical schools were more likely to work in rural areas than the students from private medical schools (Diwan et al., 2013).

This chapter, using secondary and primary data, examines the general emergence of private medical colleges, their regional distribution, and then takes up the specific case of Maharashtra to explore the above trends and their social, economic, and political determinants. Finally it comments on the implication of this growth for universal healthcare.

Methodology

The sources used in this paper are, the Medical Council of India (MCI) records, to examine the growth, trends and regional variations in the establishment of medical colleges in India. It focuses on Maharashtra, a state with high private sector presence in medical institutions, to explore the socio-economic and political determinants to explain their growth. Data was collated from the websites of each private medical college in Maharashtra along with an extensive review of the secondary literature. In addition to understanding the regional variations and socio-political determinants of private medical colleges, seventeen in-depth interviews were conducted with different key informants. The informants were professors teaching in government and private medical colleges, students from private medical colleges and local journalists.

Rise of Private Medical Colleges in India: Time-Trend Analysis

Given that there were 19 medical colleges in the 1940s, for a population of 400 million, when only 1200 students were admitted each year and the ratio was one doctor for 6400 people, the Bhore Committee suggested that there should be, at the end of the ten years, 43 medical colleges (GoI, 1946, Vol. II: 337).

With this backdrop, we find a significant involvement of the Indian state in establishing medical colleges till the 1970s (Fig. 5.1). This trend changed however, over the early 1980s with the emergence of private medical colleges that received a boost.

Between 1950 and 1980, while government medical colleges were growing at the rate of 280%, that of private colleges was 1200% (Fig. 5.1). Since 1981 the relative growth of private colleges was much higher, especially over 2001–2010. The overall increase in government medical colleges between 1990 and 2016 was only 90%, but that of private colleges was 443%. According to some scholars, the growth of private medical colleges was largely driven by economic rather than educational objectives (Ananthakrishnan, 2010) and its acceleration is attributed to the neoliberal pressures for withdrawal of state intervention and increasing spaces for private investment.

The rapid growth of medical colleges led to faculty shortages, inadequate infrastructure, and poor quality of education (Antia, 1990; Rao et al., 2011). These shortages of faculty in the medical colleges—both in the older and newly started ones—were calculated by applying the MCI norms. The shortages were of the order of nearly 26,000 medical teachers if the 260 colleges for the MBBS course alone were to be staffed adequately (Ananthakrishnan, 2007: 25).

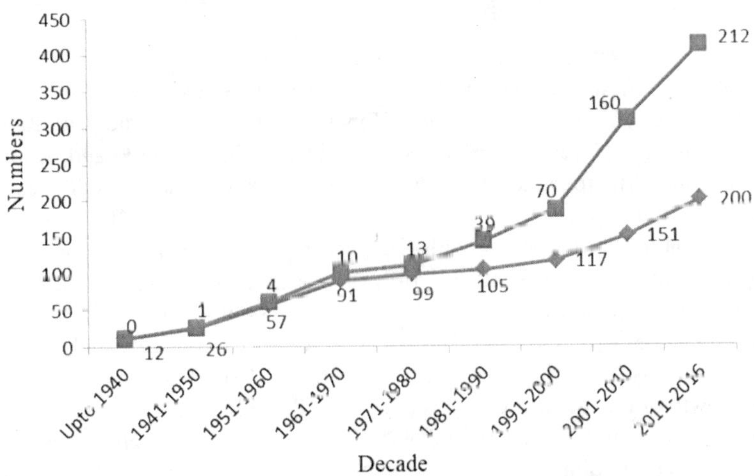

Fig. 5.1 Decadal growth of medical colleges in India (in numbers). *Source* MCI website (2016, January 15)

At the time of MCI inspection the private medical colleges fill up the empty hospital wards with patients by providing them money, and hiring doctors, who are shown as recruited by the college. Even instruments are borrowed from other colleges (Chattopadhyay, 2008). The unethical practice in private medical colleges to get recognition from MCI include putting up lists of non-existing staff, showing false records, false faculty, leaking question papers, etc. (Chattopadhyay, 2008; Deshpande & Deshpande-Naik, 2009). Quality of learning through practical exposure has remained a major issue due to very few patients in private medical college hospitals compared to public medical colleges with no shortage of patients (Supe & Burdick, 2006).

Regional Distribution of Medical Colleges and Intake Capacity: Interstate Analysis

We looked at the regional distribution of medical colleges in India, using the six zones proposed by the Ministry of Home Affairs. The Southern Zone is constituted by six Indian states, has the largest number of medical institutions (44.9%) and intake capacity (44.9%), followed by the Western Zone. Taking these two zones together (eleven states), 60.9% of medical institutions have an intake capacity of 63.2%. In contrast, the Eastern and North-Eastern Zone with 12 states have only 13.1% of medical institutions and 12.2% of total intake capacity (Table 5.1). Within the Western Zone, Maharashtra has the highest number of institutions (68.5%) and an intake capacity of 64.7%. Gujarat and Maharashtra together have 98.5% of institutions having a similar intake. These medical colleges are largely located in the urban areas.

Of all private medical colleges more than half are located in the Southern Zone and 69.3% are located in the Southern and Western Zones with 72.9% of intake capacity. The Eastern and North-Eastern Zones have only 14 private institutions out of the total of 212. Moreover, the states of Goa, Chandigarh, Jharkhand, Andaman-Nicobar, Assam, Manipur and Meghalaya do not have private medical colleges. There are three states and two Union Territories without any medical college (Table 5.1). It is also notable that the states with the largest population in India possess very few medical institutions. Using the norm of one medical college for five million population, southern and western states have an excess of 4–34 medical colleges. In contrast, the states of Uttar Pradesh and Bihar, which have large populations, need 11 and 7 more institutions respectively (Choudhury, 2016: 76).

The growth of the medical colleges then, has taken place mostly in the developed states of India (Choudhury, 2016; Mahal & Mohanan, 2006). The High-Level Expert Group (HLEG) (appointed by the Planning Commission (PC) in 2010) states that there is a 'highly uneven distribution of medical colleges which has resulted in the skewed production and unequal availability of doctors across the country' (GoI, 2011: 22).It recommends 'selectively setting up (an estimated 187) new medical

Table 5.1 Distribution of medical colleges and intake capacity

Name of the zone	Name of the states	Medical institutions, numbers and percentage			Intake capacity number and percentage		
		Gov.	Private	Total zonal	Gov.	Private	Total zonal
Southern Zone	Andhra Pradesh, Telangana, Karnataka, Kerala, Tamil Nadu, Pondicherry	66 (36.4)[a]	115 (63.5)	181 (44.9)[b]	9135 (38.8)	14,355 (61.1)	23,490 (44.9)
Western Zone	Goa, Gujarat, Maharashtra (Daman & Diu, and Dadra & Nagar Haveli)	38 (54.2)	32 (45.7)	70 (16.9)	5630 (58.8)	3945 (41.2)	9575 (18.3)
Central Zone	Chhattisgarh, Uttarakhand, Uttar Pradesh and Madhya Pradesh	29 (48.3)	31 (51.6)	60 (14.5)	3499 (51.8)	3250 (48.1)	6749 (12.9)
Northern Zone	Haryana, Himachal Pradesh, Jammu & Kashmir, Punjab, Rajasthan, Delhi and Chandigarh	27 (57.4)	20 (42.5)	47 (11.4)	3900 (64.5)	2145 (35.4)	6045 (11.5)
Eastern Zone	Bihar, Jharkhand, Orissa and West Bengal	30 (71.4)	12 (28.5)	42 (10.1)	3940 (76.6)	1200 (23.3)	5140 (9.8)
North Eastern States	Assam, Manipur, Tripura, Sikkim, Meghalaya (Arunachal Pradesh, Mizoram and Nagaland)	10 (83.3)	2 (17.1)	12 (2.9)	1076 (84.3)	200 (15.6)	1276 (2.4)

(continued)

Table 5.1 (continued)

Name of the zone	Name of the states	Medical institutions, numbers and percentage			Intake capacity number and percentage		
		Gov.	Private	Total zonal	Gov.	Private	Total zonal
	Total	200	212	412	27,180	25,095	52,275
		(48.5)	(51.4)	(100)	(51.9)	(48.0)	(100)

Source for Regions Government of India (2016, January 15). Data: MCI website (2016, January 15)
Note The states mentioned in brackets are without any medical college
[a]In each zone the percent share of government and private medical colleges is out of the total zonal colleges
[b]In each zone the total zonal percentage of medical colleges is out of the total Indian medical colleges. The same applies to intake capacity

colleges over the next 10 years in currently underserved districts with a population of more than 1.5 million' (Ibid.). However, it does not comment on the problems in the private medical colleges such as low quality of education, lack of infrastructure, corruption, lack of regulation, charging of capitation fee, and the powerful lobbies behind this growth pattern and the private investments in medical education. It is these that we explore in our case study.

The Case of Maharashtra State

We have undertaken an in-depth analysis of the growth of medical colleges in Maharashtra by tracking the emergence of the dominant caste[1] of Marathas and the Maratha-Kunbi[2] caste-cluster, exploring their economic and political power, linkages with the cooperative sector and the influence on trends and specificities of regional distribution of medical colleges. This is done by examining the economic and political dynamics behind their growth and providing insights into the social characteristics of the owners of private medical colleges.

Brief Profile of the State

The state of Maharashtra was formed in 1960. It is the second largest state in terms of geographical area and population, with 45.2% people residing in urban areas. The agricultural sector contributes 12.9% and the industrial and services sector together contribute about 87.1% of the state's income. It ranks fifth in the Human Development Index (HDI) (Government of Maharashtra (GoM), 2013a: 1–2). Currently it has 35 districts divided into six administrative divisions. Amarawati and Nagpur divisions (Vidarbha region) and Aurangabad Division (Marathwada region) constitute the two regions that are relatively the most backward with lower levels of urbanisation and significant tribal populations. Konkan and Pune divisions in contrast (western Maharashtra region) are relatively highly industrialised, agriculturally developed, and urbanised. Nashik division (northern region) developmentally falls between these two regions with two tribal districts among its six districts.

Pune Division is known as the highest sugar-producing region and, with Konkan, it is also the prominent industrial area. In the Vidarbha region only Amravati and Nagpur districts are urban and have industries, the rest are not very developed and large parts are tribal. Konkan division has the highly urbanised Mumbai as well as poorly developed Sindhudurga and Raigarh districts. The northern division has a mix of industry (including sugar) and agriculture (GoM, 2013b).

The Emergence of Marathas as the Dominant Caste in Maharashtra

Historically, the Maratha dominance existed through kinship networks and had several sub-group such as the Patils, the Watandars, the Deshmukhs and the cultivating Kunbis. The latter were not landlords but paid out of their produce to the Watandars along with the other poor castes. Brahmins (Deshpande, Kulkarni) constituted the other powerful section of priests, accountants, and landlords and the two were joined by a growing class of moneylenders who migrated from Gujarat and Rajasthan (Marwaris). During the British rule in the nineteenth century, the Maratha lineage was undermined with indebtedness due to strict revenue demands of the British and changes in rules, while the Marwaris and the 5–6% Brahmins acquired land and wealth to become the dominant caste (Carter, 1974; Omvedt, 1976; Lele, 1982; Gore, 1989a).

The British brought in liberal thoughts, new knowledge, and egalitarian values into Indian society but did not eliminate the feudal authorities, especially at the village level (Gore, 1989b). New opportunities came up in the form of government jobs in the executive and judiciary and in this period, the Brahmins were among the first to benefit from these opportunities. They dominated, along with castes such as Kayasthas and Prabhus, the newly established educational institutions in Bombay and Pune. The Marathas and the Kunbis were largely left out of the educational opportunities and government jobs.

In the late nineteenth century they started realising the importance of education and some of them did take advantage of education (Ibid.). This realisation among the backward caste people about their own deprivation and denial of rights led to the emergence of the anti-Brahmin movement in Maharashtra.

Jyotirao Phule (1827–90), a Mali by caste, was the pioneer of social reforms through education and he established the first school for girls in Pune and later for the untouchables. He also founded the Satyashodhak Samaj (Truth Seeking Society) to provide a common platform for all the non-Brahmin castes to unite and fight for religious reform and for their own emancipation. Phule insisted that the movement's primary focus should be on social, religious, and cultural revolution rather than political (Gore, 1989a).After him, however, the lack of support by the colonial government and the elite-dominated national movement, that did not want any hindrance in mass participation due to any social revolution, changed to some extent the direction of the movement (Omvedt, 1976).

Chhatrapati Shahu Maharaj (1874–1922), from the Maratha caste, formally became the Maharaja of Kolhapur and promoted education for all sections of the society, especially the lower socio-economic groups who were denied education. His resentment of the Brahmins and the Vedokta[3] controversy in 1902 led him to adopt a policy of recruiting non-Brahmins in the government service through a 50% reservation. His opposition to Brahmins got him recognition among the backward communities (Gore, 1989b). He was proud of his Maratha lineage and he attempted to restore its glory (Copland, 1973) through a policy of inclusion of Marathas in education and employment and setting up a school for the training of Patils in 1911 (Omvedt, 1976).

The Satyashodhak Samaj movement spread but it underwent a change from being a movement for cultural revolution to being a movement for political power (Gore, 1989b). Even though Shahu Maharajhad supported inter-dining and inter-caste marriage practices, he did not fully accept the radical stand of the Satyashodhak Samaj. In 1920 he established the Shivaji Kshatriya Vedic School for the training of Maratha priests and split the anti-Brahmin movement. Later Shahu Maharaj joined the Arya Samaj and it has been argued that, "in the state of Kolhapur between 1900 and 1920, a mutual influence of a Kshatriya-oriented aristocratic anti-Brahmanism and the mass-based radicalism of the Satyashodhak movement took place" (Omvedt, 1976: 130). The increasing unity among the Marathas and the Kunbis gave them a numerical advantage (Gore, 1989b). The Marathas, mainly peasants in the villages, took a central place and participated in the anti-Brahmin movement as they could see the return of power through it. The shift of the anti-Brahmin movement from social reforms in the late nineteenth century to a struggle for political power in the early twentieth century led to the rise of the Maratha caste and the peasantry (Pol, 2008). In Maharashtra the peasant class comprises the Maratha- Kunbi caste-cluster which was numerically strong. To acquire political power and to retain it in the Congress-dominated state, they projected themselves as one (Deshpande, 2004). This mobilisation of the intermediate peasant caste for political power exists till today as a dominant feature of Maharashtra despite the official recognition of the Kunbis as a backward caste.

Economic and Political Power in Maharashtra

An empirical study conducted by the scholars from the University of British Columbia has also pointed out the local economic and political dominance by the Marathas in the three regions of Western Maharashtra, Marathwada and Vidarbha.

This is borne out by the fact that in 59% of the villages studied, Marathas own most of the land. Also Marathas comprise 40% of the population but they are the Sarpanch (village head) in over 60% of the villages (Anderson et al., 2011: 10, 13). "Estimated as about 40% of the population, the Marathas have controlled nearly 80% of the positions of political power" (Lele, 1982: xii). Several scholars see the Maratha-Kunbi caste-cluster as an agricultural land-owning dominant caste-cluster in Maharashtra (Carter, 1974; Lele, 1982, 1990; Omvedt, 1976). It explains the dominance of the Congress Party in the state, as power remained in the hands of the Maratha-Kunbi caste-cluster (Datar & Ghotale, 2013; Lele, 1990), whose numerical strength and dominance facilitated their entry into the Party since 1930 and its hold over the rural masses. Till 1990 this political power has been strengthened by the Maratha-Kunbi caste-cluster's control of the cooperative sectors, especially sugar cooperatives (Datar & Ghotale, 2013: 37).

A study of 16 Cabinets in the government since 1960–2010 to quantify the Maratha dominance in politics shows that out of 173 sampled Cabinet Ministers, 78 ministers belonged to the Maratha-Kunbi caste-cluster. Since the inception of Maharashtra, Marathas occupied the largest group in the State Cabinets, except in 1995 when the Shiv Sena–BJP formed the government. Out of the 16 Chief Ministers since the state was formed, ten have been from the Maratha-Kunbi caste- cluster (Datar & Ghotale, 2013: 38–39). This reflects their dominance in state politics. The growth and regional variations of medical colleges, especially private medical colleges, is closely linked to this power structure as we see in the following sections.

Link Between the Cooperative Sector and the Ownership of Private Medical Colleges

The control over the cooperative sector in Maharashtra, that was the base of rural industry, mainly sugar, has been one of the important means to acquire political power by the dominant caste-cluster of the Maratha-Kunbis. It is observed that more than 72% of cooperatives are controlled by Marathas (Deshpande, 2014). The prominent Chief Ministers in Maharashtra who came from the Maratha caste were Yeshwantrao Chavan from 1956 to 1962, Vasandada Patil, who was elected twice; and Sharad Pawar, who was elected three times (Damodaran, 2008)

In an interview, one of the Professors of a private medical college in Pune mentioned that the trend towards private medical education was started by the cooperative movement. He stated that:

> …In Maharashtra there was an ongoing wave of co-operative movement, especially sugar factories, but after a point there was saturation in this sector and now they had to find new avenues, so they saw opportunities in higher education. There was no great vision in establishing medical colleges. (Interview conducted on August 9, 2013)

The role of politics of cooperatives and rural development in Maharashtra and the transformation of sugar cooperative societies to educational trusts is explained as follows:

> The leaders in co-operative societies set up educational trusts and foundations in their own areas and compelled the sugar factory members to 'donate'. However, they cleverly kept these trusts legally separate from the co-operatives. They appointed themselves and their family members as life-long trustees and thus ensured that the trusts remained under their control even if they lost control over the sugar co-operatives or allied organizations. In this way, trusts controlling crores of rupees came into existence all over Maharashtra. Corruption in this manner became an open and integral feature of co operatives in Maharashtra with the silent approval of all concerned. With the money collected from ordinary members of co-operatives, the leaders set up big educational enterprises. They charged heavy capitation fees for admission to their engineering, medical, computer and management colleges. Yesterday's 'Sahakar Maharshi's' (co-operative bosses) thus transformed themselves into 'Shikshan Maharshi's' (education barons). All transactions were 'under-the-table' and without any receipts and audit, there was no record of the capitation fees. (Baviskar, 2007: 4219)

It also explains that most of the cooperatives are led by a single family member and the power is being transferred from generation to generation. For example, Dr. Vithalrao Vikhe Patil, was the first pioneer of a sugar co-operative society in Asia, established in 1950–51. Later on this legacy was transferred to his son Balasaheb Vikhe Patil and then to his grandson Radhakrishna Vikhe Patil (Ibid.). Thus for three generations power has been retained by this family.

A local political leader and a journalist by profession in Karad (district Satara) explained and reiterated the politics of co-operative societies in building up the educational institutions in Maharashtra:

> …initially what they (leaders of co-operatives) did, they collected money from the members of the factory as in terms of shares and told them that we are opening up a hospital, they showed a dream to the people and likewise they collected money from the members. However, they registered as a trust and created their ownership of the trust. It was not on the principle of co-operative— the hospital was built up through people's money. On paper they created a separate trust and all trust members belong to their own family and now the whole hospital and college ownership is in their family name. (Interview conducted on August 5, 2013.)

The emergence of this new moneyed class is reflected in the ownership of private medical colleges which is presented in the next section.

Growth of Medical Colleges: Time Trends, Spatial Distribution and Social Basis

Time Trends: Among the total of 27 private medical colleges, 37.03% colleges come under deemed universities, and 62.9% were private medical colleges. The state government set up colleges only between 1950 and 1970. By 2016, only 43.75% of the total colleges were under the state. In contrast, from barely one private college in 1970, by 1990 the number increased to 14.

Over 1981–2016 the private colleges increased by 92.8%, whereas government colleges increased only by 40.0% (Fig. 5.2).

Except from 1995–99, when the Shiv Sena was in power, the party in power remained the Indian National Congress. Of the thirteen new private medical colleges established during the decade of 1981–90, three came up in 1984, when Vasantdada Patil was the Chief Minister, and ten over just two years (1989–90) when Sharad Pawar was the Chief Minister. Over the next decade (1991–2000) as well, all four new private medical colleges were established when Sharad Pawar was the Chief Minister. Both these Chief Ministers belong to the Maratha caste and most of the private medical colleges established in the two decades were founded by Marathas. Dahiwale (1995) states, "the Maratha Mahasangha (founded in 1980) congratulated Vasantdada Patil, the former chief minister, for granting permission to medical and engineering colleges on the non-grant basis. These colleges accept a huge amount of capitation fees during admissions" (Ibid.: 340).

High growth of private medical colleges has adverse consequences for the nature and quality of medical practice; as an alumnus of one of the private medical colleges in Maharashtra explained:

> …the wards were always empty, there were very few patients and at the time of inspection they used to rent healthy people by paying them some amount to show patients load in the college hospital...practical learning was very bad and even theoretical learning was not up to the mark. (Interview conducted on July 23, 2013)

Another professor teaching in a private medical college mentioned that,

> …there is no assurance whether that particular institution is really going to give them the so-called scheduled education or not, because many medical colleges are very substandard in their teaching and the clinical material, meaning availability of patients. (Interview conducted on August 8, 2013)

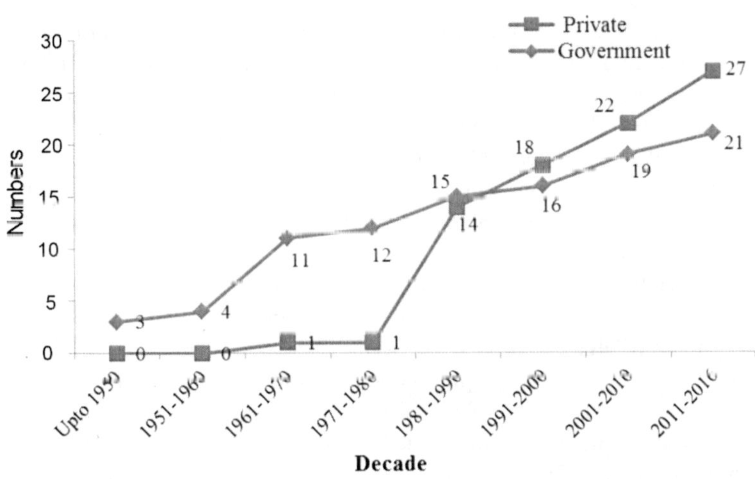

Fig. 5.2 Decadal growth of medical institutions in Maharashtra (in numbers). *Source* MCI website (2016, January 15)

Two other respondents were in favour of Public Private Partnerships (PPP) so that district hospitals could be attached to private medical colleges to fill in the gaps.

Hence, from our interviews it appears that clinical exposure for students in private medical colleges was inadequate or lacking, raising serious questions and concerns regarding the quality of education provided by these colleges.

Spatial Distribution of Medical Colleges

Pune, Mumbai and Mumbai suburban alone had 15 medical colleges (31.2% of the colleges in Maharashtra); while Pune and Konkan Divisions taken together (ten districts), had more than half of the state's medical colleges (52.08%) as well as the intake capacity (53.26%). Pune (Western Maharashtra) and Konkan were the most privileged divisions when we look at the average distribution of medical colleges per district, having more than two medical colleges. This average was 1.4 for Nashik (North Maharashtra) and just one for Nagpur (Vidarbha region). Only in Aurangabad (Marathwada region) and Amravati (Vidarbha region) this average fell below one medical college per district (Table 5.2).

In Konkan Division, Mumbai had nine of the 11 medical colleges, with the largest intake capacity. Thane and Ratnagiri had one college each (Ratnagiri college had come up only in 2015), and Raigad and Sindhudurga had none. Amravati division of Vidarbha region, comprising five districts, had just three medical colleges—all in urban locations. Similarly, three out of six districts of Nagpur and two out of five in Amravati had no medical colleges. Thus within Divisions also, there were huge inequities (Table 5.2). Amravati division had the lowest number of institutions and enrolment capacity, while Pune division had the highest institutions and intake.

The share of government medical colleges in total annual intake capacity for the state was 46.8%; that of private colleges was 53.1% (Table 5.2), pointing to the relative importance of private colleges. Interestingly, Nashik division stood out with 85.7% of its medical colleges being private. This was followed by Pune, Nagpur, Konkan and Aurangabad Divisions, where the share of private colleges was 64.2, 50.0, 45.4 and 42.8% respectively. Amravati had the lowest proportion of 33.3% private colleges. Nashik stood out as its six private colleges were in the urban and sugar-producing areas. It thus emerges that the growth of the medical colleges is largely either in the developed districts or the richer urban parts of relatively less developed districts. These are the wealthier industrial and cash crop producing areas, whereas Marathwada and Vidarbha are the most backward regions of Maharashtra, much of it being tribal as well.

The officially measured per capita income of Marathwada and Vidarbha as ratio to per capita income of the rest of Maharashtra is revealing.

It is observed that the per capita income of Marathwada is 40% lower than that of the rest of Maharashtra. Similarly per capita income of Vidarbha is 27% lower than that of the rest of Maharashtra. This ratio has gradually deteriorated in both regions during the past 10 years (GoM, 2013b: 2–3).

Table 5.2 Regional distribution of medical institutions and intake capacity in Maharashtra

Name of the division	Name of the states	Medical institutions, figures in brackets are percentages			Intake capacity figures in brackets are percentages		
		Gov.	Private	Total div.	Gov.	Private	Total div.
Pune (Western Maharashtra)	Pune, Sangli, Satara, Kolhapur, and Solapur	5	9	14	740	1250	1990
		(36.7)	(64.2)[b]	(29.1)[c]	(37.1)	(62.8)	(32.1)
Konkan	Mumbai, Thane, Ratnagiri, (Raigad and Sidndhudurga)[a]	6	5	11	810	500	1310
		(54.5)	(45.4)	(22.9)	(61.8)	(38.1)	(21.1)
Nashik (North Maharashtra)	Nashik, Dhule, Jalgaon and Ahmednagar (Nandurbar)[a]	1	6	7	100	645	745
		(14.2)	(85.7)	(14.5)	(13.4)	(86.5)	(12.0)
Aurangabad (Marathwada)	Aurangabad, Jalna, Nanded, Beed and Latur (Parbhani, Hingoli, Osmanabad)[a]	4	3	7	500	350	850
		(57.1)	(42.8)	(14.5)	(58.8)	(41.1)	(13.7)
Nagpur (Vidarbha)	Nagpur, Wardha, Chandrapur (GadchiroliBhandara, Gondiya)[a]	3	3	6	450	450	900
		(50)	(50)	(12.5)	(50)	(50)	(14.5)
Amaravati (Vidarbha)	Akola, Amaravati, and Yavatmal (Buldhana Washim)[a]	2	1	3	300	100	400
		(66.6)	(33.3)	(6.2)	(75.0)	(25.0)	(6.4)
	Total	21	27	48	2900	3295	6195
		(44)	(56)	(100)	(47)	(53)	(100)

Source for Data: MCI Website. (2016, January 15)
Source for Regions: Government of Maharashtra (2013, May 4)
[a]Districts mentioned in brackets are without any medical college
[b]In each division the percent share of government and private medical college is out of the total of divisional colleges
[c]In each division the divisional percent of medical colleges is out of the total state medical colleges. The same applies to intake capacity

The *Maharashtra Human Development Report* (GoM, 2012) shows that Sangli, Kolhapur, Pune, Mumbai, Thane, Nashik and Nagpur districts are very high HDI; whereas Hingoli, Usmanabad, Washim, Nandurbar, Gadchiroli, Jalna, Nanded, Latur and Dhule have low HDI. As Table 5.2 and Map 5.1, clearly show, Hingoli, Usmanabad, Washim, Nandurbar, Gadchiroli do not have a single medical college, not even a government college. Growth of private medical colleges is significant only in Pune, Mumbai, Satara, Nashik, Ahmadnagar, Sangli, and Kolhapur.

Since 2011 seven new medical colleges have been established, two by government and five by private entities. Three private colleges came up in the districts of Solapur, Satara and Nashik where medical colleges already existed, and the other two in

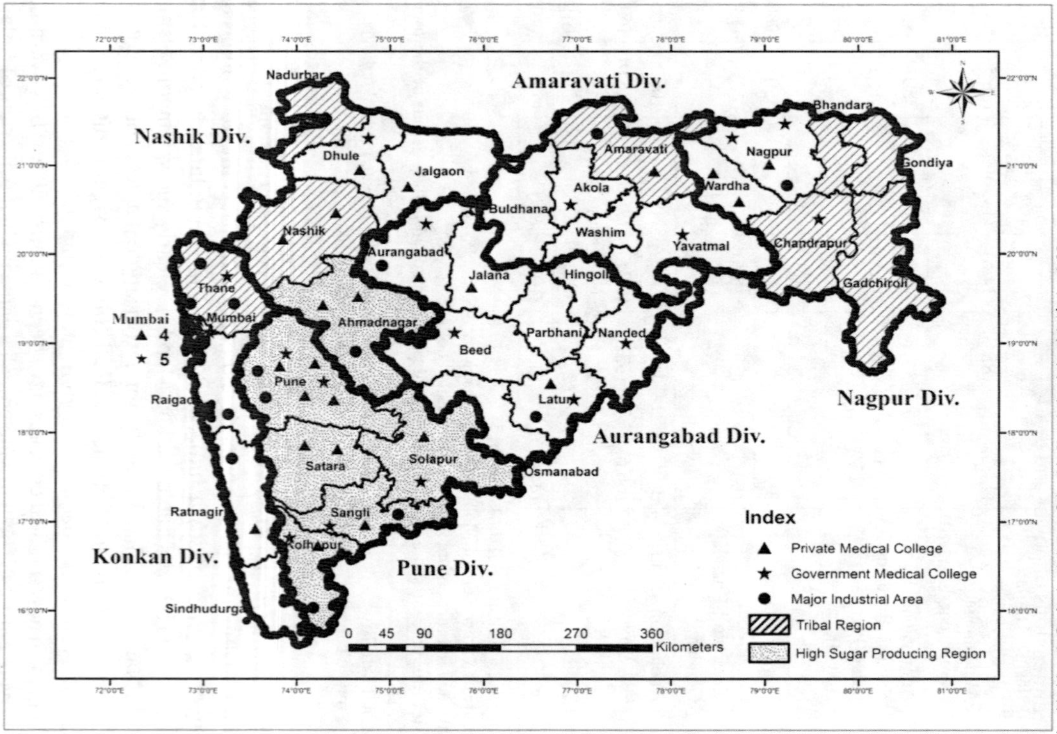

Sources for Medical Colleges Data: MCI Website (2016, January 15).
High Sugar Producing Region: Vasantdada Sugar Institute, Maharashtra Statistics. Available at http://www.vsisugar.com/india/statistics/maharashtra_statistics.htm Accessed April 17, 2016
Tribal Region: GoM (2013b:471)
Major Industrial Area: Available at <http://4.bp.blogspot.com/-OG9WkJt2yOA/UHc_BvGcl1I/AMA/xMHXeDZGtDM/s1600/majorIndustrialRegions.gif> Accessed April 17, 2016

Map 5.1 Division-wise distribution of medical colleges in Maharashtra

Ratnagiri and Jalna where there was none. One of the government medical colleges came up in Chandrapur (which had none), the other was in Mumbai with several medical colleges. The neglect of underserved and relatively backward districts, the continuation of regional disparities, and the dominance of private sector is thus evident.

Social Basis of Private Medical Colleges

The multiple dimensions of power and the emergence of medical colleges, especially private medical colleges, is reflected in the regional development of Maharashtra (Map 5.1 and Table 5.3). One of the 25 private colleges all owners were Hindus except one, who was a Muslim. Among Hindu owners, 72% of medical colleges were established by open caste categories, 16% by OBC and 8% by Vimukta Jati and Notified Tribes (VJNT). However, when seen in terms of the political domination of Marathas and Maratha-Kunbi caste-cluster, their ownership of private medical colleges was 72% (Table 5.3).

Most of these owners are politically affiliated to the Congress Party or to the Nationalist Congress Party. Seventeen colleges were owned by twelve people and these owners had occupied political positions such as Member of Parliament, Member of Legislative Assembly (MLA), and Member of Legislative Council (MLC), and have been Ministers at the state and central level. Of these, eight owners at some point were linked to sugar cooperatives. This link has already been discussed. Their

Table 5.3 Social background of the founders of private medical colleges in Maharashtra: (total 25)[a]

Number of colleges	Religion	Caste
15 (60%)	Hindu	Maratha (open)
1 (4%)	Hindu (Gujarat)	Patidar (open)
1 (4%)	Hindu (Gujarat)	Kutchi-Lohana (open)
1 (4%)	Hindu	Khatri Caste (open)
3 (12%)	Hindu	Kunbi (OBC)[b]
1 (4%)	Hindu	Mali (OBC)
2 (8%)	Hindu	Vanjari (VJNT)
1 (4%)	Muslim	–

Source The list of the names of the founders has been compiled from each college website. Data of caste and religion of the founders was gathered from local key informants and academicians

[a]In 2016 there were 27 private medical colleges, however the data was collected in 2013; two medical colleges were established after 2013; the caste background of founders of these two colleges could not be obtained

[b]One medical college was established by a trust, set up by a person who was politically strong and belonged to the Kunbi caste. However, currently it is not clear as to who is leading the trust

political leadership at the local level had either evolved through sugar cooperatives or helped them acquire it. Some till date have a strong hold on the sugar cooperatives. The nexus between the caste associations and political linkages at the local and the state levels indicates the hegemony of the Maratha-Kunbi caste-cluster in establishing private medical colleges in Maharashtra.

Implication of the Growth Pattern of Medical Colleges for Universal Healthcare

Universal healthcare is defined, as access to key promotive, preventive, curative, and rehabilitative health interventions for all at an affordable cost, thereby achieving equity in access and coverage (WHO, 2005). Even from a limited clinical perspective, this would require a fair distribution of medical colleges for tertiary care and availability of professionals. The story of medical colleges in Maharashtra, especially the private colleges, reveals their inequitable distribution and concentration in urban and economically developed areas. Private colleges emerged as a tool for wealth generation through diversification of capital produced in the agriculture sector. This capital in Maharashtra was routed through the sugar cooperatives, where political power of caste groups helped capture wealth produced for private use. The logic of profit from education and service is inbuilt in the mal-distribution of these colleges.

The historical Maratha-Kunbi caste-cluster alliance that holds political power in Maharashtra till today makes it easy for the moneyed of these castes to influence and interfere with policy implementation. Setting up of state medical colleges, though less mal-distributed, is not necessarily unaffected by this influence. This is evident from their concentration in urban areas and the neglect of more needy districts.

The nature and quality of medical education is another aspect of the challenge. While the requirement is for a need-based education that emphasises the national disease pattern and the medical care needs of the majority with emphasis on preventive, promotive, curative aspects of care and managerial dimension of healthcare systems, most private medical colleges are tuned to curative care. As it is, medical education in India is highly influenced by the Westernised models that shaped medical institutions, curriculum, and, most importantly, the value system of the medical professionals (Banerji, 1973). Specialisation in curative medicine, practice in urban areas and in hospital settings, and an individualistic perspective are the hallmarks of this professional enterprise. Its focus is on Western technology and income-generating medical industry as a lucrative business, without consideration for social aspects of the illness or community as a whole (Antia, 1990). This orientation perpetuates disparities in the health system and creates urban-oriented mindset-seeking specialisations (Ministry of Health and Family Welfare (MoHFW), 2007). These maladies are only heightened in private medical colleges.[4]

The high level of capitation fees in the private medical colleges (over INR 35 lakhs for a medical degree), pushes students to prefer practice in the private sector to recover costs and earn well (Qadeer & Nayar, 2005; Rao et al., 2011). Evidence shows that the increase in the number of private medical colleges has resulted in increase in the cost of healthcare, but not in access (Joy et al., 2007; Qadeer, 2006). Questions arise about merit too, since almost half the medical colleges in the country admit students on the basis of their ability to pay high fees, rather than their marks. What then, is the merit of these students?

It appears that the increasing numbers of private medical colleges in several states are not a very helpful trend for universalising healthcare. Despite their large production every year, there is a shortage of doctors in the country's public health system. This shortfall is 10.3% at the Primary Health Centre (PHC) level, especially in Bihar, Chhattisgarh, Madhya Pradesh, Orissa and Uttar Pradesh where this shortfall is 20.7%. At the Community Health Centre, the shortfall of specialist doctors was of the order of 62.8% for surgeons, 55.2% for obstetricians and gynaecologists, 72% for physicians and 69.5% for paediatricians (MoHFW, 2010). The high rate of migration abroad adds to the problem. Maharashtra is no different despite its high share of medical colleges; institutions in backward and tribal areas of the state remain without doctors (GoM, 2013b).[5]

The socio-economic and political basis of the emergence of private medical colleges as instruments of profit is the very reason why these colleges are not a solution for taking us towards universalisation of healthcare. Their prime objective puts a question mark on their ability to contribute to resolving the crisis of access to medical care. These institutions and their products are not inclined to participate in expanding medical care systems. The notion that their partnership with the state can cover the unreached is highly misplaced due to the reasons discussed above. Maharashtra's Maratha-Kunbi caste cluster based social and political power structure, with its economic roots and vested interests help us to understand the intricate threads of the national political economy that supports international pressures for reforms and privatisation in the health sector. Investing in medical education is in fact a profitable venture as the state permits high capitation and regular fees. It also gives prestige and power in society (Kaul, 1993). The interest of the majority of private college owners is accumulation of wealth, not necessarily in providing quality education. They will therefore fuel the medical market and not cater to the needs of partnerships for rational and affordable universal healthcare.

Notes

1. The concept of Dominant Caste is evolved by Srinivas (1955) as "a caste may be said to be "dominant" when it preponderates numerically over the other castes, and when it also wields preponderant economic and political power. A large and powerful caste group can be more easily dominant if its position in the local caste hierarchy is not too low" (Srinivas 1955 as cited in Srinivas, 1959: 1).
2. There is huge complexity in defining the terms Kunbi and Maratha. There was a distinction between Kunbi and Maratha until 1911; however, this was based on class rather than caste as, traditionally, 'Marathas' were landlords and chiefs of the villages', whereas Kunbis were the cultivators of the land. Around 1911

Kunbis were merged with the general Maratha community (Enthoven 1922 as cited in Carter, 1974). However Lele (1990) emphasised the fact that the Maratha-Kunbi caste-cluster is politically strong since independence and till today they continue to be so. Today the Maharashtra government has reversed to considering them as separate castes and Kunbis are considered as Other Backward Class.

3. The Vedokta controversy emerged around 1900 when the Brahmins opposed the acceptance of Kshatriya status for Marathas and hence, to Shahu Maharaj, thereby denying the palace the privilege of performing Vedic rites at religious ceremonies (Gore, 1989b).
4. It is being argued that private colleges tend to bring quality down by focusing on fee and capitation and corrupt practices (Singh & Devi, 2015).
5. It is said that there is a shortage of 4000 doctors in the public health system in Maharashtra (Iyer & Thomas, 2013).

References

Ananthakrishnan, N. (2007, January–February). Acute shortage of teachers in medical colleges: Existing problems and possible solutions. *The National Medical Journal of India, 20*(1), 25–29.

Ananthakrishnan. (2010, May–June). Medical education in India: Is it still possible to reverse the downhill trend? *The National Medical Journal of India* 23(3), 156–160.

Anderson, S., Francois, P., & Kotwal, A. (2011). *One kind of democracy*. (Working paper). Department of Economics, University of British Columbia. Accessed on June 15, 2015. http://faculty.arts.ubc.ca/fpatrick/documents/marathacirculate.pdf

Antia, N. H. (1990, July 21). Medical education: In need of cure. *Economic and Political Weekly, 25*(29), 1571–1573.

Banerji, D. (1973, March 3). Social orientation of medical education in India. *Economic and Political Weekly, 8*(9), 485–487.

Baru, R. (1987). *Factors influencing inter-regional variations in health services: A study of selected districts of Andhra Pradesh*. Unpublished M.Phil Diss., Centre of Social Medicine and Community Health, Jawaharlal Nehru University.

Baviskar, B. S. (2007, October 20). Co-operatives in Maharashtra: Challenges ahead. *Economic and Political Weekly, 42*(42), 4217–4221.

Carter, A. (1974). *Elite politics in rural India: Political stratification and political alliances in Western Maharashtra*. Vikas Publishing House.

Chandrasekhar, C. P., & Ghosh, J. (2002). *The market that failed: A decade of neoliberal economic reforms in India*. Leftword Books.

Chattopadhyay, S. (2008, January–March). Black money in white coats: Whither medical ethics? *Indian Journal of Medical Ethics, 5*(1), 20–21.

Choudhury, P. (2016, January 16). Role of private sector in medical education and human resource development for health in India. *Economic and Political Weekly, 51*(3):71–79.

Copland, I. (1973, March). The Maharaja of Kolhapur and the Non-Brahmin movement 1902–10. *Modern Asian Studies, 7*(2), 209–225.

Dahiwale, S. M. (1995, February 11). Consolidation of Maratha dominance in Maharashtra. *Economic and Political Weekly, 30*(6), 336–342.

Damodaran, H. (2008). *India's new capitalists: Caste, business, and industry in a modern nation*. Permanent Black.

Datar, A., & Ghotale, V. (2013, September 7). Maharashtra Cabinets: Social and regional profile 1960–2010. *Economic and Political Weekly, 48*(36), 37–42.

Deshpande, R. (2004, April 3). Kunbi Maratha as OBC: Backward journey of a caste. *Economic and Political Weekly, 39*(14/15), 1448–1449.

Deshpande, S., & Deshpande-Naik, G. (2009, October 30). Crass commercialisation and corruption of the Indian Medical Education system and the resultant decay of the Indian Health Education in the last two decades: A case for urgent international review and monitoring. *Electron Physician, 1*, 9–16.

Deshpande, V. (2014, June 28). PIL challenges Maratha reservation in Maharashtra. *The Hindu.*

Diwan, V., Minj, C., Chhari, N., & Costa, A. (2013, September 15). Indian medical students in public and private sector medical schools: Are motivations and career aspirations different? Studies from Madhya Pradesh, India. *BMC Medical Education* 13(127). Accessed December 23, 2013. http://www.biomedcentral.com/1472-6920/13/127

Gore, M. S. (1989a, April 29). Social movements and the paradigm of functional analysis: With reference to the non-Brahman movement in Maharashtra. *Economic and Political Weekly, 24*(17), 928–936.

Gore. (1989b). *Non Brahmin movement in Maharashtra.* Segment Book Distributors.

Government of India. (2016). Interstate Council Secretariat, Ministry of Home Affairs, Zonal Councils Composition, January 14. Accessed January 17, 2016. http://interstatecouncil.nic.in/zonal_composition.html#subnav2_2Source

Government of India. (1946). *Report of the health survey and development committee: Bhore Committee Report* (Vol. I–IV). Manager of Publications.

Government of India. (1961). *Report of the health survey and planning committee. Mudaliar Committee Report*. Ministry of Health.

Government of India. (2011). *The high level expert group report on universal health coverage for India.* Planning Commission of India.

Government of Maharashtra. (2013, May 4). Accessed September 15, 2013. https://www.maharashtra.gov.in/1128/Districts

Government of Maharashtra. (2012). *Maharashtra human development report 2012: Towards inclusive human development*. Sage Publications.

Government of Maharashtra. (2013a). *Economic survey of Maharashtra 2012–2013.* Directorate of Economics and Statistics, Planning Department.

Government of Maharashtra. (2013b). *Report of the high level committee on balanced regional development issues in Maharashtra.* Planning Department.

Iyer, M., & Thomas, S. (2013, July 11). Maharashtra faces massive shortage of 4k doctors for public health system. *Times of India.* Accessed April 20, 2016. http://timesofindia.indiatimes.com/india/Maharashtra-faces-massive-shortage-of-4K-doctors-for-public-health-system/articleshow/21010016.cms

Joy, S., Raveendran, R., Vijayan, S., & Ugargol, A. P. (2007). Mushrooming of private medical schools in India, the present student profile and cost of medical education and its impact on equity, healthcare accessibility, cost and perceived quality of healthcare. Paper Presented in IHEA 2007, *6 World Congress: Explorations in Health Economics.* Accessed April 14, 2012. https://doi.org/10.2139/ssrn.992143

Kaul, R. (1993). *Caste, class and education: Politics of the capitation fee phenomenon in Karnataka.* Sage Publications.

Lele, J. (1982). *Elite pluralism and class rule: Political development in Maharashtra.* Popular Prakashan.

Lele, J. (1990). Caste, class and mobilisation in Maharashtra. In F. Frankel & M. S. A. Rao (Eds.), *Dominance and state power in modern India* (Vol. 2), Oxford University Press.

Mahal, A., & Mohanan, M. (2006, November). Growth of private medical education in India. *Medical Education, 40*(10), 1009–1011.

Mathew, T. (2002). *India betrayed: Globalisation and realignment.* In T. V. Sathyamurthy (Ed.) (pp. 75–96). Touchstone and Centre for Social Studies.

Medical Council of India. (2016). Information Desk, Colleges. January 15. Accessed January 15, 2016. http://www.mciindia.org/InformationDesk/CollegesCoursesSearch.aspx

Ministry of Health and Family Welfare. (2007). *Report of the working group on medical education.* National Knowledge Commission. Accessed April 14, 2012 http://www.Knowledgecommission.gov.in/downloads/documents/wg_med.pdf

Ministry of Health and Family Planning. (1973). *Report of the committee on multipurpose workers. Kartar Singh Committee.* Ministry of Health and Family Planning.

Ministry of Health and Family Planning. (1975). *health services and medical education a programme for immediate action. Shrivastav Committee Report.* Ministry of Health and Family Planning.

Ministry of Health and Family Welfare. (2010). *Rural Health Statistics Bulletin.* Ministry of Health and Family Welfare.

Omvedt, G. (1976). *Cultural revolt in a colonial society: The non-Brahmin movement in Western India: 1873 to 1930.* Scientific Socialist Education Trust.

Omvedt, G. (1981, December 26). Capitalist agriculture and rural classes in India. *Economic and Political Weekly, 16*(52), A140–A159.

Pol, P. (2008). *Journalism of early twentieth century Maharashtra: Examining journalistic writings of non-Brahmin and untouchable movements, 1920–1930.* Unpublished M. Phil Diss., Centre for Historical Studies, Jawaharlal Nehru University.

Qadeer, I. (2006, September). The real crisis in medical education. *Indian Journal of Medical Ethics III, 3*, 95–96.

Qadeer, I., & K. R. Nayar, (2005, January–February). Politics of pedagogy in public health. *Social Scientist, 33*(1/2), 47–75.

Rao, M., Rao, K., Shiva Kumar, A. K., Chatterjee, M., & Sundararaman, T. (2011, February 12). Human resources for health in India. *The Lancet, 377*(9765), 587–598.

Rutten, M. (1986, March 29). Social profile of agricultural entrepreneurs economic behaviour and life-style of middle-large farmers in Central Gujarat. *Economic and Political Weekly, 21*(13), A15–A23.

Singh, M. M. & Devi, R. (2015). Quality of medical education and private medical colleges in India. *British Medical Journal* 350:h237. Accessed April 10, 2016. http://www.bmj.com/content/350/bmj.h237/rr-3

Srinivas, M. N. (1959, February). The dominant caste in Rampura. *American Anthropologist, 61*(1), 1–16. New Series.

Supe, A., & Burdick, W. (2006, December). Challenges and issues in medical education in India. *Academic Medicine* 81(12), 1076–1080.

Upadhya, C. (1988, July 2). The Farmer-Capitalists of Coastal Andhra Pradesh. *Economic and Political Weekly, 23*(27), 1376–1382.

WHO. (2005). *Sustainable health financing, universal coverage and social health insurance report by the Secretariat, fifty-eighth World Health Assembly.* WHO Accessed April 17, 2016. http://www.who.int/health_financing/documents/cov-wharesolution5833/en/

Part II
Evidences and Experiences of Public–Private Partnerships and Health Insurance Schemes

Chapter 6
A Critical Look at Public Private Partnership for Health Services in Karnataka

Sylvia Karpagam, Akhila Vasan, Elangovan Gajraj, Bijoya Roy, and Imrana Qadeer

Introduction

The Planning Commission (PC) in 2012 mentions two models of Public Private Partnership (PPPs) which 'can be considered wherever appropriate for replication and upscaling'. One is the Rajiv Gandhi Super Speciality Hospital (RGSSH), Raichur, Karnataka for tertiary care, a joint venture between the Government of Karnataka (GoK) and Apollo hospitals to provide management of the hospital and super-speciality clinical care services, with free outpatient services for Below Poverty Line (BPL) patients. The second model is a contracting arrangement with a non-government organisation (NGO), Karuna trust and the state government to manage primary health centres and provide rural healthcare delivery. (Government of India (GoI), 2013).

This chapter looks at how these two models of healthcare delivery have failed in Karnataka and why the possibility of replication and upscaling as recommended by the PC is not a viable option in the interest of comprehensive and cost-effective health service delivery with functioning grievance redressal mechanisms.

S. Karpagam (✉)
Urban marginalized communities, Karnataka, India

A. Vasan
Activist with the Karnataka Janaarogya Chaluvali, Karnataka, India

E. Gajraj
National Institute of Clinical Excellence (NICE), London, England

B. Roy
Centre for Women's Development Studies, New Delhi, India

I. Qadeer
Council for Social Development, New Delhi, India

I. Qadeer et al. (eds.), *Universalising Healthcare in India*,
https://doi.org/10.1007/978-981-16-5872-3_6

Background of RGSSH

The GoK, Department of Health and Family Welfare with financial aid of INR 60 crores from the Organisation of Petroleum Exporting Companies (OPEC), undertook a project for the setting up of a super specialty healthcare facility at Raichur, in North Karnataka. The construction of the 350-bedded hospitals was started in 1997 on a 73 acre campus within the city limits of Raichur (Buradikatti, 2013a; TV9, 2013). The Department of Health and Family Welfare (DoHFW) considered various options to manage the hospital; as a departmental hospital, an autonomous institution, as a joint venture with the private sector, or managed either by the for-profit or non-profit sector. A Cabinet meeting in August 2000 approved the option of inviting the non-profit private sector to run the 350-bed hospital. A committee was formed to work out the modalities of the hospital through a government order- GO No. HFW (PR) 292 WBA 2000 dated October 25, 2000. Finally, Apollo Health Enterprises Ltd. (AHEL), Hyderabad, signed a partnership agreement with the Department of Health and Family Welfare as represented by the Commissioner. A governing council was set up with representatives from the DoHFW and AHEL (vide GO No. HFW (PR) 292 WBA 2000 dated August 8, 2001).

This long-term partnership came into effect in 2002 and was to expire in June 2011, at which time, the state government decided to study the outcome of the joint venture project. It constituted an evaluation committee with five officers including the director of the State Institute of Health and Family Welfare (SIHFW), the Joint Director of the DoHFW, the Chief Finance Officer of the National Rural Health Mission, the deputy Chief Financing Officer and healthcare financing consultant of the Karnataka State Health Systems Resource Centre (KSHSRC). The main objective of the evaluation was to review the functioning of the hospital and the outcome of the PPP. The team visited the hospital and reviewed the service contract, data on utilisation of the facility, audited financial statement, government orders, base files and documents including the initial proposal. The team also looked at the overall functioning of PPP as a model of tertiary care. They looked specifically at whether the services were provided as per the MoU, compliance of AHEL with the terms and conditions of the contract, the inventory and stock register for equipment provided by GoK as well as those procured by AHEL, whether AHEL has provided a statement about services provided to Below Poverty Line (BPL) patients, the cost of services to BPL patients and subsequent claims reimbursed by the government. They also specifically looked to see if there were instances of Above Poverty Line (APL) charges being levied on BPL patients and any instances of denial of services to BPL patients. An analysis was also done on the revenue generated to the hospital from the treatment of APL patients, the average monthly operating cost and whether any financial loss had been incurred by the RGSSH. This evaluation report has been unavailable in the public domain and had to be obtained by filing a Right to Information (RTI) application. (GoK, 2011).

Salient Points from the Evaluation Report of the State Government (Government of Karnataka, 2011)

1. **Absence of Third-Party Evaluations**. No third party evaluations have been conducted on this hospital for the previous 10 years by either of the partners—GoK or AHEL, and neither is there any baseline data to assess if there had been any change in the project performance or the quality of services.
2. **Absence of Equipment Inventory**. The Gok as per the agreement had procured and handed over several items of medical and non-medical equipment including furniture, fixtures and computers to AHEL to operationalise the hospital. The report states that the hospital has not maintained an inventory of assets. A total of 70 items of equipment had been procured by the hospital authorities at a total cost of INR 3,46,47,243 and a total of 40 non-medical equipment at INR 1,02,76,140 from the One Time Grant (OTG). Twenty-eight items of computers and related items worth INR 1,00,31,033, 11 items of furniture worth INR 46,33,331and 3 vehicles at a cost of INR 20,85,459 were also procured. The hospital had however not maintained a log book for equipment, furniture or fixtures. Of the 84 items of equipment available in the hospital, 10 had not functioned since 2007 and there has been no structured system of conducting Annual Stock Verification in the hospital. These observations were also brought out in an earlier inspection carried out by the then Chief Administrative Officer (CAO), Karnataka Health Systems Development and Reforms Project (KHSDRP) on June 12–13, 2007 (GoK, 2011 Annexure 13).
3. **Poor Utilisation Rates by BPL**. One of the key objectives of establishing the RGSSH by the Government of Karnataka was to provide quality healthcare to patients below the poverty line in the districts of the Gulbarga Division, where the BPL population has been identified by the Food and Civil Supplies department to constitute the majority (67 percent) of the population. However data on utilisation of the hospital services reveals that not more than 25 percent of the In- Patient (IP) services and 15 percent of the Out-Patient (OP) services have been used by the BPL patients over the period of 10 years.

   As seen in Figs. 6.1 and 6.2, the utilisation of IP and OP services by BPL patients has not been successful in achieving its primary objective of providing services to BPL patients.
4. **Poor Bed Occupancy Rates**. As per Clause 2.5 of the Service Contract Agreement (SCA), RGSSH is required to earmark 140 beds (40 percent) (out of 350 bed strength) as general ward beds. (GoK, 2011: 38)

   The evaluation team found that only 154 of the total bed strength of 350 were operational. Of these, only 40 beds were available for the BPL patients. This works out to only 11.4 percent of the total bed strength of 350 and 25.9 percent of the total operational beds of 154. The evaluation report states that "this sub-optimal capacity utilization has seriously affected the sustainability of the hospital, thereby leading to serious questions on the commitment towards the PPP model of functioning." (Ibid.: 46).

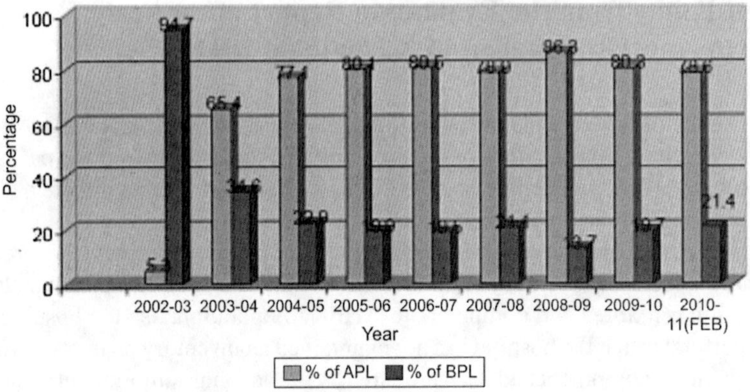

Fig. 6.1 Utilisation of In-Patient Services by BPL and APL 2002–03 to 2010–11 (February 2011). (*Source* Government of Karnataka, 2011)

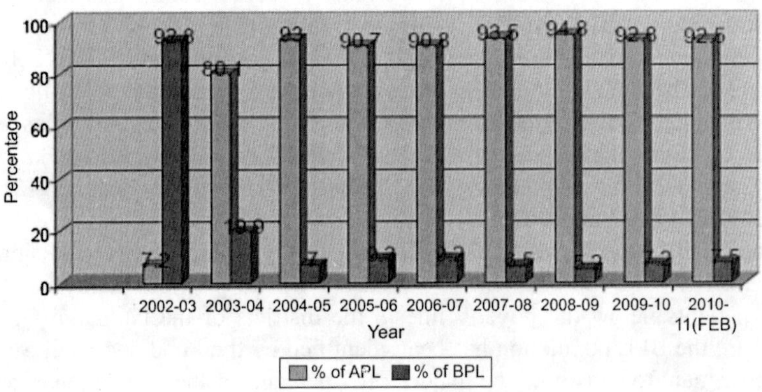

Fig. 6.2 Utilisation of Out-Patient Services by BPL and APL 2002–03 to 2010–11 (February 2011). *Source* (GoK, 2011)

5. **Poor Income Generation.** The proposal submitted by AHEL to the government as part of the Expression of Interest had indicated 70 percent occupancy at year one and moving towards 100 percent occupancy in the tenth year. The Income and Expenditure statement indicates that the hospital has not been generating any profit since its inception.
   According to the audited statement of the hospital, no profit has been generated by the hospital from the period 2002–10. (Ibid.: 27) A previous government order (GoHFW/64/CGM/2002), dated March 21, 2002 stated that in the years when no net profits are earned, the governing council can allow payment of annual service charge to the contractor out of the surplus pool account. It was then resolved that, INR 241.64 lakhs for 2002–03 and INR 858.65 lakhs for 2003–04 shall be released by the government for revenue loss incurred (Ibid).

6. **Speciality and Other Services Provided by the Hospital.** According to Clause 2.4 of the SCA, speciality services were to be mentioned in the annexure. However this annexure was not available either with the hospital authorities or anywhere on the hospital premises. There is no clarity on what speciality services are expected and what have been actually delivered.
   The contractor had outsourced maintenance, security and housekeeping services. It is observed that the large private provider who is entrusted to manage and provide services brings about multiple small local private contractors nested under it, that further challenge the process of evaluating the performance, and accountability of the sub-contracted party.
7. **Governance and Accountability.** Although the governing council was expected to meet every six months, they had met only 10 times in the last 10 years. The approval of the governing council had not been sought as stipulated in the service contract to engage a chartered accountant firm for the hospital accounts.

The service contract was initially drafted by the committee for operationalisation of the OPEC hospital, in accordance with a government order number—Go No. HFW (PR) 292 WBA 2000 dated October 25, 2000. The finance department had made certain observations and suggested amendments to the service contract. However, this amendment had not been signed by both parties. Subsequently, Apollo Hospitals objected to amendments made in the past leading to a deadlock between Apollo hospitals and the GoK.

The monitoring of hospital equipment lies with the Karnataka Health Systems Development and Reforms Project (KHSDRP); BPL claims by the Deputy Commissioner, Raichur and other hospital administrative issues are monitored by the Commissioner, Health and Family Welfare. The hospital did not have any grievance redressal mechanisms in place. Although the Deputy Commissioner of Raichur, as a representative of the owner (GoK), is expected to monitor adherence to the contract, the minimum assured beds and the payment of BPL claims have not been monitored.

An analysis of the hospital BPL claims submitted by the Local Audit Circle (LAC) of Raichur to the visiting evaluation team reveals that there is a discrepancy in the total number of BPL claims for out-patient and in-patients between the details provided by RGSSH authorities and that of the admitted claims by the LAC. For instance, the number of BPL OP as per the hospital authorities for the year 2002–03 and 2003–04 is 7,888 and 1,775 respectively. While the BPL claims admitted by LAC are 10,806 and 36,427 respectively. Similarly the in-patient number as per the hospital authorities is 1,844 and 786 while the claims by LAC are admitted for 485 and 2,310 respectively. The evaluation report states that "BPL claims submitted by RGSSH is critical for the objective for which the hospital was established and the inconsistency in the data between the hospital authorities and that provided for reimbursement to the local audit circle of Raichur is alarming" (Ibid.: 36).

The evaluation team also states that in such partnership models, the private partners should be responsible for achieving service quality benchmarks and assume the risks for delays and cost overruns in the project, including issues related to human resources and efficiency in service delivery. The Service Contract Agreement (SCA) makes no mention of measurable outcomes to assess effectiveness of clinical and ancillary services.

Community Response to Apollo-Managed RGSSH

According to a fact-finding team from Karnataka Jana Arogya Chaluvali, as early as 2007, the Karnataka Rajya Raitha Sangha[1] had formally lodged a complaint about how the hospital services were inaccessible to BPL patients and the sudden mushrooming of brokers and middlemen who were bringing in patients for a commission. By then several complaints had emerged from BPL card holders as reported by a fact finding team. They reported harassment in the name of card verification. They were frequently told by the hospital administration that their card was invalid on the pretext that their names were misspelt. Till such a time that the cards were verified, the hospital administration demanded that BPL patients pay an upfront amount of INR 25,000, which they said they would reimburse once the card was regularised. The BPL patients were later told that their cards had been cancelled while actually submitting the valid BPL card for claiming reimbursement from the government. Such large-scale fraud was exposed by the local sanghatans which accessed 144 BPL cards along with their registration number, date of admission, treatment, bill and deposit paid. The details were submitted to the Principal Secretary, Health and Family Welfare. The latter instituted an enquiry into the issue which merely directed Apollo to reimburse the deposit amount collected but there was no disciplinary action for the fraud committed. The fact finding report states that the year 2007 also marked a shift in the functioning of RGSSH. The one time grant reserves were nearly spent. Apollo had to generate its own revenue to bear the risks of delay and problems with cash flow. However 'revenue generation' was poor. Salaries started getting delayed for one month initially and soon employees had to wait for three months to get their salaries and led to the exit of several doctors whose retention had anyway been a problem. Importantly Apollo as a principal employer had not made any provision for Provident Fund (PF) or other benefits through its ten- year contract period as mandated by labour laws.

On May 31, 2012, the contract with the Apollo management was terminated by the state government, and all 285 employees on the rolls of Apollo were summarily dismissed. A year long struggle ensued with the workers demanding that the hospital be re-opened (Buradikatti, 2013b).

Instead the government handed over the hospital from the Department of Health and Family Welfare to the Department of Higher Education with intent to convert it into a teaching hospital for the Raichur Institute of Medical Sciences (RIMS) which was under risk of losing its Medical Council of India (MCI) recognition if it failed to show association with an equipped teaching hospital (Buradikatti, 2013a). The Workers Union of RGSSH staged a long protracted struggle to be reinstated in the hospital under the new administration of RIMS (Staff Correspondent, 2012).

The evaluation team who visited the hospital in 2011 mention in their report, that.

> the project initially has some concerns raised by the local people on taking over the management of the hospital by a private player. Citizens Forum of Raichur had raised concerns over, however they were not taken into consideration as Cabinet decision for outsourcing of the hospital functioning to a reputed private provider was already taken and a GO to that effect was already issued. The major concerns raised by local representatives that the cost of healthcare for the poor people would go high (GoK, 2011: 52).

In summary, the mega project of setting up a super speciality healthcare has led to more than financial losses. For the ten years, that the project had been in place, there had been no form of evaluation of the hospital. From the findings of the evaluation report, it is evident that there has been dissatisfaction regarding privatisation and increased of costs for the poor.

The poor utilisation rates of the hospital by BPL patients and in fact even by APL patients are an indication of huge expenditures that have not led to any benefit even to paying patients. The utilisation rate by BPL patients for in-patient as well as out-patient care has dropped to less than 50 percent and no serious attempts have been made either by the hospital or the state government to address this serious concern. Even as an income-generating initiative, there has been failure with no profits being generated over an 8-year period leading to the government investing more funds to sustain the hospital. The regulatory mechanisms have been dysfunctional and even those recommendations that were made have not been given due cognisance. The state government did not consider it important to include community experiences in their evaluation of the RGSSH, nor did it consider it important to have a dialogue with local people's organisations, which had been raising a voice against several irregularities particularly in management of BPL patients. Apollo as a principal employer had not made any provision for provident fund or other benefits through its ten year contract period as mandated by labour laws. However, worker's rights figure nowhere in the 'evaluation framework'. The inclusion in the evaluation report of large-scale labour law violations and financial irregularities by RGSSH would have given a more realistic picture of the fallouts of the PPP model.

Karuna Trust Model of Primary Healthcare

The other example cited in the context of PPP in the Twelfth Five Year Plan, is that of a PPP between an NGO, Karuna Trust and the Government of Karnataka for the management of primary health centres.

The Trust claims to manage 80 Primary Healthcare Centres (PHCs) in 7 states—Karnataka, Andhra Pradesh, Orissa, Arunachal Pradesh, Manipur, Meghalaya and Rajasthan. It has partnerships with different state governments, the Nuclear Power Corporation of India Limited, BOSCH Foundation, Population Foundation of India, Sightsavers, India Development Foundation (IDF), MacArthur Foundation, Karnataka Health Promotion Trust (KHPT), American Service to India, India Friends Association, etc. According to the prototype Memorandum of Understanding (MoU) for PPP between State and Not-For-Profit Organisations signed by the NGO and all state governments, it is clear that any contribution will be made by donors to the Arogya Raksha Samiti (ARS) which will take a decision on such contributions, if it is without attached conditionalities (except conditionality of proper use). If conditionalities are attached, it will be referred to the District Health Society. All contributions for civil works will be decided by the ARS if within INR 1 lakh or referred to the District Health Society if higher. (GoK, 2008) However, the NGO has directly signed MoUs with several donors and funding agencies without even a token involvement of members of the Arogya Raksha Samiti. This is a clear violation of the terms of agreement with state governments for generating funds for PHC function. The organisation has received funds for mobile health, dental health, telemedicine, management of non-communicable diseases, traditional medicine, emergency medicine, drugs, eye care, reproductive and child health, HIV/AIDS, etc. bypassing the ARS completely. Karuna Trust is registered under Sect. 12A of the Income Tax Act, 1961 and obtained certificate of exemption under Sect. 80G on the Income Tax Act, 1961. It is also registered under the Foreign Contribution (Regulation) Act, 1976. The Financial Review Report of Karuna trust by Sri Dorabji Tata Trust (SDTT) for the period of February 2008 to January 2011 shows that the NGO received INR 106.5 lakhs. The audit report criticises Karuna Trust for financial lapses. In April 2009, an amount of INR 12 lakhs had been given as a loan by the NGO without prior permission from SDTT. Expenses unrelated to the project fund, such as travel to Andhra Pradesh, Orissa and Tamil Nadu were billed to SDTT as also the Bangalore headquarters office expenditure. There were also other 'unexplained' expenses for flight tickets, audit fees, salaries, drugs, etc. without production of bills or supporting documents. An amount of INR 85,000 had been made to the sister organisation of Karuna Trust called Vivekananda Girijana Kalyana Kendra (VGKK) for 'trainings' without any evidence of training and INR 94,433 for taxi costs. (Rozmin NA, 2011).

In December 2010, 286 inmates of the Beggars' Home, Bangalore died at the primary health centre run by Karuna Trust, with subsequent disappearance of several bodies raising serious concerns. The PHC had stocks of expired drugs and was managed by a doctor whose degree itself was in doubt. The death certificate of the inmates had been signed by the nurses and pharmacist and there was no correlation between the death records maintained by the PHC and those maintained by the administration. An inquiry report ordered for a detailed inquiry regarding unaccounted dead bodies to ascertain whether organs have been traded or dead bodies have been sold. This doubt arose because death certificates had been issued without any record in the PHC registers. (Chandrashekhar, 2010a and 2010b). In a letter published in *The Lancet*, a trustee described the PPP model of Karuna Trust and posed a question to experts whether "similar partnerships should be scaled-up to cover the country's entire health sector" (Karpagam et al., 2012: 1195). It was only when the failure to disclose conflict of interest was raised that the author acknowledged the 'lapse' that, she was in fact a trustee of the NGO (Ibid).

On September 16, 2014, the Department of Health and Family Welfare held Karuna Trust, responsible for the spread of dengue fever in some of the villages covered by the PHC in Chandrabanda village under the PPP model. The District Health and Family Welfare officer is reported to have stated that,

> The maintenance of Chandrabanda Primary Health Centre, which covers 20 villages, including Naganadoddi where two confirmed dengue deaths were recently reported, has been outsourced to Karuna Trust for 10 years, from 2006 to 2016. As per the terms and conditions, the government provided all the facilities and funds to the trust, including salaries for the staff and additional funds for implementing various health-related schemes. However, the trust has not fulfilled its obligations paving the way for the spread of deadly diseases such as dengue (Buradikatti, 2014: unpaged).

The Trust has, he added, received over INR 50 lakhs annually for the maintenance of the PHC. He said that he would submit a detailed report to the commissioner, Health and Family Welfare Services recommending the termination of outsourcing agreement from the next financial year. (Ibid.).

A visit was made in 2014, by a team of researchers from Karnataka Jana Arogya Chaluvali to the PHC Hudem in Karnataka which is under the PPP project of the Karuna Trust and the Government of Karnataka. On arrival, at 11.30 am, 10–12 patients were waiting in the Out Patient Department (OPD), but the doctor had not yet arrived and the pharmacy and lab were locked. One of the staff interviewed said that the doctor did not conduct any deliveries at the PHC and most of the cases were managed by the staff nurse. The doctor did not stay at the PHC but travelled up and down from the city 18 kms away. Staff who received salaries directly from the NRHM budget were paid on time, however, those receiving salaries through the NGO had not been paid for the previous 6–8 months. By the time the research team left at 12:30, the doctor had still not arrived and the pharmacy and lab were still shut.

A public hearing in VK Salgar, brought out critical failures in the PHC run by the Karuna Trust; poor quality of antenatal care leading to death of mother and infant, poor infrastructure, charging patients anywhere between INR 5,200–10,000 for deliveries, lack of basic amenities like drinking water and toilets, poor documentation and management of children with Severe Acute Malnutrition (SAM) (Mahila Mattu Makkala Hakkugala Samrakshna Vedike (MMMHSV) 2014).

It was only as late as January 6, 2016 that the Karuna Trust was asked by the Government of Karnataka to return all the PPP PHCs. On January 6, 2016, the government passed an order (HSP (3)/25/ 2015–16), doing away with the Arogya Bandhu Scheme, under which it had partnered with non-governmental organisations, charitable trust and private medical colleges to run two of its PHCs with financial assistance from the government. It decided to take the PHCs back that had been handed over to the Karuna Trust and other non- government organisations, charitable trusts and private medical colleges, following a series of complaints of non-compliance of rules, misuse of funds, lack of accountability, and failure to provide quality service to patients by the organisations running these PHCs. To quote the health minister "on evaluation, we have also found that there is no accountability, and some of the NGOs do not even have the required number of doctors and paramedical staff. The NGOs have employed AYUSH doctors and untrained nurses in some PHCs." (Yasmeen, 2016: Unpaged).

Following the decision of the GoK to scrap the Arogya Bandhu PPP scheme, a public hearing was held at the Karuna Trust run PHC in VK Salgar in Aland taluk of Kalburgi district with the district administration. Indubai shared how her daughter had lost her first born baby two weeks ago due to delay in referring her to the general hospital, following which there was a discussion on how the PHC had failed to pick up high risk pregnancies even in the past. The Taluk Health Officer (THO) said all neonatal deaths will be audited and remedial actions undertaken immediately. People demanded that the audit report and action taken report be made public. Complaints were made about PHC staff that was collecting money for conducting deliveries. In spite of repeated complaints to the management, there was no running water in the facility and women had been bringing water from homes for drinking and cleaning up after delivery. The Zilla Panchayat of the area had sanctioned money to the Karuna Trust for a bore-well; however there was no information on what the funds had been used for. Antenatal women were regularly referred to private labs for abdominal and pelvic scans. There was no ambulance facility in the hospital.

Discussion

It has become a trend in India to talk about 'evidence-based policy'. It is not at all infrequent for one or two 'models' to be projected as a basis for large-scale implementation. The RGSSH at Raichur is projected as a model of privately managed tertiary care services while the Karuna model is projected as a model of NGO managed primary healthcare. The PC has made no effort to present any supporting evidence in favour of these two models. Neither has it taken into consideration the evidence against these kinds of models.

Over the last few years, PPP has been at the centre of debates on health service delivery. On the one hand, they have been aggressively supported by international organisations, bilateral/multilateral institutions, financial institutions and national bodies. (Deloitte and AIMA 2012; Price Waterhouse Coopers and ICC, 2012), on the other hand, it is argued that there are better and safer alternatives if we are serious about the protection, respect, facilitation and fulfilment of people's fundamental right to the highest attainable standard of health (Richter, 2004).

Concerns regarding such partnerships have been expressed as early as in 1994, by Bennet, who has argued that these partnerships are related to the use of illegitimate or unethical means to maximise profit, lower concern towards public health goals, lack of interest in sharing clinical information, creating brain drain among public sector health staff, and lack of regulatory control over their practices. In spite of an array of regulatory and incentive setting structures, with basic legislation for regulation, most developing countries have difficulty in enforcing such controls (Bennet, 1994). In India, although much is talked about evidence-based policy, except for the initial period of planning where Nehru and Mahalanobis attempted to introduce the rationale of welfare into a scientific methodology in planning (as reflected in the Second Five

Year Plan), rational planning for welfare has become a victim of neoliberal market ideology (Qadeer, 2008).

The National Coordination Committee(NCC) of the Jan Swasthya Abhiyan (JSA) in their booklet on *Health System in India: Crisis and Alternatives* give an example of the Indraprastha Apollo Hospital, New Delhi which is a PPP and the fourth largest corporate owned hospital in the world, constructed at a cost of $ 44 million in 1996 on 15 acres prime land worth an estimated $ 2.5 million given by the Delhi government free of cost (at a token lease rent of one rupee per annum). Apart from this, the Delhi government invested $ 3.4 million in construction of the hospital and contributed $ 5.22 million as equity capital apart from tax and duty waivers. In lieu of this public subsidy, the agreement was that treatment for one-third of the beds would be made available free of cost to poor patients (JSA, 2006). The Justice Qureshi Committee, which reviewed the working of 27 private hospitals in Delhi including Indraprastha Apollo, found that this hospital provided free in-patient care to only two percent of its patients. The Committee was of the view that these corporate partnerships use the tag of 'efficiency' as a promotional strategy and for pushing technology and prices. The Report of NCC of JSA further indicated that only two percent of indoor cases in 1999–2000 in Apollo Hospital were treated free and most of these were relatives of staff, bureaucrats and politicians. There are at least 500 such hospitals across the country and the public subsidy at stake would be in the range of at least ten thousand crore rupees. (Ibid.). Also, the term 'poor' and free treatment have not been clearly defined making it easy for institutions to get away with restrictive definitions according to their convenience. In fact, despite being a high level committee set up by the Government of the National Capital Territory, this Report itself was never tabled by the Delhi Government (Kumar, 2009; Qadeer & Reddy, 2010).

The Qureshi Committee Report states that the existing free treatment facilities extended by charitable and other hospitals who have been allotted land on concessional terms/rates are inadequate, erratic and far from what was desired. There are 500 such hospitals in the country and the public subsidy at stake is in the range of at least INR 10,000 crore (High Court of Delhi, 2009; Kumar, 2009). In fact this very chain of the Apollo Hospitals Enterprises Ltd was invited to help manage the RGSSH, in Raichur Karnataka.

The GoK evaluation of the RGSSH had identified sub-optimal utilisation of beds, poor cash flow management, incorrect and unrealistic assumptions for designing the revenue model, weak management and weak monitoring of the RGSSH. Although the report had raised concerns about the operation, management, coverage (population and service), quality, cost-effectiveness and risk management by this model of PPP, the GoK still went ahead and brought out a PPP policy for the state and guidelines on implementation. This PPP policy of Karnataka makes no mention of the roles, duties and obligations of the private player. Instead the government commits to provide all the essential state level clearances to enable implementation of PPP and to formulate specific policies for coordination with the Infrastructure Development Department (IDD) and other government agencies involved in PPP implementation and also to set up suitable mechanisms for facilitating efficient acquisition of land for such projects (KSHSRC & Deloitte, 2012).

The evaluation report had also suggested that the MoU should not be renewed and the super-specialty hospital be handed back to the government. This concern has been further strengthened by a community-led protest against Apollo Hospital managing the tertiary hospital. Following the community pressure, the hospital has been handed back to the Government of Karnataka and the MoU with Apollo has been terminated.

Many of the lapses highlighted by the evaluation report are serious and would be even more disastrous if implemented on a large scale at a nationwide level as envisaged in the Twelfth Five Year Plan. The fact that evaluation reports prepared by the government itself are being ignored and false gains are being projected by the PC only adds to the puzzle. It is possible that promotion of the PPP model holds more importance for policy makers than the objective use of evidence.

With regard to the Karuna Trust also, there has been growing evidence that all is not well. However there has been absolutely no oversight of the functioning of the PHCs under the Trust despite reports of serious violations. There has been no independent evaluation of the performance of Karuna Trust and yet it has been promoted as a model of PPP for primary healthcare. There have been several objections to this model of PPP in Karnataka by activists and community groups. The media in Karnataka has highlighted several instances of violation, denial of care and negligence by Karuna Trust run PHCs. The trust currently 'manages' 80 PHCs in 7 states and has mobilised huge amounts of funds and other resources from the state and central government, Indian and international donors. Though there have been complaints of financial irregularity and poor service delivery by the NGO, however they continue to be promoted in several fora.

The role of the Arogya Raksha Samiti has been completely underplayed by Karuna Trust with itself becoming the receiver of all funds in the name of donations for PHC. This is in complete violation of the PPP agreement.

What the two examples illustrate is, the way principles of 'evidence- based policy-making' are violated. The nature of what constitutes 'evidence' is itself either suspect or distorted and claims of being 'people- centric' or 'patient-centric' are merely window dressings, used to hide policies that are anti-poor.

The official promotion of PPP-based model like the RGSSH or contracting out to non- governmental institutions like Karuna Trust as models of tertiary and primary level care respectively are now being projected as the only way forward for healthcare in the country. The absence of any serious effort to generate independent and objective evidence within the policy framework is a matter of concern. It raises issues about the very nature of planning which is becoming a highly subjective and biased process in favour of private partners. It is evident that critical evidence provided by the state's evaluation report has not informed the decision of the erstwhile PC or the newly constituted National Institute for Transforming India (NITI) Aayog. It is important for policy makers who are, in principle, responsible for the rich as well as the poor of the country to understand what is meant by 'evidence' and, take a good and hard look at the quality of evidence to ensure that they make informed choices while planning for health. Till then, the motives of the policy makers in pushing for these models of tertiary healthcare will remain unconvincing.

Notes

1. The Karnataka Rajya Raitha Sangha is a farmers' movement that is fighting the sale of seeds by multinational companies such as Monsanto.

References

Bennett, S., Dakpallah, G., Garner, P., Gilson, L., Nittayaramphong, S., Zurita, B., & Zwi, A. (1994). Carrot and stick: State mechanisms to influence private provider behavior. *Health Policy and Planning, 9*(1), 1–13.

Buradikatti, K. (2013a). "Is OPEC Hospital Being Reopened to Save RIMS?." *The Hindu*, August 4. Accessed January 29, 2017. http://www.thehindu.com/todays-paper/tp-national/tp-karnataka/is-opec-hospital-being-reopened-to-save-rims/article 4987831.ece.

Buradikatti, K. (2013b). "A Super-speciality Hospital Lies in Coma." *The Hindu,* Raichur, June 10. Accessed January 29, 2017. http://www.thehindu.com/news/national/karnataka/a-superspeciality-hospital-lies-in-coma/article4797818.ece.

Buradikatti, K. (2014). "Karuna Trust Failed to Check Spread of Dengue in Raichur Villages." *The Hindu.* Raichur, September 16. Accessed January 29, 2017. http://www.thehindu.com/todays-paper/karuna-trust-failed-to-check-spread-of-dengue-in-raichur-villages-official/article6414261.ece.

Chandrashekhar, N. (2010b). "When a rehab centre turned into a house of horrors" *Deccan Herald*, December 27.

Chandrashekhar, N. (2010a). "Doc signed death certificate indiscriminately: A report." *Deccan Herald*, October 15.

Deloitte and All India Management Association (AIMA). (2012). "Innovative and Sustainable Healthcare Management: Strategies for Growth." August. (Conference background note). Accessed January 29, 2017. https://www2.deloitte.com/content/dam/Deloitte/in/Documents/life-sciences-healthcare/in-lshc-innovative-healthcare-noexp.pdf.

Government of India. (2013). *12th Five Year Plan 2012–2017, Social Sector, Volume III,* Planning Commission of India. New Delhi, Sage Publications.

Government of Karnataka. (2008). "Prototype MOU for Private Public Parternship Between State and Not For Profit Organisations, Scheme for Involving Not for Profit Agencies in the Management of Secondary (Community Health Centres) and Primary Healthcare Facilities (Primary Health Centres and Sub Centres)".

Government of Karnataka. (2011). "Rajiv Gandhi Super Specialty Hospital, Raichur: Review of PPP Project." Department of Health and Family Welfare in Collaboration with Karnataka State Health System Resource Centre (KSHSRC). (obtained through RTI application to Health Commissioner).

High Court of Delhi. (2009). "All India Lawyers Union vs Government of NCT of Delhi and Others." September 26. Accessed October 12, 2012. http://www.indiankanoon.org/doc/1508125.

Jan Swasthya Abhiyan National Co-ordination Committee Report. (2006). "Health system in India: Crisis and alternatives." *Towards the National Health Assembly II Booklet* 31–32 (October): 2. New Delhi, National Co- ordination Committee, Jan Swasthya Abhiyan.

Karpagam S., Premdas, E., Vasan, A., Dabade, G., Kilaru, A., & Bheemappa, O.B. (2012). "Failure to disclose conflict of interest", Letter to the Editor. *The Lancet*, 379(9822): 1195–96. March 13.

KSHSRC and Deloitte. (2012). PPP Health Policy for Karnataka: Collaborative Study between State Health Resource Centre (SHSRC), Karnataka and Deloitte, India. Circular Issued by the Government of Karnataka.

Kumar, P. (2009). "Apollo fined Rs 2 lakh for not treating poor patients." *India Today*, September 23.

Mahila Mattu Makkala Hakkugala Samrakshana Vedike. (2014). *Report of the Public Hearing Held at the Village VK Salgar, Aland Taluk, Kalaburgi District*. December 30. Unpublished Report (Available on request).

Price Waterhouse Coopers and Indian Chamber of Commerce. (2012). *Healthcare Infrastructure and Financing Services in India: Operations and Challenges.* Accessed January 29, 2017. https://www.pwc.in/assets/pdfs/publications-2012/healthcare_financing_report_print.pdf.

Qadeer, I., & Sunita, R. (2010). "Medical care in the shadow of public private partnership." *Social Scientist* 34, 9/10(September–October), 4–20.

Qadeer, I. (2008). "Health planning in India: Some lessons from the past." *Social Scientist* 36, 5–6(May-June), 51–75.

Richter, J. (2004). "Public–private partnerships for health: A trend with no alternatives?" . *Development 47, 2*(April), 43–48.

Rozmin, N. A. (2011). "Financial review report of karuna trust: Implementing primary healthcare through public private partnership in the states of karnataka and arunachal pradesh." Sri Dorabji Tata Trust.

Staff Correspondent. (2012). "Bandh in Raichur Total, Peaceful." *The Hindu*, June 19. Accessed January 29, 2017. http://www.thehindu.com/todays-paper/tp-national/tp-karnataka/bandh-in-raichur-total-peaceful/ article3545007.ece.

TV9. (2013). "Problem of OPEC Hospital in Raichur." June 6. News Report in Kannada. Accessed January 28, 2017. https://www.youtube.com/watch?v=f2pQsHPiEyA.

Yasmeen, A. (2016). "PPP in Public Health Suffers Setback." *The Hindu*, February 18. Accessed January 28, 2017. http://www.thehindu.com/news/national/karnataka/ppp-in-public-health-suffers-setback/article8253276.ece.

Chapter 7
Role of Public Private Partnerships in Ensuring Universal Healthcare for India

Bijoya Roy

In the early 1990s Health Sector Reforms (HSR) undertaken as part of structural adjustment programmes proposed a range of changes in governance, provisioning, financing and resource generation. In India, these reforms contributed to shifts in structural, organisational and managerial aspects of the public sector healthcare system which has undergone complex organisational rearrangements (Bennett and Muraleedharan, 2000; Baru and Nandy, 2008). Public Private Partnerships (PPPs) are very much a part of these rearrangements. When, over a decade, the reforms actually increased catastrophic expenditures in the developing countries, the concept of Universal Health Coverage (UHC) and ways of achieving it was offered to rescue the HSR. India's National Health Policy (NHP) 2017 proposes to provide "universal access to good quality healthcare services without anyone having to face financial hardship as a consequence" (GoI, 2017: 1). Despite this new approach, the public health system continues to weaken, state investment in public sector health is stagnating, and the unregulated private sector in health has come to play a vital role in the provisioning of care. In this scenario, even to achieve UHC with efficiency and effectiveness seems an enormous task. Nevertheless, to attain it, PPP is seen as a viable health policy option both nationally as well as internationally. International bilateral and multilateral bodies, financial institutions and consulting companies have particular interest in it.

Introduction

Built on the foundations of New Public Management, PPPs have made inroads into the public health facilities at various levels, establishing a contractual relationship

B. Roy (✉)
Centre for Women's Development Studies, New Delhi, India

I. Qadeer et al. (eds.), *Universalising Healthcare in India*,
https://doi.org/10.1007/978-981-16-5872-3_7

between the public and private sectors; transforming the provisioning and financing pattern of institutions and initiating cultural shifts in the public health system.

PPPs are driven by the rationale of cost containment with increasing monetary efficiency in the delivery of services, and with a heavy dependence on the private sector for quality of care. A wide range of PPPs have evolved over the past two decades, expanded, got refined and gained permanence.

Prior to the 1990s the state directly procured and provided the majority of the healthcare and its supportive services. In the mid-1990s the nature of procuring and provisioning of non-clinical and clinical services changed, paving the way for contractual services. PPPs gradually became a public policy objective in India, blurring the boundaries between the two sectors and impacting people using the public health system. Emerging evidence from studies of types, implementation and functioning of PPPs is beginning to reveal their functioning, efficiency, political and economic significance and ability or otherwise to reach out to the marginalised, as well as their value for public money invested. This chapter explicates the process of embedding PPPs within the public policy in two phases and reviews the studies of PPPs in India's healthcare services over a period of two decades— 1995–2015. The first and second sections chart out their nature and scale of proliferation, and identify the policy milestones that promote PPPs. These policies are well thought out mechanisms for institutionalising PPPs and grounding them structurally and legislatively; they are not simple coping strategies. The third section of the chapter examines the evidence of their utility in terms of coverage, cost, quality, efficiency and the risks they introduce for the state. A discussion at the end looks at their role in achieving UHC.

Types of PPP and Structural Issues: 1995–2015

Like concessions in land acquisition, subsidies in imports to the private sector, and state led insurance systems, PPPs are also one of the institutional mechanisms to promote commercialisation of health services. During 1995–2015, the traditional public sector procurement and provisioning of services has seen alterations through PPPs that emerged in different forms, such as service contracts, management contracts, lease contracts, concessions and build-operate-transfer contracts. Across these forms of PPPs, a distinction needs to be made between those that provide services (non-clinical and clinical) within healthcare facilities or National Health Programmes[1]; those which operate and manage health facilities and services; and those where the private sector builds health infrastructure, manages and provides services. Table 7.1 lays out the types of PPP models in healthcare.

The evolution of these PPP models is based on the range of available Private Providers (PP). Each type, depending upon its complexity, has varying degrees of responsibilities for the public and private sectors. These models have 'created opportunities' for different types of PPs within the healthcare landscapes "which were once the preserve of public sector organisations" (Buse & Harmer, 2004: 50). Gradually,

Table 7.1 Function based models of PPP in India's health sector

Types of functions	Public and private responsibility	Examples
Outsourcing of supportive non-clinical services	Public Sector: Provides the space, pays for the contracted services Private Sector Provides the service, appoints the staff	Diet, security, cleanliness, solid waste management in healthcare facilities; Ambulance Service (108 Ambulance Service)
Outsourcing of Supportive clinical services	Public Sector: Provides the space, pays for the contracted services Private Sector: Provides the service, appoints the staff	Pathology and Radiology, Diagnostics within National Health Programmes (like sputum collection centres and also to act as microscopy and treatment centres within Revised National Tuberculosis Control Programme (RNTCP)
Outsourcing of clinical services	Public Sector: Provides the space, pays for the contracted services Private Sector: Provides the service, appoints the staff	Dialysis, Maternity Care Services (Institutional Birthing); Cataract surgeries under National Blindness Control Programme, Private Providers in RNTCP_DOTS
Purchasing of medical services	Public Sector: Calls for Tender and Empanels the Private Operators, Pays for the Contract Private Sector: Provides the Service	Central Government Health Services, ESIS, RSBY, Yeshasvini, Rajiv Arogyasri Scheme, Kalaignar; Voucher Schemes
Social franchisee	In which the developer of a successfully tested social concept (franchiser) enables others (franchisees) to replicate the model using the tested system and brand name to achieve a social benefit	Social marketing of condoms under Family Planning Programme
Operate and manage	Public Sector: Owns the healthcare facility, pays for the contracted services, regulates and monitors Private Sector: Manages the healthcare facility, provides the non-clinical and clinical services, appoints the staff	Primary healthcare facilities by NGOs (rural and urban), super speciality hospitals
Building, designing, operating and facility management (BOT/BOOT/ DBFOT)*	Public Sector: Provides land, finances Private sector: Designs, builds, finances, operates and transfers the healthcare facility	Diagnostic Centres, Hospitals (projects in pipeline)

*BOT (Build Operate and Transfer)/BOOT (Build, Own, Operate, and Transfer): BOT/BOOT is a PPP model to develop a public infrastructure project with private funding. DBFOT (Design, Build, Finance, Operate, and Transfer): These projects involve designing and building the infrastructure, operating them for a specific time period and transferring the ownership of the project to the government after a specific time frame, which runs normally between 10 and 30 years.

they are reconfiguring the national healthcare scenario through policy discourse and fast changing structures of public sector healthcare, and enabling the private sector "to exercise power and influence" (Ibid.: 50).

Our review shows that a wide range of PPs (for profit/not for profit; local/national/multinational corporates), are entering into partnership with the state for scaling up healthcare provisioning without the state expanding public services. It also reveals that local private nursing homes/hospitals participated in the PPP-based institutional delivery programmes, even when the scheme was not attractive. Under the Mamta Scheme in Delhi, around 45% of PPs became part of the scheme since it enabled them to develop collaboration with the state government and around one-third saw it as a means to expand business and acquire a certain credibility in the local market, even though it did not provide any financial incentive, and the release of funds was often delayed (Bhat et al., 2007; Nandan et al., 2010). Ancillary services like diet, security, sanitation also bring in non-health PPs. This creates a multiplication of authorities and loss of control of health facility staff.

Corporate companies too (national and multinational) are beginning to participate in the PPPs. For example, in the case of Rajiv Gandhi Super Speciality Hospital in Raichur district of Karnataka, Apollo Health Enterprise Limited from Hyderabad had an agreement with the Karnataka Health Department to operate and manage the Raichur government hospital and provide services. The state evaluation of this experiment was critical of its functioning (Karpagam et al., 2013). In Maharashtra and Punjab multinational corporate entities have joined hands with the respective state governments for operation and maintenance of radiological diagnostic services[2]. This trend raises concerns, as private partners often tend not to comply with the agreed terms and conditions and thus weaken administrative authority (Qadeer & Reddy, 2010).

This opening up of public institutions to markets through a plurality of private partners creates a diverse set of interest groups and restructures the relations of power and authority between the public and private sectors. PPPs, particularly in the field of supportive clinical services (i.e. hi-tech diagnostics), and curative care (dialysis) shows that public sector healthcare is now beginning to be linked to the medical-industrial complex and these two areas are good examples of high end markets. Given this it is doubtful if PPPs can safeguard the public sector's interests. This restructuring also leads to significant shifts in the financing of complex PPP models that have evolved over time and are discussed in later sections.

Policies Enabling PPP

Tracking polices in the health sector reveals that there are definite policies that enable PPPs to gain space and permanence in the health sector. These policies change the relationships and domains of influence of the state and the private sector, and favour the private sector by empowering it. They do so by encouraging involvement of different types of PPPs that have evolved with or without the support of international organisations, and, by setting up institutions and supportive legislative frameworks for enhancing PPPs. The evolution of these policies can be divided into two phases.

First Phase (1995–2005)

The Eighth Five Year Plan (1992–97) recommended targeting health for underprivileged within the strategy of 'Health for All' (HFA) and privatising services in the public sector through user charges (Government of India (GoI), 1994). It advocated the need to regulate the private sector, not out of necessity, but because the government wanted to promote the private sector (Ibid.). The Ninth Five Year Plan (1997–2002) reinforced the need for public sector healthcare institutions to generate revenue by charging supportive and diagnostic services and increasing 'the involvement of voluntary, private organisations and self-help groups in the provision of healthcare and ensure inter-sectoral coordination in implementation of health programmes and health-related activities' (GoI, n.d.). Thus, the 1990s marked a shift towards a new public and private mix whereby the public sector was sent on the path of being privatised from inside and outside. Initially the PPPs emerged through the outsourcing of first level referral services from the Primary Health Centres (PHCs) and of non-clinical and clinical support services in hospitals, national health programmes, and private management and operation of health facilities. This transition towards PPP could be traced in the government policies from the early 1990s, with the implementation of the State Health System Development Project II in the States of Karnataka, West Bengal, and Punjab in 1995 (World Bank (WB), 1996). Subsequently, the second National Health Policy, 2002 emphatically supported the private sector by recognising its increasing presence at all levels of care and how it needs to address the economic restructuring that is ongoing in the country through statutory regulation, and monitoring of minimum standards (GoI, 2002). The Tenth Five Year Plan emphasised the need to develop standard treatment protocols and to improve area-specific public- private-voluntary collaborations for the marginalised sections of the population (GoI, 2002a). At the same time, it cautioned about the success of NGO involvement at the primary healthcare level mainly due "to the commitment of individuals and credibility of NGOs, which is difficult to replicate" (Ibid.: 87).

The National Macro Economic Commission too, marked PPPs as one of the innovative ways to increase access to and delivery of comprehensive healthcare services caused by shortages of specialists, high end technology and ancillary services within the public system (GoI, 2005). Across all these recommendations policy makers adopted PPP as a solution to manage the problems within the public health sector but without adequately examining PPP's effectiveness. Within the health department, Regional Resource Centres were created and one of their activities was to provide technical support for the state level PPPs. West Bengal was the first state to draft a PPP policy[3] in the health sector, in 2004. It stated that,

> The Government of West Bengal will proactively engage with the Private Sector in Public Private Partnerships in Tertiary and Secondary Level of Healthcare, … and proper safety net for the poor, such engagements at Primary Level will be carefully decided and shall generally attempt at providing alternative modes of healthcare delivery in underserved, remote and difficult to reach areas (Government of West Bengal (GoWB), 2006: 4).

Second Phase (2006–2015)

The second phase is characterised by the expansion of PPPs through private investment and state financing for addressing infrastructure gaps (construction of public health facilities) in the health sector. The Planning Commission in its reappraisal report on PPP in healthcare recommended promoting PPPs in areas like infrastructure, health manpower, Information-Education-Communication (IEC), capacity building and managerial services besides service delivery and ways to make them cost-effective (GoI, 2006). The Report proposed partnerships with branded clinics (primary care units of corporate hospitals) and involvement of the corporate sector under Corporate Social Responsibility (CSR), through the Confederation of Indian Industry (CII) and Federation of Indian Chambers of Commerce and Industry (FICCI) and other industrial associations, for advocacy and funding NGOs (Ibid). It neither specifies the role of branded clinics for the unreached populations nor the use of CSR funds for strengthening public infrastructure.

Over the same period, the health committee of CII, in collaboration with International Finance Corporation and World Bank Institute worked to lay out areas for PPP interventions and their promotion. It prepared a white paper which primarily viewed PPPs as one of the most promising integrated initiatives in developing capital4 and infrastructure, wherein the private sector consortium designs, builds, finances, and provides the services (CII-HOSMAC, n.d.).

Creation of PPP Cells

For enabling and institutionalising PPPs across sectors, centre and state level policies, institutional mechanisms and legislations have been introduced. In 2006, a PPP cell was established under the Union Ministry of Finance. Creation of PPP cells within the public sector facilitated the framing of policies, technical assistance, capacity building and in the proliferation of PPPs across sectors. This was a turning point as these cells accelerated the process of setting up PPPs through managing tenders, drawing up MoUs, liaising between departments, etc. under the overall guidance of the state. Several PPP cells have already been set up in West Bengal, Haryana, Punjab, Andhra Pradesh, Karnataka, Assam, Rajasthan, Madhya Pradesh, Tamil Nadu, Gujarat, Orissa and Uttarakhand, within different departments including health. These cells would enable streamlining of PPP projects and deepen its penetration.

Infrastructure-Based PPP Projects

To use private finance in public service infrastructure, the government created financial intermediaries like the Infrastructure Finance Development Company (IFDC) (1997) and India Infrastructure Finance Company Limited (2006). In infrastructure projects the private sector raises the money on behalf of the government and in return the private sector is awarded with the contract to design, construct, maintain and operate during the concession period. The hospital bears the responsibility to pay back the debt along with the interest including the cost escalation if it takes place. This experience from UK shows that it creates an affordability gap. As a measure to keep such projects attractive for the private sector, the Indian government in 2006, issued guidelines for Viability Gap Funding (VGF). The gap in VGF is the difference between the revenue needed to make a project commercially viable and the revenue generated through user fees. Under this scheme the government funds maximum of 20% of the total project cost. However, the financing state department or the ministry can give assistance restricted to another 20% of the project cost.[5]

The Eleventh Plan proposed to grant 'private players' infrastructure status so that the private sector could participate in provisioning of public services through PPPs with access to various government incentives, subsidies and tax benefits. Thus, it legitimised private players' access to certain concessions like, "land at concessional rates, increasing floor area ratio and ground coverage, tax holiday, and loan at concessional rates" (GoI, 2008: 82). The draft National Health Bill, 2009 set the stage for PPPs by ensuring affordable 'coverage' of services to people. The state's role was restricted to providing this economic access to the very poor. For the rest, its role remains ambiguous. The Bill then is a legislative draft that, like the Five-Year Plans, avoids ensuring tax- based state provisioning of healthcare (GoI, 2009) and encourages private providers.

In PPP models like Build-Operate-Transfer/Design-Build-Operate—Transfer (BOT/DBFOT), long-term partnerships are envisaged with both sectors financing the project. These projects are sustained either through the user charges collected by the private partner or through the annual payment by the government over a period of time. Earlier in 2005, when the Cabinet Committee on Economic Affairs approved the VGF Scheme to support PPPs in infrastructure and identified health as one of the eligible sectors for financial assistance, there were no annuity provisions. The draft National PP Policy, 2011 then, addressing the need for PPPs across sectors, proposed internal restructuring and developing infrastructure through annuity-based PPP projects in sectors like health that are 'not amenable for sizeable cost recovery through user charges' (GoI, 2011). Annuity funding is another mechanism by which the government provides 40% of the project cost as loan during the construction period with a provision for deferred budgetary payment, i.e. the public sector pays when the asset is delivered, or pays in instalments during the different stages of construction (See Endnote 5). Over the multiple annual plan periods the government pays the charges (cost of the physical assets, operation and maintenance) of the sanctioned annuity projects. Such annuity projects have an impact on the future availability of resources for the new programmes and this, "may tend to increase the total cost to the exchequer" (GoI, 2010: 6). The Planning Commission (PC) expressed caution about this. Economists like Basu also cautioned against their detrimental impact on the public sector due to a long-term burden on future budgets (Economic Times, 2010).

Such health facility projects in India are at their initial stages. They generate three important concerns at this point. Firstly, infrastructure based PPPs complicate the contractual structure of organisation. Secondly, the government goes all the way to make such initiatives lucrative for the private sector and in the process, spends much higher overall amounts including the concessions granted to them. This also reflects misplaced and heavy reliance on the private sector. Finally, how much commercial benefit the private sector accrues through these long- term arrangements and concessions is barely disclosed, in the name of business confidentiality. The commercialisation of healthcare provisioning is thus guided by the need of the private sector and private capital. It is important here to learn from the UK where, despite subsidies and efforts to meet the affordability gap, annuity based Private Finance Initiative (PFI) hospitals remained underfunded and more expensive than the traditional procurement alternatives for hospital infrastructures. Consequently, many National Health Service (NHS) trusts working with long-term PFI initiatives faced financial problems (Hellowell & Pollock, 2009).

The Twelfth Five Year Plan, in the name of public spending in backward and remote areas, paucity of capital and sustaining growth, pushed further the need for private investment in infrastructure (GoI, 2013). Despite these risks, the NHP 2017 again underlines the need for purchasing services of private healthcare through contracting out and empanelling hospitals (GoI, 2017). These policies and processes push the private sector ahead but do not necessarily address the complexities and difficulties created for the public sector and the patients. PPPs claim to smoothen and reorient the structural and governance problems of public sector healthcare, but in whose interest, is left unsaid.

Evidence on Access, Quality and Processes of Implementation

PPPs are projected as designed to overcome the weaknesses of public sector health services (inefficiency, lack of coverage and access and poor quality) and work in coordination to improve them. They need to be evaluated for (i) access to their services; (ii) quality; and (iii) the processes at work, like complexity of PPs engaging in PPPs, their selection process, monitoring and regulation, and risks embedded for the public partner in the contracts. These processes are interrelated but discussed separately for convenience.

Access to PPP Services: PPP services could be for ambulatory or in- patient care and diagnostic facilities. Access to these facilities needs to be understood in physical, social and economic terms. Physical presence of providers, though necessary, is not always sufficient given caste and monetary constraints of those seeking care. The studies reviewed either do not explore all services or all the dimensions of access.

Geographical and Social Accessibility: As there is chronic shortage of functional health facilities, PPPs do bring immediate respite to the people in remote areas. Our review of literature shows that, for free services at the point of delivery through the PPP model, the specific target population groups are: pregnant women, new born children, or all irrespective of age and sex if they are from BPL families. Several studies report inability to provide free service to those with certified BPL certificates (Roy, 2007 and 2015). Often non-issuance of health insurance cards created difficulties for the patients to access free care at the point of service delivery (Jega, 2007; Karpagam et al., 2016; Nandi et al., 2016). Secondly, location and accreditation of PPs for PPP schemes was pertinent, especially in rural areas and urban slums and in remote areas. The researchers report that PPs near urban slums or in rural areas are not well trained or are mostly unqualified (Deshpande et al., 2004). Accreditation of private hospitals or nursing homes based on Janani Swasthya Yojana norms was not very encouraging in Bihar, Madhya Pradesh (MP), Orissa, Rajasthan and Uttar Pradesh. In MP, accredited hospitals were located in urban areas; and only two hospitals could be accredited in three districts out of five in Bihar (United Nations Population Fund (UNFPA) 2009). A review of PPPs for maternal health services across states shows that they did not increase physical access to services for rural women. Experiences of voucher schemes in Agra and Kanpur showed that very few PPs could be accredited, and were once again found to be concentrated in urban areas (Ravindran, 2011). Similarly, in the PPP-based maternity care services (MAMTA scheme, Delhi; Chiranjeevi Scheme, Gujarat and Janani Sahayogi Scheme, MP), the empanelled PPs were located in the economically better off districts and in the urban centres (Acharya & Mcnamee, 2009; Nandan et al., 2010 and 2008). In a study of Chiranjeevi Yojana (CY) in Surat, marginalised people found it difficult to access empanelled PPs located in developed areas (Acharya & Mcnamee, 2009). During the fifth year of its operation, in 40% of the talukas no empanelledPPs became part of this scheme. Secondly, even though the delivery per PP had increased, the number of empanelled PPs had declined. In 2008, under the extended CY, it failed to expand PP services in the 40 under- served talukas except in two districts (Government of Gujarat (GoG) 2010). Not only this, anaesthetists were available only on call since most of them lived in urban areas. They wanted money to attend such cases soon after the delivery and expressed their reluctance in attending to BPL cases (Jega, 2007). Janani Suraksha Yojana (JSY) experience in Madhya Pradesh shows that due to non-fulfilment of selection criteria, only 10% of rural PPs were empanelled and the majority of PPs included were in urban areas (Nandan et al., 2008). Lack of rural PPs limited people's access and coverage (Devaraj, 2006). Distant location of the PPs increased the cost of access for the poor in Amravati District of Maharashtra (Rathi et al., 2012). The state-level PPPs in insurance schemes are not concerned with needs, suffering or urgency for the patients as often their selection is based on their suitability for full intervention package rather than needs (Vasan et al., 2015).

In the Revised National Tuberculosis Control Programme (RNTCP) scaling up and sustaining of the PPP model has remained a challenge (Pradhan et al., 2011). The review showed that the case detection rates had increased with greater referrals to the public sector and the case notifications varied within a range of 2–26% (Dewan et al., 2006). However, in a PPP TB-DOTS project in Delhi, the majority of the patients referred by the PPs were from the middle class (Unger et al. 2010). Added issues reported were problems of neglecting standardised treatment, follow-ups and holding back information on the availability of free treatment from public institutions (Ibid.). Ramaiah and Gawde (2014) point to the fact that in urban areas where public sector healthcare is diminishing, the involvement of PPs in the detection of TB cases and referral plays, "a short-term measure to improve effectiveness of the TB Control Programme" (Ramaiah & Gawde, 2014: 370). Doctors in Bengal echoed similar ideas in the context of PPP-based diagnostic units, i.e. "the PPP units are only seen as a midway arrangement. Issues of equity and exclusion continue to persist" (Roy, 2015: 195).

The experience of contracting with NGOs for managing primary healthcare services and provisioning in tribal areas of Meghalaya showed an increase in OPD attendance. The problem however was of functioning in distant areas without the state support of regular funds, drugs and periodic monitoring (Mairembam et al., 2012).

Thus, even though it was assumed that PPP-based services will improve access and coverage, the accessibility of good qualified PPs to the poor and remote areas remains a problem.

Financial Accessibility: PPs partner with the public sector only when this is commercially viable. The user charge is linked to financial sustainability of the PPs. The PPPs charge the Above Poverty Level (APL) patients directly and the government pays for the BPL patients. Their user charges and exemption rules vary across the states and impact the poor differentially. For example, PPP diagnostic units in West Bengal government hospitals provided 10% of BPL patients' free diagnostic services per month (Roy, 2015), whereas in PPP diagnostic units of Bihar, both, APL and BPL patients were entitled to free care (Kumar, 2013). In the urban slum health project of Andhra Pradesh and Assam, managing NGOs were allowed to levy user charges in order to raise 20% of their recurring expenditure for their sustainability while keeping in mind positive discrimination. However, to make this project sustainable, continuation of the government grant- in-aid to NGOs remained critical (Raman & Bjorkman, 2006). In recent times the pre-feasibility report for the PPP-based MRI in Karnataka recommended revising the user charges every two years (Information and Crediting Rating Agency in India (ICRA), 2013). In the public sector tertiary and secondary hospitals of many states, Computer Tomography (CT) Scan and Magnetic Resonance Imaging (MRI) and other diagnostic facilities, provided under the PPP scheme, are either priced at par with the Central Government Health Services (CGHS) rate or priced lower than the market rates in consultation with the government.

Table 7.2 CT scan at the PPP unit in tertiary hospital (TH), Kolkata (2004 and 2011)

CT scan at the PPP	(A)	Percentage of waiver cases given to patients**				(B)	(C)	Total No. of patients doing
Unit in TH Years		100%	75%	50%	25%			CT scan A+B+C
2004[a]	11062 (86.85%)	n.a	n.a	n.a	n.a	1211 (9.50%)	464	12737
2011[b]	16254 (81.45%)	82	36	1982	1257	3357 (16.82%)	343	19954

Source: [a]Roy 2007; [b]Medical College Kolkata 2012. A: *Total No. of Government Patients doing CT Scan*

B: Total No. of patients doing CT Scan receiving Waiver C: Total no. of Private patients# doing CT Scan

*Cases where patient paid government rate; **Patients who received exemptions; # Patients who paid at market rates

All BPL patients availing CT scan services in the Tertiary Hospital in Kolkata did not get 100% exemption (Table 7.2). Though the share of free cases had increased over the past six years, maximum patients received only 50% concession on the actual price and very few got 100% exemption for the CT scan. Empanelled PPs for diagnostic services in rural hospitals revealed that patients requested for further concessions on the subsidised price and also requested PPs to accept the payment in instalments (Roy & Gupta, 2011). Empanelled PPs of the rural hospital of Islampur, Murshidabad accepted this practice in order to sustain the contract (Ibid.). In a PPP-based diagnostic service in Bihar, only 19 diagnostic tests could be provided free of cost to the patients referred by government healthcare institutions; the rest were charged the market rate (Kumar, 2013). Most of the patients were not aware of the cap and consequently they ended up paying. Complaints regarding extra charge by the technicians were common (Ibid.).

In addition to variations even the out-of-pocket expenditures remained high in PPPs. Under the Mamta Scheme in Delhi for antenatal checkups, three-fourths of the women had to incur the cost for Ultra Sonography (INR 750), other tests and medicines (INR 1028) and, in case of more than one postnatal check-up, the empanelled providers levied further charges (Nandan et al., 2010). Similarly, under the JSY in Madhya Pradesh, around 45% of the PPs levied user charges. These charges were higher in the districts of Indore, Jabalpur and Chhindwada (Nandan et al., 2008). Among the 100 beneficiaries only 3 reported to have availed free-of-cost maternity care services and only one tenth of them received pre-decided cash assistance for maternity care services. Out of the 32 PPs only 6 provided free OPD service to the expecting BPL women. Under the Chiranjeevi Scheme in Gujarat, empanelled PPs did not reimburse transportation charges to the beneficiaries even when it was a part of the policy (GoG, 2010). Similar Out-of-Pocket Expenditures (OOPE) were also reported in cases of deliveries through Caesarean sections in JSY PPP scheme

(Chaturvedi & Randive, 2011). Women said that the subsidy of INR 1,500 was inadequate to meet the costs of institutional births. They had to take private loans at a very high rate of interest or mortgage property (Ibid.).

Thus, it is observed that even when a PPP service aims to provide free service to the BPL patients, the problem of either indirect or partial out-of-pocket expenditure persists. Secondly, the policy of capping the number of patients who can access free services (clinical or investigative), or the limits to the number of free tests, restricts the access to free medical care and adds to the burden of cost. This stands in opposition to the principle of universal access to healthcare.

Quality of Care

The government favours the PPP over the public system under the assumption that it brings in efficiency and quality of care. The experience of Reproductive and Child Health (RCH) services through the Mother- NGO scheme revealed that the NGOs often did not have full-time personnel for the health activities and the new workload was added on to existing personnel (Bhat et al., 2007). Similarly, in Meghalaya in NGO managed PHCs, despite the availability of staff there was a lack of skilled providers (Mairembam et al., 2012). PPPs try to bring about efficiency by cutting on budget allocations on staff. Even though the ancillary contracts in hospitals specify payment of minimum wages, in practice contractual staff is under-waged with poor working conditions (Roy, 2010). The high-end diagnostic PPP units in district hospitals of West Bengal had minimum staff with poor wages and full-time radiologists were not appointed (Roy, 2015). In Bihar, the private provider could not be empanelled under JSY due to poor infrastructure facilities and the lure of unregulated Caesarean operations in the market (UNFPA, 2009). In PPP-based institutional delivery schemes, empanelled private nursing homes were not equipped to deal with emergency obstetric cases owing to lack of a blood bank facility and anaesthetists (Mohanan et al., 2014; GoI, 2008 and 2014). Likewise, JSY for Emergency Obstetric Care (EmOC) in Maharashtra among the 34 private facilities studied, showed that 10 did not have operation theatres (Randive et al., 2012). These evidences show that PPPs are plagued with problems of human resources and infrastructure that impacts the quality of care. Meal services, laundry and cleanliness play a critical role in rendering good quality of care for in-patients and out-patients both in hospitals and primary healthcare settings. There are studies to show that contracting out brings down the quality in several instances (Bhatia & Mills, 1997; Roy, 2010). The fourth and eighth National Rural Health Mission (NRHM) Common Review Meeting Report (CRM) found grossly inadequate resources for outsourced services like diet, sanitation and security and the need to improve the poor levels of these services in the government hospitals of different states excluding Kerala (GoI, 2010a, 2014). Selected PPs tended to establish collection centres6 for collecting blood/urine samples rather than diagnostic centres in rural public hospitals under the district hospital of Murshidabad (Roy & Gupta, 2011) and Bihar (Kumar, 2013; GoI, 2014). These arrangements influence the quality of tests carried out in terms of 'prolonged turn-around time and reporting time' (GoI, 2012).

The evidence reviewed shows that the involvement of PPs does not necessarily improve quality of services and care. PPPs from different states still reported lack of adequately skilled personnel, poor working conditions, along with poor maintenance.

Processes of PPP Implementation

The MoUs vary with the type of provider, complexity of services contracted out and their numbers. Also, there is a range of common operational issues that we take up in this section.

Selection of PPs and Implementation: There are a few studies that focus on the selection process of PPs. Local level process of selecting PPs for some of the PPP-based healthcare services show that it is not always based on competitive tendering (Roy, 2007). At the district level for JSY in Maharashtra, the relations of medical superintendents with the private specialists determined the awarding of contracts to PPs (Randive et al., 2012). Similarly, political connections played a role in the selection of PPs in UP while contracting NGOs for the management of primary health facilities (Heard et al., 2011). Thus, a level of arbitrariness enters the selection process and influences the efficiency of PPPs.

In the working of service-based PPPs, the roles of the partners are often not well defined. Lack of trust, blaming each other and clash of interests, delayed payment is perennial across different PPP experiences (Devaraj, 2006; Kumar, 2013). Thus, in Ahmednagar district of Maharashtra, neither the district level government health officials nor the private doctors wanted to own the scheme for EmOC in JSY through PPPs. Records of MOUs could not be traced (Chaturvedi & Randive, 2011). Implementation of this programme varied across blocks and was mostly limited to Caesarean sections. There was no referral protocol and patients could go to any of the available PPs (Ibid.). Likewise, in PPP-based diagnostic services in West Bengal, information on exemption rules were not displayed by public institutions nor did the PPs provide this information to the poor patients. To meet their revenue targets, they targeted patients and even contacted the nearby private practitioners (Roy, 2015). The study of the Global Health Initiative on HIV in India showed that when Treatment Counselling Centres (TCC) were revived in 2009 the state medical officers viewed it as a duplication of Antiretroviral Therapy (ART) centres and cumbersome for poor patients. TCC staff too had problems with state provisioning and, in order to meet their patient targets, they began poaching (Kapilshrami & McPake, 2012). Internal conflicts between the civil society and government operated services can negatively impact patient counselling, follow-up and continuity of care as in the case of Global Health Initiative on HIV in India (Ibid.). Partnerships thus demonstrate internal tensions with hierarchical arrangements.

Monitoring and Regulation: There is a constant conflict between what is endeavoured through the PPPs (public health goals) and the actual output. PPPs range from simple to complex contracts. Even in simple contracts like in PPP diagnostic units at the secondary level hospitals in West Bengal patient utilisation records were not well maintained (Roy, 2015). Similarly, the experience of PPP in TB control in Ujjain showed that urban doctors viewed record keeping and tracking default cases as 'unrewarding' (De Costa et al., 2008). The complex contracts make the operationalisation and management very critical. From the government's point of view, the nature of engagement goes beyond just implementing and administering the PPPs. Evidence shows limited preparedness in implementing and handling PPP operations by the government (Bagal, 2008; Heard et al., 2011; Kumar, 2013; Sarma, 2006). Government officials face multiple managerial challenges (of quality control and monitoring) in dealing with a wide range of PPs operating at different levels with diverse efficiency and quality. For example, in the Mother NGO scheme there were NGOs not only at different levels of efficiency and quality but with differing nature of agreements. This required differential monitoring and evaluation at each level and made the process complex (Bhat 2007). Periodic monitoring and evaluation of the empaneled PPs during the annual renewal of contracts are important as there is laxity in this process as well (Roy, 2007).

Also, the analysis of terms and conditions of contracts show that performance and outcome indicators for different kinds of PPP are not always built-in. In the Uttar Pradesh Health Systems Development Project's call for tender specifications, the staff and infrastructure requirements that a selected NGO should provide were not clearly defined (Heard et al., 2011). Regular in-house monitoring of the ongoing PPP and outsourced services were found to be weak in the public sector hospitals as they did not have adequate personnel (Roy, 2007 and 2015; Kumar, 2013; Randive et al., 2012). These PPP-related structures overstretch government's stewardship abilities.

Risks: The underlying assumption of PPP policy is inefficiency of the public sector and efficiency of PPPs. Procedurally, PPP contracts are expected to draw up possible risks at different stages of a contract's life cycle. Risks often emerge when the PP declines to undertake the agreed role by shifting the responsibility to the public sector or when the starting of services is delayed. Round 4 of the Global Fund to Fight AIDS, Tuberculosis and Malaria (GFATM) fund grant for HIV and AIDS is an example where, despite the partnership with the corporate sector, it declined to shoulder the establishment cost and forced the state to renegotiate for funding of drugs and laboratory reagents (Kapilshrami & McPake, 2012). Similarly, there were delays in meeting targets like when the corporate sector did not establish the promised number of ART centres and was not inclined to provide care to the patients in an advanced stage (Ibid.). Thus, the experience of the contractual relationship shows that it operates within a certain level of uncertainty, i.e. not always predictable, and its operation is at risk.

One risk commonly faced by the public sector is a lawsuit between the partners. This particularly interferes with the call for new tenders after the completion of the contract period. As long as the matter remains sub-judice, the old contract continues and the long drawn process impedes the administrative functioning and quality of service (Roy, 2007). The scope of risk is high in complex multiple operational contracts. Such an inherent risk questions the very logic of efficiency through the private sector in PPPs.

Several states have opted for the BOT/DBFOT model of hospital projects such as Punjab, Maharashtra and Meghalaya, expecting that through these models' large-scale infrastructure projects will be delivered on time and prevent cost overruns. Presently in Meghalaya the state government, through external agency International Finance Corporation (IFC) financing, is setting up Shillong Medical College and Hospital with Kali Prasad Chowdhury Medical College and Hospital (KPMCH) based on a '99 year concession' wherein the private sector builds and operates the institution (International Finance Corporation (IFC, 2013). The state government provided land (23.8 acres) for the project, a 40% capital subsidy for the construction phase, and an operational subsidy for the first 12 years of operations (Ibid). Added to this the private sector protects itself from risk by fixing a higher price at the competitive bidding stage and thus the government loans are used to 'sustain and subsidise' PPPs. Construction of this tertiary hospital is unlikely to meet the 2017 deadline. In such delays, the state, besides bearing a large proportion of the financial risk, may also end up paying more as the costs of construction go up. Finally, the government cannot pull itself out of these partnerships because of the complicated procurement system.

This evidence indicates that the public sector faces higher risks from the PPP MoUs, defeating the purpose of PPP policy to save immediate capital expenses for the government and transfer risk from the public to the private sector, and thereby secure better managed and lower cost of services (Froud, 2003). Such a policy remains a myth and needs to be challenged, as Froud rightly does.

Discussion and Conclusion

The emergence of PPPs in healthcare has allowed a foothold to the private sector within the public sector healthcare system. Focused policy shifts in its favour give it greater power over the public sector healthcare services leading to their gradual commercialisation. Evidence shows that PPP has by itself done little to remove inefficiencies and improve quality of the public institutions. It has in fact forced them 'to change their own practices' in its mirror image. As of now, the PPP process is characterised by poor management, monitoring and regulatory mechanisms. Yet, this development alone is not a factor in the decline of public institutions.

Other than resource crunch, there are historical factors rooted in the socio-political structure of public sector health service infrastructure in India that also contributed. Permitting the doctors in the government hospitals to do private practice was one of them that led to creeping corruption. Lack of regulatory legislation and monitoring mechanisms for minimum standards added to the decline of government hospitals over time. Public sector hospitals also bore the impact of caste and class based familial associatons between doctors of public hospitals and private clinics and hospitals owned by their relatives. Caste class hierarchy was also retained within health care workforce in the hospitals. The policies of downsizing and casualization with HSRs primarily influenced the middle and lower strata of workforce ranging from nurses to sanitary workers who came mostly from the lower social classes. These together resulted in inequities, malpractices that impacted the quality of care and work ethics.

The so-called 'Reforms' in the mid-nineties were implemented without recognising the systemic and organizational issues in the public sector. The narrow perspective of HSR leading to resource crunch, imposition of new public management model and, penetration by private capital changed the very nature of public hospitals. The means to 'Reforms' in the public sector hospitals was through permitting market-like behavior and competition among multiple providers. This altered the very ethos, and values within the working of institutions and altered the perspective of doctors (Baru, 2005). There was little policy discussion about how public sector hospitals in low-middle income countries like India can be oriented to meet the health care and the financial needs of the infrastructure and become sustainable in the long term. Strengthening of public sector hospitals found little space in these debates. Consistently, it has been implied that public sector secondary and tertiary level hospitals being weak, provisioning at this level can be left to the private sector with the state providing primary health care in developing countries. This weakened the public hospital system.

The first phase of PPPs showed that the public sector institutions in all three levels of care were facing greater pressure to govern and manage the 'new models of provisioning' which unleashed changes within the social, financial and power relations of the public sector healthcare system. It introduced monetary values and reduced service- based values of providers and changed the class background of users (Baru, 2005). While institutionalising these practices, PPPs have replaced the old direct system of provisioning by a unified structure, with a much more complex, layered, and yet fragmented organisational structure. This demands perhaps greater administrative attention than the previous public health system. In the second phase complications increased in long-term infrastructure PPP projects operated through a large number of contracts and sub- contracts. This asked for huge administrative and managerial investment. Therefore, a weak public healthcare system with declining expenditure was put under additional pressure to ensure that the private sector remained accountable.

We have seen that PPPs, across different levels of healthcare, focus on curative care and those components of it where there is the possibility of maximising profits. Being selective in approach and with their need to meet the affordability gap in long-term healthcare infrastructure projects, PPPs reinforce medical dominance and fragmentation of patient care. This drastically impacts continuum of care as well as its quality. Furthermore, this ongoing expansionary project of PPP focuses on well-endowed regions, neglecting remote areas and marginalised populations.

With budget constraints in low-middle income countries like India, the evolution of PPP from meeting incremental service gaps to healthcare infrastructural gaps necessitates a look at the importance of capital investment. This determines the access, cost, quality and planning of healthcare. Already, along with changes through

PPPs, reforms in financing healthcare are in progress. This is reflected in the NHP 2017 that recommends a shift from "input oriented to an output based strategic purchasing" (GoI, 2017: 7). This is best suited for acute care and focuses on funding healthcare institutions based on volume of activity, such as the number of surgeries done. Evidence from Canada shows that the output/activity based funding could not reduce administrative costs in hospitals; there was mixed evidence of efficiency gains; and led to treating "high-volume, low-risk patients over higher- needs, less predictable patients" (Cohen et al., 2012: 7). Thus, with the growing fragmentation in the production of services, the healthcare planning process recedes further into the institutional framework. This makes it easy for it to be gradually taken over by the market through financial performance, incentives and rationing of care in the name of efficiency.

Despite the popularity of the PPPs at the policy level, its advantage has been questioned in recent time in different states. Civil society organisations like Jan Swasthya Abhiyan (JSA), Karnataka Jana Arogya Challuvalli have resisted PPPs in healthcare and taken the issue to the public. In Chattisgarh, the PPP initiative for diagnostic services in 379 health facilities was cancelled in 2013, followed by the cancellation of the mobile medical units where doctors and technical staff complained of non-payment of salaries and non-availability of essential medicines (Bagchi, 2013). JSA also questioned the need to replace the existing diagnostic services in these health facilities with PPP arrangements. Recently, in Karnataka the health department closed down the Arogya Bandhu Scheme under which the private sector was empanelled to manage and operate 52 primary health centres, and brought it back under its direct administration and management (Yasmeen, 2016). This happened due to non-compliance of the terms and conditions by the private sector. As of now the resistance movement has been able to shut down initiatives like the Rajiv Gandhi Super Speciality Hospital, Raichur contracted out to Apollo Healthcare Limited.

At this juncture, it is important to recognise that the challenge of genuine reform of the public sector health services and its universalisation continues and requires a critical look at the shrinking space of public sector hospitals in the name of inefficiency. Shifting the role of the state from providers to purchasers of services needs to be examined. The state level initiatives (Tamil Nadu, Rajasthan, Kerala, Orissa), like provisioning of free medicine that can work if strengthened, maintaining high standards of efficiency, quality and accountability in the public systems (Tamil Nadu Medical Services Corporation Ltd. and Rajasthan Medical Services Corporation). Studies show increase in footfall in the public healthcare institutions with increased availability of essential medicines. This has come through the efficient procurement, stocking and delivery of medicines (WHO, 2014). Direct public provisioning of services does matter to the people. Critical evaluation of ongoing service-based PPPs and infrastructure-based PPPs question their claims of creating an evidence base of efficiency, value for money, and quality. The resistance by people's movements and the evidence from studies of PPPs challenge the assumptions about their efficiency and utility and show that PPPs are an unreliable means to achieve UHC.

Notes

1. Many of the PPPs which proliferated within national health programmes have been initiated through the development of global programmes like Global Alliances for Vaccines and Immunisation (GAVI), and GFATM. Global programmes have therefore encouraged partnerships at the programme implementation level between the government and NGOs, individual private providers (PP), and the corporate sector. All these increased the range of partners and, therefore, complexities of managing PPPs.
2. http://ehealth.eletsonline.com/2013/06/ensocare-and-wipro-ge- healthcare-enter-into-a-public–private-partnership-with-government- of- maharashtra-to-upgrade-district-hospitals/accessed on January 26, 2016.
3. The draft Policy for PPP in the Health Sector in West Bengal was finalised in 2006.
4. Capital means a pool of funds whereby the government builds, acquires or upgrades the physical assets such as property, buildings, technology or equipment (Klein et al., 2013).
5. www.pppinindia.com accessed on January 25, 2016.
6. Collection centres are units where only the blood/urine or other samples are collected. They are taken elsewhere for examination.

References

Acharya, A., & McNamee, P. (2009). "Assessing Gujarat's chiranjeevi scheme." *Economic and Political Weekly* 44, 48(November 28), 13–15.

Bagal, S. (2008). "Managing public private partnerships." *Economic and Political Weekly* 43, 33(August 16), 23–26.

Bagchi, S. (2013). "Another PPP project halted." *The Hindu*. August 3.

Baru, R. V., Nandy, M. (2008). "Blurring boundaries: public-private partnerships in health services in India." *Economic and Political Weekly* 43, No. 04 (January 26), 62–71.

Baru, R. V. (2005). "Commercialisation and the public sector in India: Implications for values and aspirations." In *Commercialisation of Healthcare: Global and Local Dynamics and Policy Responses,* edited by M. Mackintosh and M. Koivusalo. New York: UNRISD and Palgrave.

Bhattacharya, V., Menon, S. (2010). *Evaluation of MAMTA Scheme in National Capital Territory of Delhi: Report*. Department of Planning and Evaluation, National Institute of Health and Family Welfare.

Bennett, S., & Muraleedharan, V. R. (2000). "New Public Management' and healthcare in third world." *Economic and Political Weekly* 35, No. 1/2 (January 4): 59–68.

Bhat, R., Maheshwari, S. K., & Saha, S. (2007). "Contracting-Out of Reproductive Child Health Services Through Mother NGO Scheme in India: Experiences and Implications." W.P. No. 2007–01–05. IIM.

Bhatia, M., & Mills, A. (1997). "Contracting Out of Dietary Services by Public Hospitals in Bombay." In *Private Health Providers in Developing Countries: Serving the Public Interest?,* edited by S. Bennett, B. McPake and A. Mills. London: Zed Press.

Buse, K., & Harmer, A. (2004). Power to the partners? The politics of public- private partnerships. *Development, 47*(2), 49–56.

Chaturvedi, S., & Randive, B. (2011). Public private partnerships for emergency obstetric care: Lessons from Maharashtra. *Indian Journal of Community Medicine, 36*(1), 21–26.

CII-HOSMAC. (n.d.). “Partnerships in Healthcare: A Public Private Perspective.” Accessed October 14, 2015. http://www.cii.in/webcms/Upload/Whitepaper%20on%20Partnership%20in%20Health care1.pdf.

Cohen, M., McGregor, M., Ivanova, I., & Kinkaid, C. (2012). “Beyond the Hospital Walls: Activity Based Funding Versus Integrated Healthcare Reform.” Canadian Centre for Policy Alternatives, BC. Accessed May 16, 2016. https://www.policyalternatives.ca/sites/default/files/uploads/publications/BC%20Office/2012/01/CCPA-BC_ABF_2012.pdf, Commission of India.

De Costa, Ayesha, T. Kazmi, K. Lönnroth, M. Uplekar and V.K. Diwan. (2008). “PPM: ‘Public-Private’ or ‘Private Public’ Mix? The Case of Ujjain District.” India. *International Journal of Tuberculosis Lung Disease* 12, No. 11 (November): 1333–5.

Deshpande, K., Shankar, R., Diwan, V., Lonnroth, K., Mahadik, V. K., & Chandorkar, R. K. (2004). Spatial Pattern of Private Healthcare Provision in Ujjain, India: A Provider Survey Processed and Analysed with a Geospatial Information System. *Health Policy, 68*(2), 211–222.

Devaraj, M. (2006). “Public Private Partnership in Health Sector: A Case Study in Jhansi District of Uttar Pradesh, India.” Research Paper, MA in Development Studies with Specialisation in Public Policy and Management, Institute of Social Studies.

Dewan, P. K., Lal, S. S., Lönnroth, K., Wares, F., Uplekar, M., Sahu, S., Granich, R., & Chauhan, L. S. (2006). Public-Private Mix in India: Improving Tuberculosis Control Through Intersectoral Partnerships. *BMJ, 332*, 574–578.

Economic Times Bureau. (2010). “Annuity Based PPP Projects to Fall Under Fiscal Responsibility Act Ambit.” *The Economic Times*. December 23.

Froud, J. (2003). “The Private Finance Initiative: Risk, Uncertainty and the State.” *Accounting, Organisations and Society, 28*, 567–589.

Government of Gujarat. (2010). “Report of the Controller and Auditor General (Civil).” Accessed December 15, 2015. http://financedepartment.gujarat.gov.in/pdf/audit%20Report_9_10_Eng.pdf.

Government of India. (1994). *Eighth Five Year Plan (1992–97)*, Vol. 2. New Delhi:

Government of India. (2002). *National Health Policy, 2002*. New Delhi: Ministry of Health and Family Welfare.

Government of India. (2002a). *Tenth Five Year Plan (2002–2007) Social Sectors*, Vol. 3. New Delhi: Planning Commission of India.

Government of India. (2005). *Report of the National Commission on Macroeconomics and Health*. New Delhi: National Commission on Macroeconomics and Health, Ministry of Health and Family Welfare.

Government of India. (2006). “Draft Report on Recommendation of Task Force on Public Private Partnership for the Eleventh Plan.” Accessed November 2, 2012. https://nhm.gov.in/images/pdf/communitisation/task-group- reports/draft-report-ppp.pdf

Government of India. (2008). *Eleventh Five Year Plan (2007–2012)*. New Delhi: Planning Commission of India.

Government of India. (2009). *Working Draft: The National Health Bill, 2009*. New Delhi: Ministry of Health and Family Welfare.

Government of India. (2010). “Report of the Task Force on Ceilings for Annuity Commitments, Secretariat for Infrastructure.” New Delhi: Planning Commission of India.

Government of India. (2010a). *National Health Mission 4th Common Review Mission, Orissa*. 15–23 (December). New Delhi: Ministry of Health and Family Welfare. Accessed on October 17th, 2017. https://nhm.gov.in/images/pdf/ monitoring/crm/4th-crm/presentation/orissa.pdf *National Health Mission.*

Government of India. (2011). “Draft National Public Private Partnership Policy.” Department of Economic Affairs, Ministry of Finance, Government of India.

Government of India. (2012). *National Health Mission Report of the Sixth Common Review Mission, Bihar*.

Government of India. (2013). *Twelfth Five Year Plan (2012–17) Social Sectors*, Vol. 3. New Delhi: Planning

Government of India. (2014). *National Health Mission 8th Common Review Mission Report 2014*. New Delhi: Ministry of Health and Family Welfare.

Government of India. (2017). *National Health Policy 2017*. New Delhi: Ministry of Health and Family Welfare.

Government of India. (n.d). *Ninth Five Year Plan (1997–2002)*, Vol. 2. New Delhi: Planning Commission of India.

Government of West Bengal. (2006). "Policy for Public Private Partnerships in the Health Sector." Strategic Planning and Sector Reform Cell. Department of Health and Family Welfare, Government of West Bengal.

Heard, A., Awasthi, M. K., Ali, J. , Shukla, N., & Heard, B.C. (2011). "Predicting Performance in Contracting of Basic Healthcare to NGOs: Experience from Large-Scale Contracting in Uttar Pradesh, India." *Health Policy and Planning*, 26: 13–19.

Hellowell, M., & Pollock, A. M. (2009). The Private Financing of NHS Hospitals: Politics, Policy and Practice. *Economic Affairs, 29*, 13–19.

ICRA Management Consulting Services Limited. (2013). "Prefeasibility Report of Setting Up MRI Scan Centres on PPP Mode in Medical Colleges of Belgaum, Bidar, Hassan, Mandya, Raichur and Shimoga Districts." Submitted to the Karnataka Infrastructure Development Department Project. NOIDA: ICRA Management Consulting Services Limited.

International Finance Corporation. (2013). "Public Private Partnership Stories: India Shillong Medical College, IFC Advisory Services in Public-Private Partnerships." Washington D.C. Accessed March 21, 2016. ifc.org/ppp.

Jega, F. M. (2007). *Contracting Out to Improve Maternal Health: Evaluating the Quality of Care Under the Chiranjeevi Yojana in Gujarat, India*. Unpublished M Comm H Diss.

Kapilshrami, A., & McPake, B. (2012). Transforming Governance or Reinforcing Hierarchies and Competition: Examining the Public and Hidden Transcripts of the Global Fund and HIV in India. *Health Policy and Planning, 28*(6), 626–635.

Karpagam, S., & Akhila. Vasan, and Vijayakumar Seethappa. . (2016). Falling Through the Gaps: Women Accessing Care Under Health Insurance Schemes in Karnataka. *Indian Journal of Gender Studies, 23*(1), 69–86.

Karpagam, S., Roy, B., Seethappa, V., & Qadeer, I. (2013). Evidence Based Planning—A Myth or Reality: Use of the Evidence by the Planning Commission on Public-Private Partnership. *Social Change, 43*(2), 213–226.

Klein, D. J., Brown, A.D., Huynh, T. M., Bevan, G., Markel, F., Ottaway, S. D., Pink, G., & Zyblock, M. (2013). "Capital Spending in Healthcare: A Missed Opportunity for Improvement?" Canadian Foundation for Health Improvement.

Kumar, C. (2013). "An Exploratory Analysis of Public Private Partnerships in Diagnostic Services Under the National Rural Health Mission, Bihar." Unpublished MPhil Diss., Centre of Social Medicine and Community Health, School of Social Sciences, Jawaharlal Nehru University.

Mairembam, S. D., Lisam, S., Ved, R., Baruah, J., Goel, P., Srivastava, R., & Mokashi, T. (2012). "Public Private Partnership in Meghalaya: Delivering Healthcare in Difficult to Access Tribal Areas." *BMC, Proceedings 2012,* 6, Supplement 5: P3. https://doi.org/10.1186/1753-6561-6-S5-P3.

Medical College Kolkata. (2012). *Annual Report: 2012*. Medical College.

Mohanan, M., Bauhoff, S., Forgia, G. L., Babiarz, K. S., Singh, K., & Miller, G. (2014). "Effect of Chiranjeevi Yojana on Institutional Deliveries and Neonatal and Maternal Outcomes in Gujarat, India: A Difference-in- Differences Analysis." *Bulletin of the World Health Organisation* 92, 187–94.

Nandan, D., Pal, D.K., Toppo, N.A., Tekhre, Y. L., Das, J.K., Bhattacharya, V., & Menon, S. (2008). *An Appraisal of Janani Sahyogi Yojana in Madhya Pradesh*. National Institute of Health and Family Welfare.

Nandi, S., Dasgupta, R., Garg, S., Sinha, D., Sahu, S., & Mahobe, R. (2016). Uncovering coverage: Utilisation of the universal health insurance scheme, Chattisgarh by women in slums of Raipur. *Indian Journal of Gender Studies, 23*(1), 43–68.

Pradhan, A., Datye, V., Kielmann, K., Khilare, K., Datye, A., Inamder, V., Porter, J., & Rangan, S. (2011). Sustaining PPM-DOTS: The case of Pimpri Chinchwad, Maharashtra India. *Indian Journal of Tuberculosis, 58*(1), 18–28.

Qadeer, I., & Reddy, S. (2010). "Medical tourism in India: Progress or predica—ment?" *Economic and Political Weekly, XLV*, No. 20 (May 15), 69–75.

Ramaiah, A. A., & Gawde, N. C. (2014). Economic evaluation of a public—private mix tb project in Tamil Nadu, India. *Journal of Health Management, 17*, 370–380.

Raman, A. V., & Bjorkman, J. W. (2006). *Public Private Partnerships in the Provision of Healthcare Services to the Poor*. Indo-Dutch Programme for Alternatives in Development.

Randive, B., Chaturvedi, S., & Mistry, N. (2012). "Contracting in specialists for emergency obstetric care—does it work in rural India?" *BMC Health Services Research*, 12:485.

Rathi, P., Mukherji, A., & Sen, G. (2012). "Rashtriya Swasthya Bima Yojana: Evaluating Utilisation, Roll-out and Perceptions in Amaravati District, Maharashtra." *Economic and Political Weekly* 47, No. 39 (September 29), 57–64.

Ravindran, T.K. Sunadri. (2011). "Public private partnerships in maternal health services." *Economic and Political Weekly* 46, No. 48 (November 26), 43–52.

Roy, B., & Gupta, S. (2011). "Public private partnership and user fees in healthcare: Evidence from West Bengal." *Economic and Political Weekly* 46, No. 38(September 17), 74–78.

Roy, B. (2007). *Private Investment in Public Sector Medical Care Institutions: A Study of the Processes in Tertiary and Secondary Level Care in Six Districts of West Bengal.* Jawaharlal Nehru University.

Roy, B. (2010). "Outsourcing of service provisioning and changing employment relationship in public sector hospitals of West Bengal." *The Indian Journal of Labour Economics* 53, No. 2 (April–June), 410–422.

Roy, B. (2015). "Public private partnership in healthcare: Trajectories and experiences from West Bengal'." In *India Social Development Report 2014: Challenges of Public Health*, I. Qadeer (Ed.). Council for Social Development and Oxford University Press.

Sarma, E.A.S. (2006). "Public-private partnership: New 'Reform' Mantra." *Economic and Political Weekly* 42, No. 48 (December 2), 4956–4958.

Unger, J. P., De Paepe, P., Gilbert, P., Zocchi, W., Van Dassel, P., Qadeer, I., & Sen, K. (2010). "Privatisation (PPM-DOTS) Strategy for tuberculosis control: How evidence-based is it?." In *International Health and Aid Policies: The Need for Alternatives.* In: J.P. Unger, P.D. Paepe, K. Sen, & W. Soors (Eds.) Cambridge University Press.

Vasan, A., Karpagam, S., & Sethappa, V. (2015). "Design, Implementation, and Patient Experiences of the Rashtriya Swasthya Bima Yojana and Vajpayee Arogyashree Scheme: A Qualitative Study from Bangalore District, Karnataka." In *India Social Development Report 2014: Challenges of Public Health*, edited by Imrana Qadeer, Council for Social Development and Oxford University Press.

United Nations Population Fund, India. (2009). "Concurrent Assessment of Janani Suraksha Scheme in Selected States: Bihar, Madhya Pradesh, Orissa, Rajasthan, Uttar Pradesh." Accessed January 20, 2016. http://countryoffice.unfpa.org/india/drive/JSYConcurrentAssessment.pdf.

WHO. (2014). *Universal Access to Medicines in India: A Baseline Evaluation of the Rajasthan Free Medicines Scheme.* WHO.

World Bank. (1996). *State Appraisal Report India State Health Systems Development Project II.* Population and Human Reources Operation Division, South Asia Country Department, World Bank.

Yasmeen, A. (2016). "Arogya Bandhu Scheme Scrapped." *The Hindu.* February 18

Chapter 8
Unaccountable Deaths and Damages: An Analysis of Socio-Legal Implications of Sterilisation Camp Deaths in Bilaspur, Chhattisgarh

P. M. Arathi

Background

Bilaspur District of Chhattisgarh hit the news pages when 13 women died following tubectomy operations in a sterilisation camp. On November 8, 2014, 83 women underwent sterilisation surgery at the camp conducted at Takhtpur block in Sakri at Nemi Chand Jain Hospital. On November 10, camps were organised in Gaurella block at three Primary Health Centre (PHC) sites—Gaurella, Marwahi and Pendra, where 23, 16 and 15 women were operated respectively (Population Foundation India (PFI) et al., 2014). According to the information provided by the officials, after the surgeries, some of the women experienced burning sensation in the throat, vomiting, pain in abdomen and breathing problems and they contacted the Mitanin (Community Health Worker (CHW)) of the locality. These women were admitted to the District Hospital, Chhattisgarh Institute of Medical Sciences (CIMS) and Apollo Hospital.

There were several speculations and debates around the causes of the tragic death of these 13 women. The initial assumption was that the doctor who conducted the surgeries violated the standard operating procedures and guidelines prescribed by the Ministry of Health and Family Welfare (MoHFW). The surgeon conducted 83 sterilisations in about one and a half hours, whereas the government limit is 30 per day (Bagchi, 2015). Dr. R.K. Gupta, the surgeon at Bilaspur District Hospital, spent approximately three- four minutes per patient and did not follow the infection control protocols. He used the same laparoscope for all women without disinfecting it after each case.

The second hypothesis was about the quality of medical care provided in the camps. The camp in Bilaspur was held in an abandoned hospital with no running water and sterilisation of rusty surgical equipment was inadequate.

P. M. Arathi (✉)
School of Indian Legal Thought, Mahatma Gandhi University, Kottayam, Kerala, India

I. Qadeer et al. (eds.), *Universalising Healthcare in India*,
https://doi.org/10.1007/978-981-16-5872-3_8

"The dangerous conditions are not uncommon in sterilisation camps throughout India, claim women's health activists. They say that such tubectomy camps are favoured by the Indian government as a way to operate on many women at one go. They often exceed the prescribed limit of surgeries in a day, do not adequately sterilise the equipment used on patients, and do not provide counselling before operations or afterwards" (Pulla, 2014: 1).

The doctors at the Apollo Hospital stated to the fact finding team that, "a few cases showed raised levels of peritoneal fluid that suggests septicaemia (a life-threatening bacterial infection), indicating that the women may have had an infection during or after their operation" (PFI et al., 2014:6). The doctors who conducted the post-mortem of the first seven cases of death, at CIMS and district hospital revealed to the fact finding team that, "there was evidence of peritonitis with fluid in peritoneal and pleural cavities, and septic foci in the lungs and kidneys, suggesting sepsis leading septicaemia" (Ibid). There was plenty of evidence indicating that the surgical staff used the same hand gloves, injections, syringes, sutures on all 83 women in the private hospital (Krishnan, 2016).

The third proposition was that there was a 'problem with drugs', namely Ciprofloxacin 500 mg, the antibiotic provided in the camps along with a pain reliever. Four drugs commonly prescribed in all four camps were Diazepam, Ibuprofen and Ciprofloxacin and Povidone Iodine for external application. The press statement of the state health department, soon after the tragedy, claimed that the drugs Ibuprofen and Ciprofloxacin which were prescribed after the surgery as post-operative care were laced with rat poison. However, viscera reports from the Central Forensic Science Laboratory in Ramanathapur, Hyderabad and from the Central Drugs Laboratory, Kolkata, and State Forensic Science Laboratory in Raipur later, dismissed this argument of adulterated drugs. The tests conducted for the quality of the drugs were limited to only two drugs out of the fifteen prescribed in the sterilisation process, the rest did not go through a quality check (Ibid.).

The identification of these different causes of deaths that happened in Bilaspur gives a fragmented picture restricted to bio-medical aspects. The combination of social realities and the shifts in economic and health policies might give us a more comprehensive understanding. The recent works on this issue interrogating, mapping and challenging the experiences of women who had undergone mass sterilisation helps in that direction. Our endeavour is to understand the social, political, economic and legal contexts which enabled the brutal legal and ethical violations in the camps, to analyse how the legal interventions and policy enforcements become skewed in the domain of accessibility, availability and quality of healthcare service delivery provisions, and to explain how the coercive population policies in India along with the unmet demand for reducing family size tend to create a level of callousness that resulted in deaths in sterilisation camps in Bilaspur.

The first part of the chapter traces the transition in the agrarian economy and land holding patterns and its corresponding changes in the fertility patterns. The second part marks the shifts in population policies and changes in the approaches in India's Family Planning Programme (FPP). The third critically examines the legal and ethical standards and safeguards prescribed nationally and internationally and its limitations in the specific context of India by reviewing a couple of case laws. Finally, it is argued that the rampant privatisation and commodification of healthcare services in the name of Universal Health Coverage (UHC) is not the answer to the questions and challenges emerging out of the Bilaspur sterilisation tragedy.

Economic Transition and Fertility Changes in India

Changes in the agrarian sector in the last two decades, through neoliberal policies, have led to an acute yet unnoticed deprivation in rural India. This deprivation rooted in the growth-led developmental ideology has impacted the agrarian sector severely, reducing the size of cultivable land, migration to urban location and has influenced the fertility choices of married women. The different components of power structure and their confluence (intersectional dynamics) influence the participation of women in the decision-making process regarding the number of children. Therefore, it varies from region to region. The fact-finding team report shows that the discussion with the peripheral level staff—Auxiliary Nurse Midwife (ANM), Mitanin and Anganwadi Worker (AWW)— revealed that "women had no say in choosing their family size, contraceptive use, spacing of children, etc." (PFI et al., 2014: 12). Hence, the role of women in the decision-making process is unbound neither from the history nor from the context or social identity. National Family Health Survey (NFHS)-3 indicates that among the sterilised women, 8% were less than 20 years old, 38% were between 20 to 24 years of age and 35% were between 25 to 29 years of age. Three rounds of NFHS show a steady decline in the median age of sterilisation for women[1]. The Annual Health Survey (AHS) 2010–11 report of Chhattisgarh reports 43% of women with two children in Bilaspur wanting no more children (37.9 for rural and 54.7 for urban). In Bilaspur, family planning practices of women— 15–49 of age—showed that 37.9% currently used female sterilisation (36.8% in rural and 40.2% in urban), and use of male sterilisation was only 0.5% of total sterilisations. This report further showed that the unmet need for limiting family size was 15% and for spacing 16.8% (GoI, n.d.). This clearly shows that there is a shift in people's receptiveness and acceptability of fertility control measures over time. In the decisions of rural women to reduce their family size, one of the measures to address is their poverty. The 'unmet need' for reducing the family size is the major concern of family planning programme in India, however it does not really consider addressing the availability, accessibility, affordability and quality of the services. The reasonable expectation of the people from the state is to get quality services at an affordable price, which is not being addressed adequately.

The availability of contraceptives is limited and method of spacing became expensive due to private provision in India. Male/rich/upper caste-centric policies which are seemingly gender responsive and caste- neutral are dominant and, the camp approach for family planning is only one such policy. Institutional and structural failures and restricted demands for their resurrection contribute to the weakening of social justice mechanisms and legal capacity to resist expansion of deprivation and disparities. This has created a situation of skewed choice for rural poor women who have little option but to seek the only available method of population control, female sterilisation, and that too provided in the mass sterilisation camps often violating all the national and international prescribed standards.

The standards prescribed by the Government of India, such as Standard Operating Procedures for Sterilisation in Camps; Guidelines for Laparoscopic Sterilisation Procedure; Guidelines for Camp Services for Sterilisation and the Quality Assurance Manual were violated blatantly in Bilaspur (PFI et al., 2014). If the protocols set by the government were to be followed, a camp of 83 service seekers would need three teams[2]. The camp on November 8 at Nemi Chand Jain private hospital had violated all these protocols. The participation of private and public sector workers in conducting the camp shows the poor functioning of public private partnerships. In this model of PPP the infrastructure and some members of the healthcare delivery team belonged to the private provider and the rest of the responsibility was with the public institutions. The fact finding report indicates that the camp at the private hospital had "only four medical officers including two MBBS doctors and two Registered Medical Assistants responsible for general screening of the women and selection for the sterilisation procedure; two staff nurses (from PHC Amsena and Takhatpur) to assist in the operation theatre; two ANMs (one each from PHC-Amsena and nearby Sub Centre) to give pre-medication and inject local anaesthesia outside the OT; two dressers from PHC to stitch the wounds after procedure; two ward boys from two PHCs to bring cases outside OT, position them on the OT table and shift them after the procedure. A number of ANMs and Mitanins from the field were also present at the hospital as motivators. The Laparoscopic surgeon came with one assistant" (PFI et al., 2014: 7).

The public sector is by far the most commonly used source for both female and male sterilisation (84–85%). A further sub-division of the public sector shows, 51% of the female sterilisations were done in government municipal hospitals; 18% in Community Health Centres (CHCs), rural hospitals and PHCs, and 12% in camps (GoI, 2007: 138). In contrast, the private medical sector acts as sources for spacing methods. Utilisation of public sector for female sterilisation in Chhattisgarh is 93.3% (Ibid.).

Slightly more than three-quarters of sterilised women got their sterilisation free of cost, and 5% said they did not know the cost. For the remaining women who reported the cost, the median cost was INR 1,996. Only 1 in 10 women who used the public medical facility for their sterilisation had to pay for the operation, and even if they did, the median cost was only INR 500. Ninety-two percent of women who used the private medical sector source (including an NGO or trust hospital/clinic) had to pay for the sterilisation, and the median cost was INR 2,995 (GoI, 2007: 142).

Factors that contribute to preventable maternal deaths remain strongly embedded: anaemia, early marriage, generally poor nutritional status of women and their overall discrimination (Qadeer, 2010). Another major contributing factor for maternal deaths has been health service delivery system-systemic rupture of public health system, unaccountable private sector and its rampant activity to meet the coercive population policies through state subsidised insurances.

The Census of India 2011 recorded 2.55 crores of population in Chhattisgarh, 49.4% of which was Below the Poverty Line (BPL) and a large proportion was tribal. About 56.2% of married women had anaemia[3], Infant Mortality Rate (IMR) was 48 (113/1000 for teenage mothers)[4]. Chhattisgarh falls under one of the highest Maternal Mortality Ration (MMR) reported states (269 in 2007-09 and the Twelfth Plan aimed to reduce it to 122.395)[5]. The practice of child marriage was common and reports showed that 45.2% of women of the age group 20-24 were married before 18[6]. The unmet need for contraception was reported to be 20.9%, whereas married women using sterilisation was 41.3%[7]. Most of the women who died in the camp belong to the socially marginalised communities[8] and were economically backward. The state has a wide network of Mitanins but the lack of support from the infrastructure has made them ineffective.

Though the programme on paper envisaged full support of a strengthened primary care infrastructure, the latter was neither strengthened nor did it give importance to patients referred by the Mitanins. She was seen as technically and socially inferior and was treated more as an adjunct rather than a representative of the community. Thus the Mitanins were used for just one targeted programme—the reproductive health programme (Som, 2014). In Bilaspur also the Mitanins acted as the facilitators between healthcare delivery system and women and the district health authorities used Mitanins to reach out to women and get them to the camps.

The skewed resources and infrastructure in the public health delivery system is one of the strong factors that made the situation worse. The state lacks 1246 nurses, 293 pharmacists, 460 laboratory technicians at the PHC and CHC. The reported scarcity of doctors is 302 at the (PHC), 45 general and 525 specialist doctors (131 obstetricians and gynaecologists, 130 paediatricians) at the CHC. "Chhattisgarh's ill-equipped public health system coupled with the state's relentless pursuit of family planning targets creates an environment where deaths became inevitable" (Human Rights Law Network (HRLN), 2014: 7). The camp method for sterilising women, where quality of care is deeply compromised and ethical and legal provisions violated, itself is a reflection of systemic rupture of the public healthcare delivery system. Rather than addressing the question of how to improve public health systems to meet the requirements of the people, policy level interventions through PPPs and insurance schemes, open the door for profit making private providers and create lethal situations like the one at Bilaspur.

Family Planning Programmes: Yesterday and Today

Population policies in India have witnessed different trajectories, namely, voluntary, coercive and targeted. In this section, we discuss these trajectories and see how women become 'targets' and continue to be the targets in recent policy statements. This section shows how the dominance of Malthusian ideology in conceptualising, perceiving and drafting these policies persisted in India and stood as an iconic representation of anti-women and anti-poor strategies. FPP is one of the oldest components of the healthcare system in India and continued to be the focus of planning over the last five decades.

However, it has remained primarily a programme of controlling numbers rather than focused on reproductive and human rights that India had affirmed at the International Conference on Population and Development (ICPD) in 1994 and in its National Population Policy (NPP), 2000 (PFI et al., 2014: 3). Though as policy, both these documents speak about dispensing with targets and incentives in FPP, in practice, it still continues despite major tragedies in the past (Hartmann & Rao, 2015).

The global propaganda of 'population explosion' and the shift in the national concerns of policy makers to 'population stabilisation' as a national priority, has resulted in the promotion of permanent methods like sterilisation surgeries, which constitute 72% of the total contraceptive use in India (MoHFW, 2010). In India it is women who predominantly bear the burden of family planning, and the proportion of tubal ligation in the total annual sterilisation was 71% at the peak of implementation of the family planning programme in the early 1980s and it has increased to 98% in 2013 (MoHFW, 2013). The Chhattisgarh government alone had planned for 1,50,000 female sterilisations in 2014 while vasectomies were only 8,000 (Pulla, 2014).

The fact finding report acknowledged the state level variations within FPP but pointed out that it,

> ...remains a target and incentive driven and not a demand driven programme. The demand for sterilisation services exists, but it is essentially a false demand as there are neither other long term suitable options available on a regular basis nor is there adequate access to information and counselling on all aspects related to sterilisation. (PFI et.al., 2014: 4)

Re-Emergence of Malthusianism

After several decades of an outright Malthusian approach, ICPD became a watershed where an integrated, non-targeted and welfare- oriented approach was put forward and India apparently agreed to it. In actual practice however, notions like choice of method, focus on Reproductive Child Health (RCH), emergency contraceptives and treatment of sterility were primarily tackled through techno-centric approaches, by bringing in more dangerous and invasive contraceptives. As the Health Sector Reforms (HSR) became pervasive and infrastructure contracted with casualisation of paramedical workers and shrinking of primary care, the camps returned on the agenda and the focus on laparotomy intensified. Ultimately, the understanding that, "Family planning is critical for our nation's economic development, and is a big first step towards growth, equality and sustainable development that opens the door to opportunity and prosperity for women and families everywhere" (Nadda, 2016), re-established itself. The data produced by the NFHS-3 and AHS clearly contradicts this understanding as it shows the declining fertility rates and increasing unmet need for contraceptives does not correspond to the anticipated economic development (Sarojini et al., 2015).

Union Health Minister Nadda (2016) emphasises the importance of public- private partnership as "we will also work closely through private sector engagement, using approaches such as social marketing and franchising to help us to consistently build strong public–private partnerships to ensure that our interventions reach everyone." The withdrawal of the state from being a provider of service to the facilitator of market, adversely impacts the quality of services in the public sector service provisioning. In the financial year of 2013–14, the expenditure on FPP was INR 396.97 crores[9] and the amount spent for female sterilisation constituted 85% of the total FPP expenditure. The quality of service, defined as choice of method, dignity and comfort, privacy and confidentiality, safety procedure, follow up and referral services as well as space for feedback, ranges from low to very poor quality (PFI et al., 2014). Chapter II of the draft National Health Bill describes the obligation of government in relation to health. Section 3(a) mentions budgetary allocation that should be, "Appropriate and adequate budgetary measures, as per globally accepted norms, to satisfy, the obligation and rights set out herein, throughout ensuring transparency and equity in the allocation, planning and rational allocation and distribution of resources for health and related issues and concerns" (MoHFW, 2009: 13), but does not prescribe any minimum percentage of the Gross Domestic Product (GDP) as mandatory investment in the health sector allocation. Unless the "appropriate and adequate" allocation of the budget is clearly defined in terms of proportion of GDP, there will be no commitment to the objectives expressed. As a result, the obligation of the government towards health remains but is barely met. This shows a heightened emphasis on female sterilisation without adequate safety and security of methods.

The statement of the health minister almost condones the state for coercive population policies as he believes that the camps in Bilaspur were driven by 'demand' rather than for meeting targets (Nadda, 2016). Though the Population Policy of India has officially adopted 'target free approach', the medical practitioners and officers continued to receive targets and incentives for 'good performance' (Das & Contractor, 2014). Given the healthcare delivery system we have, the targets and quality never go together. The sterilisation camp experiences of different parts of the country affirm this.[10].

The ambitious goals of family planning policies and counting numbers, not people and their lives, pushes coercion of women and compromises on quality. India's commitment to family planning 2020 is based on the argument that, to provide contraceptive service to 48 million couples there is no other way for the policy makers but to continue with crude camp approaches, and targets more and more vulnerable women (Das & Contractor, 2014).

Legal Articulation of Rights in the Indian Context

In the face of increasing pressures of a neo-Malthusian approach, the urgency of a protective and progressive legal framework deepens. This section focuses on the analysis of international and national legal instruments applicable in India and critically demonstrates how they fail to capture the lived realities in rural India. We focus on four key issues: definitions of coercion, reproductive choices and accountability of providers, and use of camps. The international standards prescribed by the World Health Organisation (WHO) and other legal instruments which ensure right to health discuss 'forced sterilisation' in the context of coercive population policies. Erdman (2015) draws attention to lived experience, as a category to understand institutional, culture and structural injustice. This could be a possibility for inquiry in the case of sterilisation camp deaths and damages in the Indian context. The discourse on reproductive choices ignores these aspects of violations happening on an everyday basis in countries like India.

The definition of 'force' and 'coerciveness' involved in the female sterilisation deviates from the standardised legal articulation of rights and becomes complex in the specific context of rural India. The beneficiary is the focus of coercion which operates from two sides. Self-coercion of the service seekers originates from desperation due to limited access to service and a pressure to limit family size due to poverty (for lower class and caste), and aspiration to live a 'modern middle class' life influenced by the commoditisation (for lower and upper middle class). On the other side, the health policy makers and the administrators function within the larger framework that is ideologically underlined by Malthusianism/neo-Malthusianism. Malthusianism links economic growth and sustainable development with numbers in the country. This has led to intensified thrust for population control and emphasis on family planning. Since the private sector is disinterested in these services given their low profitability, family planning falls primarily in the domain of public sector health services often operating in partnership with small private providers. Public services are being undermined through unbridled privatisation, commercialisation of public health service in the name of public-private partnerships for UHC. When denied access to quality services their only recourse is to accept sterilization camps.

Just as the link between coercion and oppressive population policies is rooted in the denial of services to the poor, the felt need for birth control among rural poor women in India cannot be analysed within the reproductive choice framework of the WHO (WHO, 2014). The choice framework emerged in the Western context where choice is a function of support systems for maternal and child care, other social welfare measures and a better social environment for women to make choices. However in the given situation for the majority of women in India (both rural and urban), the 'choice' comes mostly out of necessity and desperation. Here, the affordable birth control measures mostly are permanent contraceptive methods, generally female sterilisation.

This context calls for first developing some legal safeguards which incorporate rights to equality and protection from social and material discrimination as an essential prerequisite for any demand for freedom of choice. International legal instruments which India has signed are equally considered as law of the land under Article 253 of the Constitution of India. Implementation of many of these international legal instruments[11] could have prevented the avoidable deaths in the sterilisation camps, either through setting the standard protocols for treatments or through making the state accountable and liable for the medical negligence committed in these cases. The camp approach to sterilisation continues in developing countries no matter what agreements are made in international platforms by the nation state. India is a concrete example for this. It is clear that accepting a camp approach inevitably leads to violations of medical ethics other than undermining the ethics of public health. The diminishing state investment in the social welfare sector including public health and the introduction of market rationality in the social sector resulted in inhumane treatment of the poor, lower caste, rural women in the sterilisation camps of Bilaspur. The accountability and legal regulation of the private sector is a mirage in pro- market statehood. Hence, their partnership does not necessarily contribute to efficiency but often damages more than it helps. Though the Parliament of India has passed the Clinical Establishment (Registration and Regulation) Act 2010, which governs the regulation of all healthcare institutions including the private providers, it still remains on paper.

The Working Draft of the National Health Bill (version January 2009) states that the Union of India has the mandate to legislate on matters related to population stabilisation and family planning (MoHFW, 2009: 8). This piece of law is still in the Bill format and is waiting to get passed in Parliament.

Legal Battles in India

Struggles for health justice in developing countries historically relied on judiciary through litigation, both in the form of public interest litigation as well as complaints filed by individuals based on their personal grievances. The history of public interest litigation in India marks an attempt to reframe health-related entitlements as legally enforceable claims. The individual or personal grievances were mostly around medical negligence or violation of consumer rights of patients seeking service (middle class initiatives for entitlements). Judicialisation (approaching judiciary to get relief under a law or implementation of it) of medical negligence often interprets and visualises these as pragmatic rights (recognised but not acted upon) and not as justiciable in many of the legal fights. Structural and hierarchical discrimination also reflect in the healthcare delivery system, many people who live on the periphery of society are fatally affected. Here, it is important to establish the linkages between right to life and right not to be discriminated against in health rights litigation. It demands an inclusive approach in the legal paradigm, which incorporates, individual entitlements to healthcare, re-writing intellectual property rights rules, changes in policies related to social determinants of health, influence in the health priority setting forces and drive for more budgetary allocations (Yamin, 2014).

Judicialisation of health rights cannot be seen or analysed in abstract but has to be done in specific socio-political and legal contexts. In India, this judicial process can be observed as court acts on immediately enforceable minimum core content; judging the reasonableness of government actions; granting silent sanctions to corporate hospitals and pro-corporate government actions (Baxi, 1985: 132). Yamin (2014) argues that the blatant violation of human dignity in healthcare settings continue to occur across all development levels, despite well established standards. Equity in health is a complex and multivalent topic, especially in a multilayered stratified society. This makes questions on discrimination much more complex to negotiate litigation which alone cannot be the end or beginning, or the end of struggle for justice and rights in health.

Civil society efforts with the judicial system in India on the quality of care in sterilisation camps (*Ramakant Rai* vs *Union of India* 2005) resulted in the Supreme Court directing the Government of India to frame guidelines for quality of care for these services. Almost a decade later, the Court had to be approached again as the ground situation had not changed (*Devika Biswas* versus *Union of India* 2012)[12]. Here, the petitioner sought a declaration that sterilisation camp surgeries conducted in unhygienic and unethical conditions violated fundamental rights guaranteed under Articles 14, 15 and 21 of the Constitution. The court observed in this case that there is an order from the Rajasthan government which proved that Accredited Social Health Activists (ASHAs) are trained to promote sterilisation without consideration of other forms of contraception and use a target-based coercive approach. In a mass sterilisation camp in Ratangarh, Rajasthan, the team of surgeons exceeded the limits imposed by the National Guidelines (50 sterilisations per day) and operated on 95 women and 10 men. This case clearly showed, how every single guideline was violated, like, women were forced to lie on the floor to recover because there were not enough beds for all the patients. Ration dealers (Public Distributive System) were given targets of two sterilisations per person which clearly violates the international and national norms and standards prescribed by the authorities. The court ordered compensation to the affected families. Despite the government's claim of a 'target free- approach' in family planning, Bilaspur sterilisation deaths exposes the persistence of the reality of camps. The Supreme Court of India has again extended the previous order to the Bilaspur case. Families were paid compensation as directed by its 2005 order.

> The Court also directed the state of Chhattisgarh to file an affidavit indicating the steps that have been taken to ameliorate the conditions of the persons who faced recent tragedy in sterilization camps in Bilaspur where a large number of persons are said to have died; the order said. The court further sought details on the action that has been taken against the doctors involved and what steps have been taken to educate the people in the state of Chhattisgarh with regard to sterilization (HRLN, 2015: 9).

However a report shows that the compensations are not dispersed after completion of almost one and a half years (Krishna, 2016).

In a previous case, *Ramakant Rai* versus *Union of India*, the Supreme Court of India observed that,

> A Family Planning Indemnity Scheme sometime in the year 2013 which provides inter alia for compensation in the event of death following sterilization, within 8-30 days from the date of discharge from the hospital, failure of sterilization, cost of treatment in hospital up to 60 days arising out of complication following sterilization operation and indemnity per doctor/health facilities. According to the counsel for the petitioner, the Indemnity Scheme has not been implemented in as much as it is not very clear whether the Central Government has released the funds under the aforesaid Scheme and whether the State Governments/ Union Territories have passed on the funds to the deserving persons (HRLN, 2015: 10)

The Indian legal system follows the British system of law, due to the political and administrative experience of colonisation. The criminal justice system still follows the colonial law of the Indian Penal Code, 1860. However, the kind of legal principles followed by the British Courts in medical negligence did not get evoked in any of the judicial debates in the above mentioned cases. The British system follows the notion of the tort of negligence when a patient had been injured due to the mistake by the doctor or by the system of healthcare service delivery. To establish this principle of tort of negligence in the classical notion of law there should be three conditions: the patient must be owed by a 'duty of care' by the doctor; there should be a breach of duty by the doctor (doctor's conduct must be below the standard of care prescribed by the law); and finally the breach of duty should cause harm to the patient.

In the case of the Bilaspur sterilisation deaths, the causation between the deaths and damage and breach of duty of the doctor and the healthcare delivery system is well-established with ample evidences. However, it did not become a legal question. By allowing meagre compensation to the relatives of the women who died, the administrative system tried to avoid the legal process of tort of medical negligence. It is always hard to prove a medical negligence case in the Indian judicial system, as it needs the approval of experts from the medical field to prove the breach of duty. The common practice is that none of the doctors will produce expert evidence against their fraternity. What then could define justice in the Bilaspur case? Can justice be ensured only by punishing the doctor/s? Can justice be delivered by granting meagre compensation? What was the logic behind fixing the amount for compensation? How is the value of life of women who died owing to lack of state accountability being measured? Are there any legal mechanisms which guarantee the distribution of compensation without further delay? How can one assure the quality of drugs and liability of drug manufacturers towards the consumers be established? These legal questions remain unaddressed in the context of the retreat of the welfare state during economic liberalisation. In fact the shift from being a provider of service to a facilitator of the market does not absolve the state of this responsibility. Yet, it ignores its responsibility towards developing guidelines and regulating the providers. This inability is a feature of the UHC model propagated by the Indian state which instead of providing solutions actually adds to the problem. The families of the women who died in the Bilaspur tragedy were given compensation but no responsibility was fixed.

Is India's UHC Model a Solution?

UHC is considered as a magic medicine for the healthcare needs of low and middle income countries. This section mulls over the concept of UHC and argues that the ambiguities in the prevailing model within the Indian context reflects the state's commitment to growth-oriented development and an intentional sabotage of health rights of the people. The West, which has nurtured the concept of UHC, began with social solidarity acquired through welfare measures by the state. In that context, the UHC model emerged under the pressure of demand for medical care and pressures of the private providers for autonomy under the rising expectations of the populations which had acquired a certain level of economic prosperity. These countries ultimately developed mixed models of medical care provided by public and private sectors. The former were strong partners ensuring basic care to all with market options for specialised care. The services were supported through state finances and well regulated (Qadeer, 2013).

Unlike in the West, in the context of India, the income disparities are too high, and there are various forms of discriminations based on caste-gender, religion and ethnicity, with deep historical roots. The lives of the people in the country remained divided and are of poor quality for a significant proportion. The existence of rural and urban differences in terms of infrastructure development and access to healthcare services has made the situation much more intricate to imagine a healthcare delivery system. The need was for both, welfare and medical care. However, UHC in India focuses on involving the private sector for coverage, protection from financial catastrophe, and basic medical care (without economic and social welfare). In India, PPPs, insurance, state health assurance schemes and the medical market have become pivotal. This model transforms health into a commodity and a service that responds to demands. Given the vast majority that need but are not able to demand services, their needs are to be met by the state through state-led insurances/assurance in partnership with the private sector. This only adds to the conversion of the state not only into a steward but also a client of the private sector. The shift of subsidies away from the health infrastructure leads to paucity of infrastructure and absence of regular services. This prepares the grounds for such camps and the callous treatment of poor women (Qadeer & Ghosh, 2016).

These schemes are distorting whatever little/poor public infrastructure there is, as well as provisioning of services, and Bilaspur is not an isolated example. We have to articulate our demands for health rights beyond the demand for free medical services, to ensure state accountability, to ensure justice to women of Bilaspur and such like situations., Accessibility of services that are non- discriminative will be inadequate without an assurance of quality of service. The struggle for an equitable and just health system has to be part of the larger resistances for comprehensive rights and entitlements.

Notes

1. From NFHS-1(26.6) to NFHS-2 (25.7) to NFHS-3(25.5) (GOI, 2007: 134).
2. Each team would have three staff in the operating room—one laparoscopic surgeon; one Operation Theatre Assistant and one nurse. In addition, the local PHC will have two doctors (including one lady woman medical officer) four staff nurses, one ANM and two attendants would be required (PFI et al., 2014: 7)
3. Report of District Level Household Survey 2007–2008.
4. The data on MMR and IMR is from Sample Registration System (SRS) Bulletin, 2011.

5. https://data.gov.in/resources/state-wise-targets-infant-mortality-rate-maternal-mortality-rate-and-anaemia-12th-plan/download accessed on June 8, 2016.
6. Report of District Level Household Survey 2007–2008.
7. Ibid.
8. Two are from Scheduled Tribes, 4 from Scheduled Castes, 6 from Other Backward Castes and one is unknown. See: Human Rights Law Network(HRLN) Report, http://www.hrln.org/hrln/reproductive-rights/reports/1661-fact-finding-report-on-sterilization-access-to-contraceptive-information-and-services-and-womens-health-in-bilaspur-district-chhattisgarh-14-18-november-2014.html.
9. This calculation is based on NRHM and RCH expenditure of all states for the year 2013–14, see: Report of PFI et al. 2014:0.4.
10. The experience from Malda, West Bengal in 2013 and Kaparfora Bihar, 2012 show the blatant breach of medical standards and ethics."100 Women Kept in Open Field After Undergoing Surgery in Malda District." *Times of India*. February 7. Accessed June 18, 2014. http://timesofindia.indiatimes.com/city/kolkota/100-women-kept-in-open-field-undergoijng-surgery-in-Malda-distict/articlesshow/18,380,887.cms
11. Article 25 of the Universal Declaration of Human Rights: Article 12 of the International Covenant on Economic, Social and Cultural Rights; Article 12 of the Convention on the Elimination of All Forms of Discrimination Against Women; Declaration of Alma—Ata, 1978; Programme for Action of the International Conference on Population and Development, Cairo, 1994; Platform for Action for the Fourth World Women's Conference, Beijing, 1995; and International Heath Regulation, 58th World Health Assembly, 2005.
12. Writ Petition(s) (Civil) No(s). 95/2.

References

Bagcchi, S. (2015). "Thirteen women die from mass sterilization in Chhattisgarh. *British Medical Journal., 349*, g6868.

Baxi, U. (1985). "Taking suffering seriously: Social action litigation in the supreme court of India." *Third World Legal Studies*. 107–132.

Das, A., & Contractor, S. (2014). India's Latest Sterilisation Camp Massacre. *British Medical Journal., 349*, g7282.

Erdman, J. N. (2015). Commentary: Bioethics, human rights, and childbirth. *Health and Human Rights, 17*(1), E43.

Hartmann, B., & Rao, M. (2015). "India's population programme".. *Economic and Political Weekly, L*(44), 10–13.

Human Rights Law Network. (2014). "Fact-Finding Report on Sterilisation, Access to Contraceptive Information and Services, and Women's Health in Bilaspur District, Chhattisgarh." November 14–18. Accessed February 14, 2015. http://www.hrln.org/hrln/reproductive-rights/reports/1661-fact-finding-report-on-sterilisation-access-to-contraceptive-information-and-ser vices-and-women's-health-in-bilaspur-district-chhattisgarh-14-18-november-2014.html#ixzz44ZXaYP00.

Krishnan, V. (2016). "Victims of the number game." *The Hindu*, March 25. Accessed April 23, 2016. http://www.thehindu.com/opinion/op- ed/victims-of-the-numbers-game/article8393771.ece.

Ministry of Health and Family Welfare. (2009). "GoI Working Draft Version 2009 The National Health Bill 2009." Accessed March 19, 2015 http://www.prsindia.org/uploads/media/Draft_National_Bill.pdf.

Ministry of Health and Family Welfare. (2010). "District Level Household and Facility Survey 2007–08. Fact Sheet." Accessed March 20, 2015. www.rchiips.org/pdf/rch3/state/ijndia.pdf.

Ministry of Health and Family Welfare. (2013). "Health and Family Welfare Statistics." Accessed March 20, 2015. https://nrhm-mis.nic.in/PubFWStatistics%202013/Section%20B%20-Family%20Planning.pdf.

Nadda, J. P. (2016). "Family planning is critical for our nation's development." *The Indian Express*. April 5. Accessed May 25, 2016. http://indianexpress.com/article/opinion/columns/family-planning-child-mortality-planning-the-future/.

Population Foundation of India, Parivar Seva Sansthan, Family Planning Association of India and Common Health. (2014). "Robbed of Choice and Dignity: Indian Women Dead After Mass Sterilisation: Report of Situational Assessment of Sterilisation Camps in Bilaspur District, Chhattisgarh." New Delhi.

Pulla, P. (2014). Why are women dying in India's sterilization camps? *British Medical Journal, 349*, g7509.

Qadeer, I. (2010). "New reproductive technologies and healthcare in neo-liberal India: Essays." *Monograph*, 1–73. New Delhi, Centre For Women's Development Studies.

Qadeer, I. (2013). Universal healthcare: The trojan horse of neoliberal policies. *Social Change, 43*, 149–164.

Qadeer, I., & Ghosh, S. M. (2016). "Public Health's in the Infirmary" Accessed April 23, 2016. http://www.thehindubusinessline.com/opinion/public-healths-in-the-infirmary/ article8486437.ece.

Sarojini, N., Sri, S. B., Ambhore, V., & Venkatachalam, D. (2015). "Bilaspur sterilisation deaths: Evidence of oppressive population control policy." *Indian Journal of Medical Ethics* 12(1) (January- March), 2–5.

Som, M. (2014). "Women as primary providers of healthcare in the mitanin programme: Gender, social and organisational constraints." In *Samyukta-Special Issue on Dynamics of Women's Health in India* 14, No. 2 (July): 153–67.

WHO. (2014). "Ensuring Human Rights in the Provision of Contraceptive Information and Services." Accessed June 18, 2014. http://www.who.int/reproductivehealth/publications/family_planning/human-rights-contraception/en/.

Yamin, A. E. (2014). Promoting equity in health: What role for courts? *Health and Human Rights, 16*(2), 1–9.

Chapter 9
Universal Healthcare and Universalising Health Insurance: Examining the Binary Through the RSBY/MSBY in Chhattisgarh

Rajib Dasgupta, Sulakshana Nandi, Kanica Kanungo, Madhurima Nundy, Ganapathy Murugan, Samir Garg, Dipa Sinha, Sangeeta Sahu, and Reeti Mahobe

Introduction

The Rashtriya Swasthya Bima Yojana (RSBY) is a state-funded health insurance scheme in India, targeted at families living Below Poverty Line (BPL). Operationalised in 2007–08 it is designed as an innovative and pro-poor scheme for providing equitable healthcare and cushioning from catastrophic health expenditure, it has created considerable interest among both public health scholars and practitioners. The scheme provides coverage for a family of up to five members with a cap per year of INR 30,000 ($ 600). It provides standardised packages for surgical procedures as well as reimbursements for hospital admissions for medical causes. The state invites bids from private or public insurance companies (licensed by the Insurance Regulatory Development Authority (IRDA) for providing the insurance

R. Dasgupta (✉)
Centre of Social Medicine and Community Health, Jawaharlal Nehru University, New Delhi, India

S. Nandi
Co-convener of Public Health Movement, New Delhi, India

K. Kanungo
Public Health Resource Network (PHRN), New Delhi, India

M. Nundy
Institute of Chinese Studies, New Delhi, India

G. Murugan
Executive Director, Public Health Resource Network (PHRN), New Delhi, India

S. Garg
State Health Research Centre, Chattisgarh, India

D. Sinha · S. Sahu · R. Mahobe
Ambedkar University Delhi, New Delhi, India

I. Qadeer et al. (eds.), *Universalising Healthcare in India*,
https://doi.org/10.1007/978-981-16-5872-3_9

cover. Enrolment and annual renewal of cards is the responsibility of Third Party Administrator (TPA)[1], selected by the insurance company.

Other state-supported insurance schemes have been in operation for several years and provide insights on issues of enrolment, empanelment of hospitals, utilisation and cost of hospitalisation, Out of Pocket Expenditure (OOPE), insurance premium, adequacy and appropriateness of the packages, issues in access, and systems of monitoring, transparency and grievance redressal. Many of those had limited effectiveness due to poor policy design, lack of clear accountability, lack of sustained efforts in implementation, weak monitoring and evaluation, unclear roles and responsibilities of stakeholders, and poor awareness among beneficiaries (Das and Leino, 2011; Mahal & Fan, 2011; Nundy et al., 2013; Rajasekhar et al., 2011).

There has been a growing tendency to pass off health insurance as Health for All. As the Jan Swasthya Abhiyan (JSA) (2012) argues, this has a 'critical implication for both the diminishing meaning of health for all and the role and responsibility of the government in ensuring that it is truly achieved (Ibid.) A recent article claimed that by extending health insurance coverage through RSBY to the entire state, Chhattisgarh would attain 'Health Cover for All' from 2012.

This chapter illustrates some key issues through two studies from Chhattisgarh, socio-economically one of the weakest among the states of the Indian union, with a high proportion of tribal population. The first study is unique in being a qualitative study (most studies focus on beneficiary experiences, both quantitative and qualitative) undertaken to gain an understanding of the provider perspectives in order to focus on design issues that have relevance for both policy and practice. The second study makes use of the state offering a 'natural experiment' scenario in this context. In addition to RSBY, the state government launched the Mukhyamantri Swasthya Bima Yojana (MSBY) in 2012 for the non-BPL families with identical provisions as the RSBY, thereby universalising health insurance coverage. This Universal Health Insurance Scheme (UHIS) is being promoted as the strategy to attain Universal Health Coverage (UHC) in Chhattisgarh. Private and public hospitals have been empanelled for providing services under both RSBY and MSBY.

Provider Perspectives

We present key findings of the qualitative study that focused on provider perspectives and design-related issues. We sampled three districts in Chhattisgarh from among those in the second phase of RSBY implementation and included empanelled private-for-profit (small 10–20-bedded nursing homes and multi-specialty corporate hospitals), public (medical college, district and sub-district hospitals) and not-for- profit (low-cost and Christian missionary) institutions; state level administrators were also interviewed (Dasgupta et al., 2013). The study sought to capture opinions, motivations, behaviours and attitudes of key stakeholders within their organisational and socio-cultural matrix. The unique feature of this study was identifying design-related issues that could affect treatment procedures and implementation of

Table 9.1 Typology and numbers of institutions

Units	Numbers
Districts	3 [Raipur, Dhamtari and Balod]
Private hospitals	9
• Super specialty	2
• Nursing homes	7
Public hospitals	5
• Medical colleges	1
• District hospitals	1
• Community health centre	2
• Primary health centres	1
• Not-for-profit hospitals	4
• Mission hospitals	3
• Trust hospital	1

the universal insurance scheme. Open-ended semi-structured in-depth interviews (with pre-defined topic guides) were conducted with a range of providers. Detailed notes were taken by research team members and analysed to assess similarities and differences in perceptions across stakeholders. We did not find differences in observations between the districts. Tables 9.1 and 9.2 detail the institutional and respondent profiles.

We present our thematic findings below. Issues of enrolment, settlement and related technological glitches are cross-cutting issues. A unique feature of this study is the documentation of contrasting experiences of public (government) hospitals, for profit (private—both individual owned as well as corporate) and not for profit (mostly but not exclusively missionary) hospitals.

Table 9.2 Respondents' profile

Units	Numbers
Doctors-cum-RSBY in-charges [hospitals]	9
Doctors	8
Hospital managers	5
Medical college officials	1
Block level officials	6
RSBY Data Entry Operators	10
District level officials	6
State level officials	3

Technology

The internet-based technology involves swiping the beneficiary card and doubly verifying the thumb impression with a scanner. Some rural areas of the study districts lack reliable internet connectivity; there are options for offline operations though, a provision hardly being used.

It was often not possible to swipe the card within 24 h of admission or discharge. This along with the lack of training to the implementers was leading to rejection of claims. Another critical limitation that emerged was the inability to swipe the card more than once in 24 h; this would be a necessity for changing the category, for example (and fairly commonly) from normal delivery to the caesarean section and, referral to a higher-level institution. Some of these drawbacks have been resolved in the subsequent years.

Annual renewal of cards was consistently reported as affecting the providers as much as the beneficiaries. The software at the institutions needs to be changed with the change of TPA. Following the change of the TPA from E MediTek in 2010–11 to MedSave in 2011–12, three out of four Primary Health Centres (PHCs) in Raipur district did not have the software updated and was unable to treat RSBY patients till the first few months of 2012. State level administrators considered enrolment of beneficiaries through TPAs as a conflict of interest as the insurance company—for whom the lesser usage of insurance translates into more profits—contracts the TPA both for enrolment and for processing the claims.

This was corroborated by two studies undertaken in Chhattisgarh during 2011–12 on enrolment and coverage in tribal and remote areas. The studies found that no enrolment was done in remote and inaccessible villages (Nandi et al., 2012a, b).Enrolment was low (32%) among the Particularly Vulnerable Tribal Groups (PVTGs).

Settlement of Claims

Settlement was irregular except for the claims at the medical college (located at the state capital, Raipur). The TPA in 2012 was unanimously reported to be more responsive than the previous one, notwithstanding the delays. Private hospitals were of the view that at least some reimbursements kept coming in. Delays were reported to be up to six months to two years. About 10–15% of the settlements were rejected. The bigger private institutions explained that the claims were resolved when a detailed explanation was provided. The reason most cited for rejection was that the number of days of stay exceeded that given in the package. 10% tax was deducted at source as per standard government regulations. Not-for-profit institutions claimed that they were exempted from this tax; this was a provision not being implemented. There was no functioning grievance redressal system. The providers met once a month with the officials of the State Nodal Agency (SNA) to discuss these issues; there was unanimity in their opinions that much of their problems remained unresolved.

For-Profit (Private) Hospitals

Small nursing homes, typically owned by specialist husband-wife partnerships have made the most of the scheme. Patients with chronic conditions, complications or requiring prolonged and costly treatment were mostly referred to government institutions. Patient volumes have increased considerably in these hospitals and incomes have gone up. Most institutions reported up to 50–70% occupancy on account of RSBY patients. The corporate hospitals reported only 5–10% of occupancy on account of RSBY smart card holders. They were also empanelled with other public and private insurance companies; and in addition had a large clientele who paid out-of-pocket.

As the institutions were not accredited for specific services, institutions/doctors could pick and choose conditions that have profitable package rates. Doctors reported treating mostly simple/ uncomplicated conditions. Thus, most of the hospitals were providing an extremely narrow and selective band of services. Gynaecologists preferred hysterectomy that offered a reasonable margin but not caesarean section. In ophthalmology, it was cataract that was being performed more than any other procedure.

Packages were unanimously reported to be priced considerably lower than those charged to the paying patients. The packages did not cover for treatment of complicated ailments which often entail multiple conditions that the packages did not account for. High end procedures, onco-surgeries and complicated orthopaedic surgeries for example, were few and far between as packages were reported to be too low. In order to limit RSBY patients several institutions reported earmarking a fixed number of beds. One super-specialty hospital, treating patients from different districts of the state, reported difficulty in reimbursement in cases of patients from districts with other TPAs.

Public Hospitals

Across levels (primary-secondary-tertiary), about 80–90% of the claims were for medical conditions. Surgical conditions/procedures formed a minuscule proportion of the claims, except in the medical college where a multitude of conditions were being treated; the most frequent ones included cancer chemotherapy and animal bites. Minor surgeries (such as incision/drainage of abscesses), closed reduction of fractures and tubectomies were commonly being performed under this scheme.

There were no packages for specific medical conditions; they were claimed at the rate of INR 750 per day of hospitalisation. Within this limit, it was not possible to provide for conditions that require long- drawn hospitalisation and cost-intensive treatment such as snake bite, poisoning (commonly, organo-phosphorus poisoning) and burns. Conditions such as psychiatric illnesses and suicidal attempts were not covered. Cases of animal bites were often admitted for anti-rabies vaccination.

Analysis of samples of claims (for different seasons) revealed that common conditions such as diarrhoea and respiratory infections formed about half the admissions. The other half consisted of conditions such as anaemia and weakness (innovatively billed as 'weakness and hypocalcaemia'). Patients were typically admitted for three to five days, investigated (for anaemia and other chronic conditions, say blood sugar) and provided a stock of medicines such as haematinics and anti-diabetics. An analysis of costs of treatment (using Standard Treatment Guidelines of the state and current prices of generic medicines available through outlets run in government hospitals) revealed that cost of medicines for treating common morbidities such as diarrhoea, malaria, respiratory infections and viral fevers was about INR 100, whereas hospitals were admitting patients for up to five days and charging INR 3750.

Twenty-five percent of the package cost was earmarked for incentives to all categories of personnel (in public institutions) including administrative staff; no institution reported disbursing it. State level administrators explained that the purpose of the incentive was to prevent patients being diverted to private facilities by the hospital staff. The administrator at one of the public hospitals said that there has not been any significant increase in revenue being earned by them due to RSBY. This is also because some of the funds earlier given for maintenance have been withdrawn after RSBY was introduced.

Not-For-Profit Hospitals

These institutions provided a natural 'control', located somewhere in the middle of the spectrum of experience of private and public institutions. The three sampled hospitals had bed strengths ranging from 75 to 200. The larger of these institutions performed a fair range of services including general surgeries, orthopaedic procedures and chemotherapy. Many of the RSBY packages were priced higher than their rates. The pattern was opposite in the smaller 75-bedded mission hospitals. They reported incurring losses if they had to hire a surgeon or gynaecologist not on their staff; this phenomenon was also reported by smaller for-profit nursing homes. These bigger institutions reported a sizeable increase in the number of patients. One of the mission hospitals had a separate RSBY medicine counter to keep accounts of the costs incurred. While not compromising on the quality of services, certain cost-cutting measures were commonly resorted to; for example, cheaper silk sutures were used rather than the absorbable.

Beneficiary Perspectives

The second study was conducted in the slums of Raipur, the capital and largest city of Chhattisgarh (Nandi et al., 2016). Chhattisgarh ranks second amongst all Indian states in terms of proportion of slum population in urban areas (31.9%) and

Raipur ranks sixth among cities with the highest slum population (nearly 40%) (CRISIL, 2014). There are 282 slums listed in Raipur city with more than 80,000 households. Under the National Urban Health Mission (NUHM) there has been introduction of urban Mitanins (Community Health Workers), Swasthya Suvidha Kendras (SSKs) led by Auxiliary Nurse Midwives (ANMs) and an increase in the number of Urban PHCs. Free transport service for general emergencies (108) and for pregnancy-related emergencies (102) are also operational. Various government programmes and schemes related to reproductive health (for example, the Janani Suraksha Yojana (JSY) and the Janani Shishu Suraksha Karyakram (JSSK)) and national disease control programmes are also operational. At about the same time, the MSBY was introduced to make the state-supported insurance scheme available for people Above the Poverty Line (APL).

Private and public hospitals have been empanelled for providing services under both RSBY and MSBY. The total number of families enrolled under RSBY and MSBY in the state, in 2011, were 2.14 million and 1.67 million ("Chhattisgarh Sasan" n.d)respectively. Enrolment was 57% in Raipur district; data was not available for Raipur city separately. Raipur had the highest number (136) of empanelled facilities of the total empanelled hospitals (628) in Chhattisgarh, 56% of these were in the private sector. Significantly, 93% of the empanelled facilities in Raipur city were in the private sector.

As per available data ("District-wise Claims" n.d.), private facilities had made 62% of the total number of claims in 2011, amounting to an average claim amount of INR 7,532. On the other hand, public facilities made an average claim amount of INR 4,443. Private facilities in Raipur district accounted for 80% of the claims with an average claim amount of INR 7,291 and the average claim amount by public facilities was INR 4,662. Significantly, 72% of the rejected claims in the district were from the public sector.

This quantitative study was undertaken to understand the extent to which women in slums of the urban areas of Chhattisgarh were able to access the intended benefits of UHIS for hospitalisation care in public and private health facilities. The specific objectives were:

- Assess coverage of women under UHIS in terms of enrolment, medical conditions and utilization.
- Assess the extent to which cashless treatment was available under UHIS and to examine OOPE incurred.
- Compare differences between the public and private health facilities in the above aspects

The sample constituted of people who had been hospitalised in the last six months prior to the study in 2012. In order to select the sample, 50 (urban) Mitanins (community health workers) were selected through simple random sampling out of 1,010 Mitanins in Raipur city. The sampled Mitanins were asked about all hospitalisations in the last six months in the respective populations that they served and a line list was drawn up. The surveyors interviewed all the listed cases. In addition, surveyors also used the snowball technique to expand the sample size.

Under the Mukhyamantri Sheheri Swasthya Karyakram, one Mitanin covers approximately 500 slum population. It was expected that as the rate of hospitalisation/population as per the National Sample Survey (NSS) 60th round was 2.4% in 365 days, i.e. 1.2% in six months, the slum population covered by 50 Mitanins (i.e. 25,000) would provide at least 300 respondents. The number of families finally sampled was 323. The total number of patients that emerged was 367 (284 females and 83 males) and all of them were included. This chapter documents the experience of women patients. In the current analysis, data of two women patients were removed as they had accessed health facilities outside the state.

A structured interview schedule was used that had three parts.

Part A listed the number of family members and documented which member was enrolled under RSBY/MSBY and how many times each member was hospitalised in the last six months. This was done to re- check information provided by Mitanins.

Part B documented the profile of the family, and, experience of enrolment in RSBY/MSBY and renewal of the insurance smart cards. The profile included components like entitlement under PDS, type of housing, fuel, source of drinking water, availability of electricity and toilet.

Part C documented specific events and experiences of hospitalisation in the last six months.

Women comprised the largest proportion of beneficiaries; the relevant findings are summarised below.

Demographic and Socio-Economic Characteristics of the Female Patients

The highest proportion of female patients belonged to the Other Backward Castes (OBC) (65%), followed by Scheduled Castes (SC) (17%), General Category (13%) and Scheduled Tribes (ST) (4%).The highest percentage (85%) of the female patients was in the age group of 18 to 45 years. Eight percent were below 18 years of age while 7% of the women were above 45 years of age.

The main sources of income for the families of the women patients were labour (47%); followed by service (30%) generally in the informal sector; and, small business/self-employment (19%). More than half (56%) the families of the women patients were entitled to receiving highly subsidised grain, while 19% did not have a ration card.

This profile corresponds well to the profile of slum population surveyed in the urban baseline survey on health by the State Health Resource Centre, Chhattisgarh (SHRC, 2013) and the census data, thus confirming a fair degree of representativeness.

Enrolment

Among 323 sampled families 66% of the family members were enrolled. There was no gender differential in the overall enrolment. A slightly higher percentage of women (68%) were enrolled than men (65%). Disaggregated by age, more boys (81%) in the 6–18 years age group were enrolled than girls (74%). A slightly higher percentage of men (90%) were enrolled than women (88%) in the age group over 45 years.

In a sample of 282 women patients chosen from among the 323 families; 57% reported that their families were enrolled. Disaggregated by social categories, enrolment patterns conformed to the expected social gradient: highest among General Category (63%) followed by SC (57%) and OBC (57%). The lowest enrolment was reported among ST (44%).

Of the families who were enrolled, enrolment under RSBY (42%) and MSBY (43%) was nearly the same; 15% of the beneficiaries could not specify the scheme in which they were enrolled. They were included in the enrolled category and data analysed as they were able to answer all the other questions related to enrolment and benefits.

Reasons for non-enrolment were reported to be: not having information regarding the enrolment drive (35%); name missing from the list (16%); certain family members being not available at the time of enrolment drive (13%); unaware of the scheme (10%). Eight percent reported not receiving the card despite enrolment. Other reasons included being refused enrolment, not having an identity card and not interested in enrolling.

Among the enrolled families, 57% had enrolled in 2013 for the first time while 24% had first enrolled in 2011. Of the families who had enrolled in 2013, 69% were MSBY card holders while 17% were RSBY card holders and the rest were not aware of the type of card. Significantly, of the 65 families enrolled before 2013, only 46% had renewed their cards in 2013. Fifty-seven percent of those enrolled received the insurance smart card on the day of enrolment (the norm), 31% received between 1 to 5 days and another 8% by 15 days. INR 30 was charged for enrolment; 97% reported paying the stipulated amount. It was stipulated that the list of empanelled hospitals had to be given along with the smart card; only 5% reported receiving it.

Hospitalisation

Conditions for Which Women Were Hospitalised

Seventy-eight percent of women were hospitalised for obstetrics and gynaecological conditions, including 72% for delivery. Among men, respiratory conditions and water/food-borne diseases (including jaundice and typhoid) were the most common conditions for hospitalisation. Of the total number of hospitalisations for non- gynaecological conditions, women constituted 43% while men constituted 57%. Table 9.3 details the profile of conditions for which female and male respondents were hospitalised.

Table 9.3 Profile of Conditions for which Female and Male Respondents were Hospitalised

	Female (n)	Female (percent)	Male (n)	Male (percent)	Total (n)	Total (percent)
A. Pregnancy-related	205	72			205	56
Delivery	202	71			202	55
Miscarriage/ANC	3	1			3	1
B. Other gynaecological	17	6			17	5
Uterine problems	3	1			3	1
Tubectomy	14	5			14	4
C. Non-gynaecological	62	22	83	100	145	40
Accident	1	0	2	2	3	1
Respiratory diseases	5	2	10	12	15	4
Weakness/anaemia/malnutrition	5	2	3	4	8	2
Cancer	3	1	0	0	3	1
Cataract	5	2	6	7	11	3
Diarrhoea and vomiting	7	2	5	6	12	3
Fever/malaria/dengue	3	1	3	4	6	2
Fracture	6	2	4	5	10	3
Heart-related	3	1	5	6	8	2
Gastroenteritis	1	0	6	7	7	2
Mental illnesses	0	0	1	1	1	0
Paralysis/nerve/brain related	1	0	6	7	7	2
Sickle cell disease	3	1	1	1	4	1
TB	1	0	4	5	5	1
Jaundice/typhoid	5	2	10	12	15	4
Leprosy	1	0	0	0	1	0
Appendicitis/Appendectomy	1	0	2	2	3	1
Burn	2	1	0	0	2	1
Hernia	0	0	2	2	2	1
Hydrocele	0	0	2	2	2	1
Kidney Problem	3	1	1	1	4	1
Pancreatitis	0	0	1	1	1	0
Others	6	2	9	11	15	4
Total (A + B + C)	284	100	83	100	367	100

In the aggregate, 57% of women accessed the public sector for the conditions reported, 37% the private sector and 5% accessed both. A higher proportion of women whose families were not enrolled went to the public sector for all conditions. The women accessed the public sector more for pregnancy (63%) and other gynaecological conditions (76%); the trend was opposite for non- gynaecological conditions, 55% accessed the private sector.

A total of 325 visits were made by 282 women during the recall period. 234 (72%) visits were to a facility empanelled under UHIS. While most of the public facilities visited were empanelled (90%), only half of the private facilities used were UHIS empanelled (47%).

The main reasons for selection of the facility included: familiarity with the facility (38%), suggestion or referral by someone (46%) and proximity to place of residence (6%). More than half the women (58%) went to the public sector because somebody had suggested to them to go there or referred them. Fifty% of the women going to the private sector reported that they usually accessed that particular facility. 'Choice' of a provider, one of the hallmarks of the insurance schemes seemed to be a determinant for only 8% of women going to the public facility and for 5% of women going to the private facility.

A higher proportion of visits were made to empanelled public facilities than to private facilities. While 58% of the visits to private facilities were to an empanelled one, 42% of the visits were to a non-empanelled facility (Table 9.4). Out of 325 visits, empanelment status for 12 facilities could not be determined.

Utilisation of the UHIS

About a fifth (21%) of the sampled beneficiaries were able to use the insurance card at least once for treatment during the recall period. Only about a third (36%) of the women, who had insurance cards (161), used it for treatment. Forty-one percent of the men who had insurance cards (51) used it for treatment at least once during this period. For women, the card was least used for pregnancy-related conditions (33%) and most for non-gynaecological conditions (44%) (Table 9.5). In terms of visits to facilities, 18% (59 women) of the total 325 visits to facilities involved usage of insurance cards.

On disaggregating the data into utilisation of public and private providers, the usage of cards was found to be higher for the private sector (49%) for all conditions when compared to the public sector (24%), (Table 9.5).

Fifty percent of those who underwent hospitalisation were not enrolled for either scheme and therefore could not use the card. This is significant as this is a 'universal' insurance scheme and receives considerable commitment and support from the state. Sixteen percent women accessing the public sector reported that the hospital did not ask for the card and another 13% reported that the card was not renewed. The principal reason for non-utilisation of the card for those accessing private institutions was that the hospital was not empanelled. In 7% of cases, the patient was not enrolled

Table 9.4 Choice of empanelled versus non-empanelled facilities

Enrolment status	Public		Private		Combined	
	Empanelled	Non-empanelled	Empanelled	Non-empanelled	Empanelled	*Non-empanelled*
Enrolled	*97*	*3*	*58*	*42*	*78*	*22*
Not enrolled	*89*	*11*	*33*	*67*	*70*	*30*

Table 9.5 Utilisation of cards in public and private sectors*

Conditions	Public		Private		Went to both		Combined	
	Card used atleast once by cardholder	Card not used by cardholder	Card used atleast once by cardholder	Card not used by cardholder	Card used atleast once by cardholder	Card not used by cardholder	Card used atleast once by cardholder	Card not used by cardholder
Pregnancy-related	23	77	48	52	33	67	33	67
Other gynaeco-logical	0	100	100	0	0	0	25	75
Non-gynaecological	35	65	48	52	50	50	44	56
Total	24	76	49	51	43	57	36	64

* Numbers of women patients

Table 9.6 Reasons for non-utilisation of the RSBY/MSBY Cards

Reason for not using card	Public (%)	Private (%)	Combined (%)
No smart card	55	42	50
Hospital staff did not ask for smart card	16	7	12
Card was not renewed	13	6	10
Services under RSBY/MSBY card not provided there	0	22	9
Patient not registered under smart card	7	7	7
Hospital authority refused to treat under RSBY/MSBY smart card	2	7	4
Others	6	7	6
Don't Know	0	4	1
Total	100	100	100

as part of her family's card. In 2% of cases in public facilities and in percent of the cases in private facilities, the hospital refused to treat under the insurance scheme; the reasons were not shared with the patient and the family (Table 9.6).

Out of the total number of visits to empanelled facilities (234), 61% had cards; nearly two-thirds to public facilities. Of these cardholders who went to an empanelled facility, only 41% could use the card for treatment. The usage was least for gynaecological conditions and the highest for non-gynaecological conditions. Card usage in empanelled private facilities (71%) was higher than in empanelled public facilities (25%). The reasons for non-utilisation of cards in empanelled facilities were that either the card was not renewed, or the hospital did not ask for the card. The latter was more so in the case of public facilities.

Nearly two-thirds of the women with cards were not aware of the toll free number for complaints and grievance redressal; only one woman had filed a complaint.

Oope

Ninety-six percent (271 women) of the women reported incurring out OOPE. The average OOPE was INR 9,947. More than half of the OOPE (52%) was on account of fees charged by the facility. Expenditure incurred on medicines contributed to 18% and investigation and tests contributed to 15% of the expenditure.

Of the women who incurred OOPE, 90% had to spend on transportation, followed by medicines (76%). Nearly half of the women reported paying money to the doctor/nurse and pay for fees charged by the hospital.

Disaggregating by clinical conditions, the highest expenditure was incurred for heart related conditions (INR 1,22,800), followed by cancer (INR 52,828, appendectomy (INR 52,980), fracture (INR 44,000) and kidney conditions (INR 40,780) (Table 9.7).

Table 9.7 Average OOPE for Different Clinical Conditions

Clinical Condition	*Average OOPE*	*n*
Pregnancy related	10,352	3
Respiratory diseases	26,794	5
Weakness/anaemia/malnutrition	9,770	5
Cancer	52,828	3
Cataract surgery	8,810	5
Delivery	6,646	200
Diarrhoea and vomiting	3,936	7
Fever/malaria/dengue	5,467	3
Fracture	44,000	6
Heart related	1,22,800	3
Sickle cell disease	15,433	3
Jaundice/typhoid	1,898	5
Burns	22,650	2
Kidney problem	40,780	3
Uterus problem	4,235	3
Tubectomy	480	14
Total	9,947	282

When average OOPE is calculated for the total number of visits made (n=325) to a facility it works out to an average INR 8,624 per visit. The average OOPE for women in the private facility was more than six times higher than in the public facility.

Women incurred OOPE despite using the RSBY/MSBY card for treatment. The average OOPE incurred was much higher for women who have used the card in private facilities (INR 10,733) than in public facilities (INR 2,518).

More than one-third of the women (37%) borrowed money in order to pay for treatment. Sixty-one percent used their savings. Four women had to sell jewellery or some other valuable items while three women had to mortgage valuables in order to pay for treatment.

Childbirth

The single most important cause for hospitalisation of women was childbirth; 200 deliveries were reported from among 282 women users. About 145 were normal deliveries, while 55 women (28%) had caesarean section (C-section). Sixty-three percent accessed public facilities for childbirth, principally the District Hospital and Medical College in Raipur. Forty-two percent of women accessing private facilities had C-section compared to 19% in public facilities. Cards were used in 17% of the cases; 28% in the private sector and 10% in the public sector. The utilisation of insurance was higher for C-section than for normal deliveries, with a higher proportion in private facilities (32%) than in public ones (21%). Of the cardholders accessing empanelled facilities 73% used it in private empanelled facilities and 23% in public facilities.

The average amount booked under insurance for normal deliveries in private hospitals was more than twice the amount booked for the same in the public sector (INR 7,607 versus INR 3,775). However, for C-section, the average amount booked in the public sector was slightly higher than the average amount booked in the private sector (INR 13,333 versus INR 12,388).

Current Concerns

Chhattisgarh provides universal health insurance through the RSBY and MSBY schemes. While the RSBY coverage is restricted to BPL families, MSBY seeks to make the scheme universal. The introduction of the MSBY in 2013 increased the insurance coverage. However the study found 43% of the urban slum population in Raipur city continued to lack coverage, though enrolment was not very different for men and women as well as for different social groups.

While awareness of the schemes is high, many were unable to enrol due to problems in the enrolment process such as lack of information regarding enrolment date, name not being listed for enrolment, enrolment not being possible without certain family members and not being given the insurance smart card on the same day of enrolment (as is the norm). Similar findings have emerged from other studies (CTRD, 2012; Das and Leino, 2011; Grover and Palacios, 2011; Rajsekhar et al. 2011).

We found that while most of the accessed public facilities were empanelled (90%), only half of the private facilities used were UHIS empanelled (47%). In our study, of the enrolled women who visited private facilities, 58% visited empanelled facilities while 42% visited non-empanelled facilities. Of the 5% beneficiaries who did receive a list of the empanelled hospitals, half of the women went to private empanelled facilities, but that too because they usually visited that particular hospital. This implies that the patients may not be convinced about the utility or efficacy of UHIS and therefore other considerations carry more weight.

The main objective of the UHIS is to protect beneficiaries from catastrophic health expenditure. It is therefore restricted to medical care. We found that despite the limited roll out of UHIS, women were continuing to incur very high expenditure for hospitalisation, an average of INR 9,947. Only 4% of women did not incur OOPE. Nearly all had to spend money on transportation, two-thirds had to spend on medicines and nearly half had to pay money to health personnel and pay fees charged by the facility. Various schemes have been introduced in recent years for the promotion of institutional deliveries such as JSY (for providing monetary incentives), JSSK (for providing free services during pregnancy, delivery and post-natal period) and 108 and 102 for emergency transport and referral. Under UHIS too, there are packages for Ante Natal Care (ANC) and deliveries (normal and C- section). Despite this myriad of schemes and entitlements, we found that women incurred high OOPE in both public and private facilities, with an average of INR 6,240 per visit for delivery. Only 2% of visits did not entail OOPE. Studies on JSY and JSSK have found that women continue to incur high OOPE for delivering in public facilities (Bonu et al., 2009; NHSRC, 2011; SHRC, 2013; Tripathi et al., 2014).

Such high expenditure can be catastrophic for the poor with more than one-third (37%) of the respondents reporting that they had to borrow money in order to pay for the hospitalisation expenses. Other studies on publicly funded insurance schemes have also found that people have to incur expenses in spite of using insurance (CTRD 2012; Grover and Palacios, 2011; Nandi et al., 2012; Rajasekhar et al., 2011). Moreover, the emerging evidence on irrational procedures and prolonged hospitalisation for normal procedures, as stated by the provider, indicates a distorted rationality in order to get more state funds through claims, including the threat of an artificial increase in healthcare costs.

Global evidence on the efficacy of these schemes on financial risk protection and health outcomes is far from encouraging. There is adequate evidence that health insurance schemes for the informal sector in low and middle income countries suffer from several drawbacks: low uptake, and, no strong evidence of impact on utilisation, financial protection or health status (Acharya et al., 2013). Undeniably, few insurance schemes provide protection for high level of OOPE, but this impact is weaker on the poor. Our study on experiences of utilisation of the RSBY/MSBY in the context of urban poor women is no departure from this trend. Universal insurance is clearly no guarantor of universal access and not a reliable route to universal healthcare.

Notes

1. TPA is the agency employed by the insurance company to undertake enrolment and to process the claims by the empanelled hospitals. The change was on account of the contract of the previous firm coming to an end and another firm appointed in the next year.

References

"Chhattisgarh Sasan—Rashtriya Swasthya Bima Yojana, Mukhyamantri Swasthya Bima Yojana." n.d. Accessed September 14, 2014. http://cg.nic.in/healthrsby/.

"District wise Claims Chhattisgarh Sasan—RSBY MSBY." n.d. Accessed September 9, 2014. http://rsbycg.nic.in/healthrsby/reports/Distwiseclaims.aspx.

Acharya, A., Vellakkal, S., Taylor, F., Masset, E., Satija, A., Burke, M., & Ebrahim, S. (2013). "The impact of health insurance schemes for the informal sector in low and middle-income countries: A systematic review." Policy Research Working Paper Series 6324, The World Bank.

Bonu, S., Bhushan, I., Rani, M., & Anderson, I. (2009). "Incidence and correlates of 'catastrophic' maternal healthcare expenditure in India." *Health Policy and Planning* 24, 6(November), 445–56.

Centre for Tribal and Rural Development. (2012). *Final Report on Evaluation of the Rashtriya Swasthya Bima Yojana Scheme in Chhattisgarh.* Chhattisgarh: CTRD.

CRISIL. (2014). *Revised City Development Plan: Raipur (Interim Report).* Accessed September 14, 2014. http://nagarnigamraipur.nic.in.

Das, J., & Leino, J. "Evaluating the RSBY: Lessons from an experimental information campaign." *Economic and Political Weekly* 46, No. 32(August), 85–93

Dasgupta, R., Nandi, S., Kanungo, K., Nundy, M., Murugan, G., & Neog, R. (2013). "What the good doctor said: A critical examination of design issues of the RSBY through provider perspectives in Chhattisgarh, India." *Social Change* 43, No. 2(June), 227–43.

Grover, S., & Palacios, R. (2011). "The first two years of RSBY in Delhi." In *India's Health Insurance Scheme for the Poor: Evidence from the Early Experience of the Rashtriya Swasthya Bima Yojana,* Palacios, R. et al. (Eds.) New Delhi, Centre for Policy Research.

Abhiyan, J. S. (2012). "Jan Swasthya Abhiyan action alert: Dangerous drift in health policy." New Delhi, Jan Swasthya Abhiyan.

Mahal, A., Fan, V. (2011). "Achieving universal coverage in India: An assessment of the policy challenge." *India Policy Forum 2011–12,* Monash University, School of Public Health and Preventive Medicine, Australia and Department of Global Health and Population Harvard School of Public Health, USA.

Nandi, S., Mishra, J. P., Kanungo, K., Manikpuri, H., Yadav, C., Paikra, G., & Upadhyay, V. (2012b). "Public health advocacy to reinstate reproductive rights of particularly vulnerable tribal groups (PTGs) in Chhattisgarh." *BMC Proceedings* (Suppl 5): P1DOI: https://doi.org/10.1186/1753-6561-6-S5-P1. Accessed 19 April, 2018. http://www.biomedcentral.com/1753-6561/6/S5/P1.

Nandi, S., Nundy, M., Prasad, V., Kanungo, K., Khan, H., Haripriya, S., Mishra, T., & Garg, S. (2012a). "The implementation of RSBY in Chhattisgarh, India: A study of the Durg District." *Health, Culture and Society (Health System Dynamics and Barriers)* 2, No. 1, 40–70.

Nandi, S., Dasgupta, R., Kanungo, K., Garg, S., Sinha, D., & Mahobe, R. (2016). "Uncovering coverage: Utilisation of the universal health insurance scheme, Chhattisgarh by women in slums of Raipur." *Indian Journal of Gender Studies* 23, No. 1 (February), 1–26.

National Health Systems Resource Centre (NHSRC). (2011). *Programme Evaluation of the Janani Suraksha Yojana.* New Delhi, NHSRC.

Nundy, M., Dasgupta, R., Kanungo, K., Nandi, S., & Murugan, G.(2013). *The Rashtriya Swasthya Bima Yojana (RSBY) Experience in Chhattisgarh: What Does it Mean for Health For All!* New Delhi, Sama.

Rajasekhar, D., Berg, E., Ghatak, M., Manjula, M., & Roy, S. (2011). "Implementing health insurance: The rollout of Rashtriya Swasthya Bima Yojana in Karnataka." *Economic and Political Weekly* 46, No. 20 (May 14), 56–63.

State Health Resource Center (SHRC). (2013). *Baseline Survey of Health in Urban Slums of Chhattisgarh.* Raipur, SHRC.

Tripathi N., Saini, S.K., & Prinja, S. (2014). "Impact of Janani Shishu Suraksha Karyakram on Out-of-Pocket Expenditure Among Urban Slum Dwellers in Northern India." *Indian Pediatrics* 51 (June 15), 475–477.

Chapter 10
Aarogyasri Scheme in Andhra Pradesh, India: Some Critical Reflections

Sunita Reddy and Immaculate Mary

Introduction

Universal Health Coverage (UHC) is currently being debated all over the world and the ruling Bharatiya Janata Party (BJP) government in India has now brought in the idea of health assurance. Only three countries have achieved UHC so far and a few others are almost reaching that goal. In 2012 China achieved 96% coverage with three insurance schemes successfully introduced. Thailand, Mexico and Turkey are almost there. Even India's neighbouring countries, like Sri Lanka, Bangladesh and Nepal, which are economically poor, are performing better in health. India committed itself to UHC under the Twelfth Five Year plan (Government of India (GoI), 2013), and the National Health Mission(NHM) is resorting to multiple health insurance schemes, like Rashtriya Swasthya BimaYojana (RSBY), Aarogyasri, Yeshaswi Scheme, etc. However, these schemes are fragmented and piecemeal as the budgetary allocation on health in India is far too low.

India is one of the few countries that have public health spending of less than one percent of Gross Domestic Product (GDP), resulting in three quarters of the expense being met by Out-of-Pocket Expenditure (OOPE) spending by individual households. The National Commission on Macroeconomics and Health, in 2005, had pointed out that 3.3% of India's population was getting impoverished every year on account of health distress (GoI, 2005: 3). India's meagre health budget is a cause of, and complicates the existing health inequities, poor quality and high costs. The Government of India has made a commitment to increase public spending on health, which includes water, sanitation and other public health facilities from less than from 1% to 2.5% of the GDP during the next five years (GoI, 2013). Financial protection against medical expenditure is far from universal in coverage with only 10% of

S. Reddy (✉)
Centre of Social Medicine and Community Health, Jawaharlal Nehru University, New Delhi, India

I. Mary
i4 Connect Foundation, Hyderabad, India

I. Qadeer et al. (eds.), *Universalising Healthcare in India*,
https://doi.org/10.1007/978-981-16-5872-3_10

the population having medical insurance. Low level of public financing led to 71% of all spending on health as OOPE causing huge economic burden on households. The government now advocates implementing health-financing mechanisms that will protect the citizens from financially catastrophic effects of illness (Ministry of Health and Family Welfare (MoHFW), 2006).

To achieve universal health coverage, India is adopting both the tax-based regime and also social health insurance. The health insurance programme started with Employees' State Insurance Scheme (ESIS) in 1952 and Central Government Health Scheme (CGHS) in 1954, for unorganised worker population and central government employees respectively. Both these insurance schemes were meant for patients to be treated in public hospitals. Post-structural adjustment reforms, states started buying private healthcare services for the CGHS. Post-2007, several health insurance schemes were started: the RSBY by the Central Ministry of Labour, the Rajiv Gandhi Aarogyasri Scheme by the Andhra Pradesh government, the Vajapayee Aarogyasri and Yeshaswini Cooperative Farmers' Healthcare by the Karnataka government and the Kalaignar Insurance Scheme by the Tamil Nadu government. The RSBY is a national effort largely for secondary level care of common diseases, covering about 3 million people. Whereas, the state social health insurance schemes cover only high end, low frequency diseases and catastrophic illness at tertiary level care and surgical care. The primary and secondary care of general illnesses are not covered by these social insurance schemes.

This chapter presents a case study of the Aarogyasri health insurance scheme also called 'RACHI' (Rajiv Gandhi Aarogyasri Community Health Insurance), launched in 2007 by the state government of Andhra Pradesh. It traces the evolution and motive behind the implementation of the RACHI scheme in 23 districts in Andhra Pradesh prior to the division of the state. The chapter probes the role of key players at different levels: public sector and private sector. It is based on secondary literature available from the Aarogyasri websites, published government reports, newspaper articles and refers to relevant case study reports of the schemes. The chapter analyses how public subsidies flow towards the private sector. It was found that the Aarogyasri scheme is skewed towards the tertiary private care with limited coverage and is run solely on the state subsidies, which is unsustainable. The treatment of the surgeries can be alternatively used to strengthen the public health system, which is more comprehensive in nature and also sustainable.

Is Public Private Partnership in Healthcare Desirable?

Under health sector reforms, one strategy has to collaborate with the private sector through Public Private Partnership (PPP).There are various definitions for partnerships in health. According to the World Health Organisation (WHO) it means to bring together a set of actors for the common goal of improving the health of a population, based on the mutually agreed roles and principles (WHO, 1999). Core elements of a viable partnership are identified as: beneficence (joint gains), autonomy (of each partner), joint-ness (shared decision-making and accountability) and equity (fair returns in proportion to investment and effort) (Venkatraman, 2014). The powerful political forces unleashed by the Structural Adjustment Programme (SAP) and Health Sector Reforms (HSR) (Pollock et al., 2001; Sen, 2001) commodify services. Using the biomedical view of health it promotes technology-based strategies and the resultant expansion of health markets. For the private sector, profitability is the bottom line, ignoring equity and rationality. Bennet et al. (1994) identified five main problems associated with private-for- profit provision of health services. They are related to the use of illegitimate or unethical means to maximise profit, with little concern towards public health goals, lack of interest in sharing clinical information, creating brain drain among public sector health staff and lack of regulatory control over their practices. These concerns caution us against ill-defined partnerships.

Growth of Private Sector

The private health sector in India has grown remarkably over the years. There has been a substantial increase in the number of hospitals under the private sector during the 1990s (Baru, 1999; Hooda, 2015). Health services in India have been tilted towards the private sector from the very beginning. However, from the 1980s onwards the trend has been towards establishing a large tertiary sector, multi-specialty and super specialty hospitals. They were started initially by professionals who, after having worked in the USA or UK, realised the potential of 'healthcare' as an industry with profitable margins. The success of this experiment was followed by scores of businessmen investing in the health sector. These big hospitals have been set up with huge public investments and subsidies by the state in the forms of tax exemptions, land subsidies, buying back services like CGHS and other insurances paying to the private sector for their services (Qadeer and Reddy, 2006). Other important issues relate to 'domestic or internal brain drain', where the doctors trained in government colleges and the mid-career reputed doctors, wooed by the corporate hospitals to serve in their hospitals with huge pay packets, found the offers hard to resist (Reddy & Qadeer, 2010). Thus, it is another way of passing public subsidy to the private sector.

Having promoted the overwhelming presence of the private sector in health, various state governments have been exploring the option of involving the private sector in order to meet the growing healthcare needs of the population. At the central level, the Tenth Five Year Plan (2002–2007) first formalised the need for private sector participation for the healthcare delivery system. At the same time, various state governments have been experimenting with partnerships with the private sector to treat the poor. The Tenth Plan document (GoI, 2002) recognised that private super-specialty tertiary/secondary care hospitals should be given land, water, electricity, etc. at concessional rates and permission for duty free import of equipment with the understanding that they will provide 25% in-patient and 40% out-patient services to poor patients free of charge. The experience in this has been varied and several problems have been reported. In 2000 the Health and Family Welfare Department of the Government of National Capital Territory (NCT) of Delhi constituted a 10-member High Level Committee under the chairpersonship of Justice A.S. Qureshi, to review the existing free treatment facilities extended by the charitable and other private hospitals that had been allotted land on concessional terms by the government. This Committee Report clearly documents the greed, corruption and mismanagement of private and corporate hospitals in Delhi, their indifference and resistance to any monitoring and regulation(Qureshi Committee Report, 2001). None of the corporate hospitals that received land at throwaway prices and tax exemptions followed the lease conditions put forth by the government.

Health Insurance: Benefits to the Private Sector

Health insurance has been accepted by the state as an important financing tool for health security of the poor. At the national level, RSBY was launched. Among the states, the Yeshasvini scheme in Karnataka, Kudumbasree in Kerala and Aarogyasri in Andhra Pradesh were launched to extend coverage to workers in the informal sector. However, most of these schemes are still in the experimental phase (Kumar et al., 2011). Table 10.1 gives a snap shot of all the insurance schemes and their distribution across public and private network hospitals. Thus, emerges a clear picture of domination of the private sector, in accruing the patients and the resources.

A study by Acharya and Ranson (2005) on four community-based health insurance schemes in Gujarat shows that only a pooling of resources, as well as regular pre-payment of received small medical expenses sustains them, otherwise, it is not viable. Thus, these schemes are sustained only due to some form of external support without which they could not have survived on their own. Further, community-based health insurance covers a very small population so has a limited impact from a public health point of view. A critical scrutiny of Aarogyasri by Prasad and Raghavendra (2012) too shows that this scheme is politically driven while, at the same time, it promotes the interest of tertiary corporate hospitals. It is pertinent to see how the RACHI scheme fairs in Andhra Pradesh.

RACHI Scheme

The Government of Andhra Pradesh took several measures to improve access to healthcare and to cut down OOPE through PPP projects. Notable PPPs are the Emergency Management and Referral Institute (EMRI), which implemented 108 Ambulance Service and Health Management Research Institute (HMRI) which provided round-the- clock helpline for medical advice and rural outreach health services. RACHI scheme is one of the outreach strategies of the Government of Andhra Pradesh (Mallipedi et al., 2009). It is the flagship scheme for all health initiatives of

Table 10.1 Distribution of network hospitals

Scheme	Networked Hospitals (2009–10)		Total
	Public	Private	
ESIS	148 (42%)	202 (58%)	350
CGHS	0 (0%)	401 (100%)	401
RSBY	2267 (32%)	4923 (68%)	7190
Rajiv Aarogyasri Scheme (AP)	97 (29%)	241 (71%)	338
Vajpayee Arogyasri Scheme (KN)	08 (5%)	86 (95%)	94
Kalignar (TN)	20 (3%)	643 (97%)	663
Yeshasvini (KN)	29 (6%)	421 (94%)	450

Source Planning commission of India 2011: 52

the state government with a mission to provide quality healthcare to the poor. The state government had set up the Aarogyasri Healthcare Trust under the chairmanship of the Chief Minister to facilitate the effective implementation of the scheme.

Coverage and Budget

The Aarogyasri scheme aims to ensure healthcare for the BPL population at the time of critical and catastrophic illness, through health insurance. Surgeries and therapies are done through an identified network of healthcare providers under the PPP model. Before setting up of RACHI, the Chief Minister's Relief Fund (CMRF) supported the poorest segment at the time of serious health crises. Part of the funds was utilised for the hospitalisation, medical assistance as per individual needs and demands.

The Aarogyasri scheme covered nearly eight crore BPL population in 23 districts of Andhra Pradesh (Aarogyasri Healthcare Trust 2011a). However, an independent study put it to 6.5 crores (Lal, 2017). This scheme provided coverage upto INR 2 lakh per family per year subject to limits in any of the network hospitals (Babu, 2009). The government earmarked INR 925 crore in the financial year (2009–10), which is almost 25% of the total health budget (Table 10.2). The state government is the sole funding agency for this health insurance scheme. The government takes care of the entire premium on behalf of the beneficiary.

Key Stakeholders in RACHI

The key stakeholders in the RACHI scheme are the state government, private insurance company (Chennai-based Star Health and Allied Insurance), Tata Consultancy Services (TCS) for ICT solution (Aarogyasri Healthcare Trust 2011b). One fifty

Table 10.2 Budget allocation for Rajiv aarogyasri community health insurance (2007–10)

Budget Head-Year	2007–08 INR in thousands	2008–09 (Revised Estimates-INR in thousands)	2009–10 (Budget Estimates. INR in thousands)	Total (INR in thousands)
Health Insurance				
for BPL Families	1,406,189	0	0	1,406,189
Aarogyasri Healthcare Trust	0	3,474,000	7,141,000	10,615,000
Tribal Plan	0	297,000	610,500	907,500
SC Plan	0	729,000	1,498,500	2,227,500
Total	1,406,189	4,500,000	9,250,000	15,156,189
Total Health Budget	25,282,162	31,517,836	37,905,004	94,705,002
Percentage of Total Health				
Budget Allocation	6%	14.27%	24.40%	16%

Source www.budget.ap.gov.in and Government of Andhra Pradesh State Health Budget Manual (2007–10)

one government and 275 private sector tertiary hospitals across the state have been involved in implementing the scheme. The hospitals get empanelled[1] for providing treatment for Aarogyasri patients based on the fulfilment of certain criteria[2] set by the trust and insurance company and all those empanelled hospitals, both private and public, are called network hospitals.

The TCS programme director oversees the IT solution[3] and ensures that all the IT needs of the scheme are being addressed on time. The RACHI scheme appointed a key link person, Aarogya Mithra (Health Coordinator), to connect people and the programme at the grass root level. The insurance company appointed Aarogya Mithras at all network hospitals to facilitate admission, treatment and cashless transactions of patients round the clock. The Aarogya Mithras played a key role.[4] The beneficiaries for the RACHI scheme were identified through the white ration cards provided as part of the Annapoorna and Anthyodaya Anna Yojana Scheme for BPL families. It is estimated that about 80% of the population of the state had BPL ration cards and were considered eligible to use the benefits provided by the RACHI scheme. The families, who were covered for specific diseases by other insurance schemes such as CGHS, ESIS, were not considered eligible for any benefits provided in the RACHI scheme. The RACHI scheme incorporated the philosophy of social inclusion in terms of the number of people covered without age limit as well as covering the pre-existing illness[5].

Patients/Beneficiaries were referred from nearby PHC/Area Hospitals/District Hospital or network hospital. Aarogya Mithras placed in the hospitals facilitate the process. The beneficiary could also be referred from health camps conducted by the network hospital in the villages and get the referral card based on the diagnosis. The Aarogya Mithras at the network hospital examine the referral card brought by the beneficiary and also verify the details of the ration card, based on the diagnosis results, admits the patient. After that they send the preauthorisation request to the insurance company and the Aarogyasri Healthcare Trust. Specialists of the insurance company and the trust examine the preauthorisation request and approve it, if all the conditions are satisfied. The network hospital extends cashless treatment and surgery to the beneficiary. Network hospital, after discharge of the patient, forwards the original bill, discharge summary with signature of the patient and other relevant documents to the insurance company for settlement of the claim. The Insurance company scrutinises the bills and approves the same for sanction. The network hospitals also provide follow-up services. The entire scheme is cashless for the beneficiary/ patients for 121 procedures, which are pre-identified (Aarogyasri Healthcare Trust 2011c). The scheme provides insurance for a specific catastrophic illness[6] that can have serious financial repercussions in the lives of the poor. There are specific diseases that are not covered under this scheme.[77] High-end diseases such as 'hip and knee replacement, bone morrow, cardiac and liver transplantation, gamma-knife procedures in neuro surgery, assisted devices for cardiac failures and diseases covered by National Programmes viz.,TB, HIV/AIDS, Leprosy, Infectious diseases, Malaria, Filaria, Gastroenteritis and Jaundice.

Till January 20, 2013, a total of 17 lakh surgeries and therapies were covered[iii]. The cost of treatment for every medical and surgical procedure is fixed by the panel of doctors, which has to be uniformly followed by all the network hospitals that implement the Aarogyasri scheme.

The government played the role of a key regulator. It streamlined the cost of private care through fixed protocols. The government ensures the timely reimbursement to the healthcare providers. It is claimed that through continuous monitoring, accountability of the private healthcare providers can be ensured.

The programme was designed in such a way that there was continuous monitoring at the grassroots level through the Self Help Group (SHG) federation and key district level officials, who carried out periodic review of the progress of the scheme. The other members in the trust were also involved in direct monitoring. The internet web-based solution enables common monitoring and evaluation framework of the RACHI scheme from any part of the state.

Achievements of the RACHI Scheme

The objective of the RACHI scheme was to improve access to healthcare for the poor. Rao et al. (2012) showed that only 111 beneficiaries per 1,00,000 BPL had used the scheme till the end of 2008. The needs of the really marginalised like the SCs and STs were less covered compared to other caste groups. It is important to look at the progress of the programme in terms of quantitative indicators, (Table 10.3).

The Aarogyasri website[iii] shows that since inception of the programme, in April 1 2007, till January 20, 2013, a total 35,718 health camps were held in villages in 23 districts. A total of 65,79,658 people had been screened; and of those 41,74,941 were treated as outpatients and 19,62,515 were treated as inpatients. Till 2013, 14 lakh surgeries were conducted on the patients. Among them only 4,41,591 underwent surgeries in government hospitals and 13,145,19 underwent surgeries in private hospitals. The preauthorised amount was INR 4,729 crore, with an annual budget of around INR 1000 crore.

As on January 20, 2013, statistical data provided in the Aarogyasri website showed that 17 lakh patients underwent surgery and therapy. Numerically, these figures might look attractive. However, if we analyse the figures to assess the extent of outreach of the care received under this scheme since its inception, the total number of beneficiaries appears to be very limited as compared to the overall figure of those insured. As per the details mentioned in the Programme Implementation Plan (PIP), the total number of families covered was 1.84 crore. However, according to the Aarogyasri Trust estimates as on April 5, 2009, insurance had been provided to 2.03 crore families. If we analyse these figures, the outreach of the scheme remains very limited. In every phase, we could see that not more than 5% of the people were screened and less than 1% actually got hospitalised and treated for the diseases for the huge amount paid from public sector to private sector (Mani, 2009).

The RACHI Scheme has been recognised as one of the largest health social security schemes implemented in India. It is acclaimed by the Planning Commission and Ministry of Health Government of India and by the Thirteenth Finance Commission, and has won the Manthan Award, South Asia 2009 and eIndia award for 2010.[3] Yet, it needs a critical evaluation. The following section does that.

Critical View of the Aarogyasri Scheme

It is important to evaluate schemes to assess their implications, sustainability and deliverables, especially as it targets the poor and the marginalised. Ideally under UHC, every citizen should be entitled for free healthcare. In Andhra Pradesh, 80% of the population has a white card, though it is called a BPL card meant for the poor. With limited resources, the question is how far the scheme is sustainable and who benefits?

Skewed Towards Tertiary Sector

The purpose of the RACHI scheme is to cut down OOPE for the BPL population and to provide financial protection for catastrophic illness.

Studies have shown that in social categories like SC and ST in the phase I, it did not affect OOPE spending as that of non- SC/ST households (Victoria et al., 2012). Another study too shows that the schemes have no impact on OOPE expenditure, which is largely determined by outpatient care and medicines (Selvaraj & Karan, 2012).In a survey in Hyderabad 58% of patients reported having incurred an average

OOPE of INR 3600 per patient (Planning Commission of India, 2011: 36). A very critical issue about the RACHI scheme is that it is skewed towards tertiary care and for a smaller population at the cost of majority and focused only on surgeries and certain chronic diseases at the cost of communicable diseases. It has, undoubtedly, created access for the rural poor for specialised health services. But there is a clear shift in focus in terms of setting priorities for providing healthcare for the poor. The scheme completely prioritises tertiary level super specialty healthcare that requires surgery and hospitalisation (Table 10.3). It is important to note that no health insurance scheme focuses on curative care that is not dependent on over medicalisation and high medical technology.

Only cardiac, cancer and neurological intervention made up to 65% (Rao et al., 2012) gets attended. Larger epidemiological healthcare needs are not addressed like mental illnesses and primary level and secondary level care for all diseases. Spatial distribution of the services also shows congregation in cities. Out of 353 participating hospitals, 30 hospitals are located in six cities, which undertake 50% interventions (Rao et al., 2012).

There are pressing concerns as the primary healthcare delivery system for the poor in rural areas is neglected and the poor continue to suffer frequently from infectious

Table 10.3 Broad activities under the aarogyasri scheme

Type of Service Activity	Institution	Since April 1, 2007-Till January 20, 2013
Health Camps		35,718
Preauthorisations	Government	502,944 (28.4%)
	Private	1,413,557 (79.8%)
	Total	1,916,501
Out-patients	Government	527,570 (12.6%)
	Private	3,647,371 (87.4%)
	Total	4,174,941
In-patients	Government	535,017 (27.3%)
	Private	1,427,498 (72.7%)
	Total	1,962,515
Patients screened and registered	Screened	6,579,658
	Registered	6,544,391
Surgeries/Therapies	Government	441,591 (25%)
	Private	1,314,519 (75%)
	Total	1,756,116
Amount Preauthorised	Government	Rs. 1073 Crores (22.7%)
	Private	Rs. 3656 Crores (77.3%)
	Total	Rs. 4729 Crores

Source https://www.aarogyasri.org/ASRI/index.jsp accessed January 20, 2013

illness, malaria fever, gastrointestinal disorders and anaemia. There is no PPP to cover all kinds of frequent illnesses afflicting the poor that lead to impoverishment, disability and premature mortality. Mahapatra (2001) analysed the leading causes of premature mortality and disability in rural and urban areas in Andhra Pradesh, and found that the leading causes of overall disease burden and mortality are lower respiratory infections, diarrhoeal diseases, low birth weight (malnutrition) tuberculosis, ischaemic heart diseases and malaria. Among the main causes of disability are accidents due to fall and fire, depression, epilepsy, schizophrenia and protein energy malnutrition among children. These are the illnesses, which hamper the daily life of the poor and have a significant impact on their economic condition. Many premature deaths and morbidity faced by the vulnerable sections in the rural areas are merely because of deficient public primary healthcare and referral system with apparent lack of qualified healthcare providers. Hence, the majority of the rural and urban poor may require basic primary healthcare services and access to facilities for proper referral services to reduce their disease burden and financial consequences.

Aarogyasri only caters to the biggest share of the catastrophic illness cases (Table 10.4) and there is no provision for out-patient treatment of everyday illnesses that affect the working capacity of the patient. The focus on tertiary healthcare to the exclusion of all other forms of medical assistance leads to an inefficient medical care model with a low level of real impact on meeting the needs of healthcare and the health of the population (Shukla et al., 2011).

State Sponsored Private Health Systems

Table 10.5 shows that the majority of surgeries (77%) are done in the private sector, taking away 79% resources as compared to only 22% treated in government with 20% resources.

The Director[8], Nizam's Institute of Medical Sciences (NIMS), Hyderabad, opined that the public healthcare system was 'limping' because of governmental neglect, while the private healthcare industry was thriving. He cited the soaring number of surgeries conducted in private hospitals as compared to the government hospitals. He was of the opinion that the health sector was 'going through a major crisis in the state' due to 'misplaced priorities of the government'; tertiary government hospitals like Osmania had been neglected (Special Correspondent, 2008).

The Aarogyasri website as of August 9, 2013, showed district performances, where in every district except one (Chittoor) preauthorised amount for treatment in private hospitals was much higher than that in government hospitals. In Hyderabad it was maximum in private hospitals, with preauthorisation amount of INR 105,670.85 lakhs, compared to INR 57,103.805 lakhs in government hospitals. Ranga Reddy district with only private share amounts to INR 40,377.023 lakhs. In the districts of Krishna, Vishakapatnam, Nellore, Guntur, East Godavari and Karimnagar, therapies in private hospitals were almost 80% of the share compared to government hospitals. The only district where government procedures were higher was Chittoor district[XII].

Table 10.4 Category-wise surgeries/therapies (January 12, 2012)

Category	Surgeries/Therapies
Surgical oncology	27,751
Medical oncology	126,193
Radiation oncology	66,616
Cardiac and cardiothoracic surgery	129,617
Neurosurgery	73,716
Genito-urinary surgeries	98,560
Poly trauma	1,241,416
General surgery	102,074
Gynaecology and obstetrics surgery	37,712
Nephrology	71,370
Cardiology	28,526
Neurology	29,488
Pediatric surgeries	16,998
Orthopedic surgery and procedure	22,053
Pediatrics	31,628
Plastic surgery	12,747
ENT surgery	30,111
Prosthesis	66
Surgical gastroenterology	6607
Ophthalmology surgery	12,759
Critical care	4956
Gastroenterology	5814
Pulmonology	5208
General medicine	2637
Cochlear implant surgery	706
Rheumatology	928
Endocrinology	451
Dermatology	423
Infectious diseases	27
Total	21,87,158

Source Procedure-wise incidence data accessed from Explore statistics, in the official website of Aarogyasri Healthcare Trust, Government of Andhra Pradesh (www.aarogyasri.org)

Since April 2007, a whopping INR 3,811 crore went into the kitty of private hospitals even as the state-run hospitals accrued a meagre sum of INR 1,142 crore out of the state-run scheme (Baseerat, 2013). After spending crores of rupees the claim still is that the current rates only provided for about 50% of the costs incurred in treatment,

Table 10.5 Sector-wise hospital distribution of surgeries/ therapies (Janauary 12, 2012)

	Surgeries/ Therapies	Percentage	Amount (INR Crores)	Percent-age
Corporate/Private Hospitals	10,11,514	77.47	2861	79.36
Government Hospitals	2,94,103	22.53	744	20.63
Total	13,05,617	100	3605	100

equipment, medicines, and other necessities and that these tariffs have to be hiked by 30%.

Under-Utilisation of Public Healthcare System

States ability to expand existing infrastructure shrank since due to new rules of financing, only specified amount is now refunded. Given the poor funding in the past, this led to increased financial burden on public institutions as no additional resources accrued from follow ups. This led to further decline in the performance of institutions in public sector and its poor usage. Even bigger government hospitals & sophisticated infrastructure and specialisation facilities–who could not generage additional resources by providing low cost surgeries—found it difficult to maintain theselves or realize their true potential. The cardiology wing of the Gandhi Hospital (a government hospital) was inaugurated on October 2008 with a capacity to perform 1,000 surgeries in a year, between January and May 2009, had performed only 85 surgeries (Singh, 2009). In spite of world-class operation theatre facilities, the hospital is not being able to function to its full capacity for want of the required pool of specialist doctors to conduct critical surgeries. The situation is similar at the level of PHCs and CHCs in rural areas and many operation theatres in government facilities remain underutilised due to lack of skilled manpower. Correction of these systemic deficiencies is essential in order to reach large number of the poor in the long term. The private/ corporate healthcare institutions are pushing costs up forcing the government to assist their strategy to maximise their monetary benefits.

Pressure Tactics and Lobbying

The PPP is not on equal footing; it is always public resources and private provisioning of services. The private sector is a powerful player, that influences policy and plays on pressure tactics. 270 hospitals are enrolled as members in the association like AP Private Hospitals and Nursing Homes (APNA) and Andhra Pradesh Super Specialties Hospitals Association (APSSHA). These associations urged the government to restore the list of 938 procedures under Aarogyasri schemes for all the network hospitals failing which they would withdraw their services, as 132 procedures have been reserved only for government hospitals. Associations form pressure group to bargain and lobby around to restore all Aarogyasri tests and 30% hike in the tariffs by the government or else threaten to stop treating the poor under the Aarogyasri. They also demanded that they were not going to cater to the government employees at the tariffs provided under the Aarogyasri plan (Restore All Aarogysri, 2013).

Finally the lobbying and pressure tactics did work and the government succumbed to APNA and ASHA by increasing the tariff by 30% in May 2013. The hike will entail an additional expenditure of about INR 250 crores by the government. At present, the yearly expenditure on Aarogyasri is about INR 1000 crore (Express News Service, 2013). This leads to a major question of sustainability of the scheme, for it will continue to encash from the government public resources and will be at the whims and fancy of the private hospitals. The moment funding stops, the free services will cease.

Issues of Sustainability

The major concerns about this social insurance scheme are its cost effectiveness and sustainability. The mean hospital expenditure of the private health insurance industry stood roughly at INR 19,637 per annum. Mean hospital expenditure in Tamil Nadu and CGHS scheme are at INR 33,720 and INR 25,000 respectively. It is reported that in publicly funded insurance scheme, where third party payment is made to private providers, supply side moral hazard appear loaded heavily in favour of private providers (Planning Commission of India, 2011). In Delhi, Andhra Pradesh and Tamil Nadu over half of all government health expenditure goes in to the tertiary care showing misguided priorities of medical professionals and medical-industrial complex (Planning Commission of India, 2011; Qadeer & Reddy, 2013).

Health insurance works best when services are available in the remote corners and poor households can actually exercise choice (MoHFW, 2005). National Family Health Survey (NFHS) 3, records high levels of BPL card holders in Andhra Pradesh, Karnataka and Kerala. In Andhra Pradesh, 86% of the population held white cards, which are the BPL cards. This is an imprecise indicator of poverty according to them as two-fifths of the BPL cards are with the non- poor households. This overestimation of BPL families leads to misuse of White cards by the non-poor (Ram et al., 2009). Ram et al. also report that 65% of the non-poor in Andhra Pradesh have white cards. Given this situation, it is very likely that those who can afford treatment are also covered under RACHI. Under UHC, this may be a welcome step. However, the concern is its financial sustainability and the neglect of primary level services. Given the huge expenditure in the private sector, incurred by the state and the present reality of under-utilisation of the public sector even when it is functional this model cannot be called efficient as it drains the state exchequers. In 2011, the state had 21 million households, out of which 19 million had BPL cards (Reddy, 2013). From 2014, these cards were being scrutinised and were to be attached to the Aadhar Card (an identity card). The former Chief Minister K. Rosaiah mentioned that the average amount claimed by the Aarogyasri beneficiaries per day is about 3.5 crores. In the fiscal year 2010–11, the government allocated INR 925 crores only. As on January 20, 2013, the total amount claimed from its inception was about INR 4,729 crores. According to the Aarogyasri scheme CEO, the state government spent a quarter of the health budget towards the scheme and wanted to approach the central government for support (GoAP, 2009), supporting the funding of Aarogyasri and extend financial support on 70:30 cost sharing basis on the ground that the burden of the scheme has put enormous pressure on the state exchequer. However, the central government turned down the proposal on the advice of the Planning Commission that recommended against partnering with states for funding any community health insurance scheme. The Planning Commission observed that these insurance schemes are turning out to be a 'cash cow' for the corporate hospitals. Even though this scheme helped poor families to undergo surgeries, the fact is that the private hospitals were making money through reimbursement by the state government (Planning Commission of India, 2011).

In the project implementation plan of NRHM (2008–09) prepared by the state government for the central government, the health insurance premium for BPL families was estimated at INR 279 (GoAP, 2008). However, the premium amount for these families until March 2009 was INR 330. From April 5, 2009, the premium worked out to be INR 439 per family. There is a likelihood that the premium amount will increase in the coming years. Since the premium insurance cost is fully borne by the state government, there is no direct financial burden on the poor. However, if the prices grow faster than the delivery capacity, the cost escalation might burden the government, raising concerns about financial sustainability. It is a huge 'burden' on the healthcare system of Andhra Pradesh (Ghosh, 2012) and is cost inefficient and points to the need for alternative social protection and health promotion programme (Sood et al., 2014). This is more so in the light of the central government denying cost sharing to support the state government in implementing this insurance scheme. This may also affect the sustainability of the scheme in the long run.

Ethical Issues

Apart from the above-mentioned critical issues, there are concerns about unethical means of practice in the empanelled private hospitals. In November 2009, the media highlighted how the health providers, the private health hospitals, were collecting consultation fees, not providing medicines and performing unwanted operations like hysterectomies for the women (Mallikarjun, 2009; Kameswari and Vinjamuri, 2011), in clear violation of the MoU they signed with the Aaogyasri Trust. It was found that the hospitals discharged the patients who underwent surgeries earlier than the stipulated time required for recovery. Some of the hospitals collected deposit amounts prior to the admission and failed to reimburse the amount, yet collected the bill.

Around 22 hospitals were suspended from their service for Aarogyasri patients for faking medical bills (In Kakinada.com, 2009). However, the government has been keenly tracking and monitoring the network hospitals and around 116 hospitals, who were indulging in malpractices or flouted rules, were de-listed[iii]. However, in the cases where the private hospitals which were blacklisted for malpractices, the associations of private hospitals, blamed the government for witch-hunting and filing criminal cases against them. TV9, a news channel in Andhra Pradesh has been raising questions about unethical practices under the Aarogyasri scheme through their news channel and Youtube films. The films online shows the malpractices, unnecessary surgeries like lumbar surgeries for simple back pain, not providing post-operative care, under aarogyasri conducted in corporate hospitals. The vigilance report 2010 by TV9 says some hospitals are charging the patients or beds, medicine, diagnostics and transportation. The media is highlighting that the doctors are like '*yamabattulu*' (Gods of death), and that the 'aarogyasri is corporate *dhanasri*' (God of Laxmi- money), 'corporate hospitals loot aarogyasri funds', 'aarogyasri has turned in to *anarogyasri* (illhealth)' 'aarogyasri is a '*Kalpavriksham*' (tree of boon) for corporate hospitals. The whole logic of spending crores of rupees under aarogyasri for surgeries/tertiary care is also referred to as '*goranthalabam, kondanthaavinithi*' meaning 'for a nail size profit it is mountain size corruption'.

Discussion

The National Commission on Macroeconomic and Health observed that increase in health spending, especially if states subsidise and buy from the private/corporate sector, will not yield commensurate results unless equal levels of investments are made in the sectors that have a defining impact on health outcomes. It advocates that poverty alleviation measures and assurance for regular employment and minimum threshold of income is a critical prerequisite of health. What is required is developing an integrated public health system that strengthens the primary, secondary and tertiary level care with due emphasis on inter- sectoral linkages: improving nutrition by ensuring food availability (by strengthening the public distribution system) ensuring safe drinking water supply, creating adequate shelter and sanitation facilities, creation of public transport facilities and road connectivity in interior and remote areas to improve access for mobility of patients, strengthening primary education (National Commission on Macroeconomics and Health, 2005). These are the primary social determinants of health that need focus to improve health and reduce inequalities. Until these needs are addressed for the large number of poor who are living in rural area, there is no chance for improving their health and getting them out of poverty.

Under the philosophy of PPP, contrary to the core ethical principles for the partnerships, beneficence (joint gains), in this case the state is bearing the whole cost, and equity is defeated, where there are no fair returns in proportion to investment, instead over-medicalisation and unnecessary surgeries are being carried out. Control is in the hands of corporate/private hospitals which lobby for the schemes' continuation and inclusion of maximum number of surgeries. This has only served the corporate/private hospitals and resulted in complete neglect of primary and secondary care. Though Andhra Pradesh is an economically forward state, still only 46% of the population has received basic immunisation. Close to 449 persons per lakh are suffering from TB, which is more than in Rajasthan and Orissa. AP is the second highest in HIV prevalence rate (0.97%) followed by Manipur. A few studies (Victoria et al., 2012; Selvaraj & Karan, 2012) have shown that these schemes have no significant likelihood of reducing OOPE. There is an urgent need for an empirical research at household level to assess OOPE on primary, secondary and tertiary level and for catastrophic illnesses after the experience with the Aarogyasri scheme. Its benefits and problems need to be captured.

To have a sustainable healthcare model, there is a need to strengthen the public health service systems and also use them to their optimum level by upgrading them rather than giving state subsidies to the private sector. It is important to strengthen drug price control by bringing all essential drugs into price control. Some have also suggested that there should be subsequent merging of all publicly-financed schemes or, at least review how else one can reduce subsidies to institutions that are excluding those whom they committed to benefit. Also ensure proper administration and management system to consolidate the fragmented supply situation (Gupta & Chowdhury, 2014). The annual expenditure of 1,000 crores, where 80% goes to private sector (Table 10.5) if spent only on the public sector healthcare system, can help better in realising the dream of 'Arogyandhra'.

In Andhra Pradesh, 74.3% households do not generally use government health facilities. The reasons are there is no nearby facility (49.2%), facility timing is not convenient (18%), health personal are often absent (12.8%), waiting time is too long (23.4%) and quality of care is poor (53.3%) (IIPS and Macro International, 2007). Further Aarogyasri focuseson high end tertiary care alone, whereas the fact that only 2.3% and 3.1% of rural and urban population, on an average, are hospitalized at any given point of time, while 8.8% and 9.9% of the population access outpatient coverage (NSSO, 2006). Corporate hospitals handle the biggest share of tertiary care, excluding all other forms of primary and secondary outpatient care. If one were to examine the expenditure pattern of households, it is again clear that outpatient expenditure far outweighs inpatient care expenditure (Selvaraj & Karan, 2012). This is an inefficient medical care model with a low level of real impact on meeting the needs of healthcare (Shukla et al., 2011).

It can be concluded that the curative services have been given priority at the cost of preventive, promotive and rehabilitative services. Neglect of public hospitals is comparable only to the private sector, which is thriving and flourishing at state expenses. Public hospitals, which have good infrastructure and medical expertise, are being underutilised. There is no mechanism to monitor the household healthcare expenditure at all levels, primary, secondary and tertiary and for catastrophic illnesses. Assuring universal health coverage will require explicit acknowledgement by government and civil society of healthcare as a public good. Only a radical restructuring of the healthcare system that promotes health equity can eliminates impoverishment due to OOPE (Patel et al., 2015). Thus, there is no alternative than to strengthen public sector, which will be sustainable and also universal.

Notes

1. The district-wise hospital empanelment records can be viewed at the Aarogyasri website, information can be accessed from the web link: http://www.aarogyasri.org/ASRI/FrontServlet?requestType=HospEmpanelRH&actionVal=ShowHospRecords&ButtonOption=true&empanelType=N&fromPage=HomePage)
2. The criterion is that it should have at least 50 inpatient medical beds with adequate spacing and supporting staff as per norms. 25% beds should be allocated exclusively for the Aarogyasri patients, Medical and Surgical facilities along with Diagnostic facilities, fully equipped Operation Theatre, fully qualified doctors, and nursing staff Using ICD and OPQS codes for Drugs, Diagnosis, Surgical procedures etc., having all the infrastructure required for cancer and orthopaedic treatments.
3. The well developed IT system helps to track, monitor and approve medical treatment for all beneficiaries under this scheme. Each and every service provided for the patient who is registered under the RACHI scheme can be monitored 24X7 through the trust's portal where the Aarogyasri workflow system can be tracked from the entry point to treatment and discharge.
4. Arogyamitras help hospitals in pre-auth, claim settlement and follow- up. They also ensure proper reception and care in the hospital and send regular MIS. The insurance company ensures that prefabricated Aarogyamithra kiosks with all additional requirements as per the design approved by the Trust is put up in all hospitals. For effective and instant communication all the Aarogyamithras are provided with cell phone CUG connectivity by the insurance company.
5. Private insurance companies like ICICI Lombard covers pre-existing illness only after four years of enrolment in the policy provided it is renewed continuously with the same company. Most Health Insurance Policies hospitalisation expenses arising from pre-existing conditions are not allowed. Most disputes between insurance companies and consumers on claims made for hospitalisation expenses arise from this point. Even the RSBY for the unorganised sector workers below poverty line and their families by Government of India covers pre- existing conditions but with minimal exclusions only (Swarup, 2008). The RACHI scheme is unique as it includes all pre-existing illness of the people below poverty line.
6. The specific insurance coverage for the systems like heart, lung, liver, pancreas, renal diseases, neuro-surgery, pediatric congenital malformations, burns, post-burn contracture surgeries for functional improvement, prostheses (artificial limbs), cancer treatment (surgery, chemo therapy, radio therapy), poly trauma (including cases covered under MV Act) and cochlear implant surgery with auditory-verbal therapy for children below 6 years (costs reimbursed by the Trust on a case-to-case basis).

7. High-end diseases such as 'hip and knee replacement, bone morrow, cardiac and liver transplantation, gamma-knife procedures in neuro surgery, assisted devices for cardiac failures and diseases covered by National Programmes, viz. TB, HIV/AIDS, Leprosy, Infectious diseases, Malaria, Filaria, Gastroenteritis, Jaundice.
8. The Aarogyasri Scheme was strongly criticised by Dr.Raja Reddy, a well known neurosurgeon and former Director of NIMS, Hyderabad, in a symposium organised by NIMS in September 2008 xii(http://www.aarogyasri.gov.in/ASRI/reportsAction.do?actionFlag=hospDistCatPer. Accessed on August 9, 2013).

References

Aarogyasri Healthcare Trust. (2011a). "Rajiv Aarogyasri Scheme Achieves Following Landmarks." Accessed January 12, 2013. http://www.aarogyasri.org/ASRI/EXT_IMAGES/documents/Note_LandMark.pdf.

Aarogyasri Healthcare Trust. (2011b). "About Aarogyamithra, Role of Aarogyamithra." Accessed January 20, 2013. http://www.aarogyasri.org/ASRI/FrontServlet?requestType=CommonRH&actionVal=RightFrame&pageName=About_Aarogya_percent20mithra.

Aarogyasri Healthcare Trust. (2011c). "Follow-up Services for Aarogyasri Beneficiaries," Accessed January 20, 2013. http://www.aarogyasri.org/ASRI/FrontServlet?requestType=CommonRH&actionVal=RightFrame&pageName=follow-up.

Acharya, A., Ranson, M. K. (2005). "Healthcare financing for the poor: Community based health insurance schemes in Gujarat." *Economic and Political Weekly* 40, No. 38 (September 17–23), 4141–4150.

Babu, A. (2009). "Aarogyasri health insurance scheme." In *Fostering E- Governance: Selected Compendium of Indian Initiatives*, Piyush Gupta, Bagga, P.K., & Ayaluri, S. (Eds.), p. 315. ICFAI University Press.

Baru, R. (1999). *Private Healthcare in India: Social Characteristics and Trends.* Sage Publications.

Baseerat, B. (2013). "Private Hospitals Lobby for Hike in Aarogyasri Tariff." *The Times of India,* March 13. Accessed August 9, 2013. http://articles.timesofindia.Indiatimes.com/2013-03-31/hyderavad/38162471_1_private_hospitals-corporate-hospitals-government-hospitals.

Bennett, S., Dakpallah, G., Garner, P., Gilson, L., Nittayaramhong, S., Zurita, B., & Anthony, Z. (1994). "Carrot and stick: State mechanisms to influence private provider behavior. *Health Policy and Planning, 9*(1), 1–13.

Express New Service. (2013). "Hospitals get 30 percent fee hike under aarogyasri." *The New Indian Express,* May 3. accessed August 9, 2013. http://newindianexpress.com/cities/hyderabad/Hospitals_get-30-%fce-hike-under-Arogyasri/2013/05/03/article1572637.ece.

Government of India. (2013). *Twelfth Five Year Plan. 2012–2017 Vol. III. Social Sectors.*, Sage.

Government of India. (2002). *Tenth Five Year Plan 2002–2007: Volume II-Sectoral Policies and Programmes.*, Planning Commission.

Government of Andhra Pradesh. (2008). "Andhra Pradesh, Project Implementation Plan-NRHM." Accessed January 13, 2013. http://www.mohfw.nic.in/NRHM/PIP_08_09/PIP_AP.doc.

Government of Andhra Pradesh. (2009). "Finance Minister's Budget Speech (2009–2010), by Mr. K. Rosaih, to the Andhra Pradesh Legislative Assembly on July 24, 2009." Accessed January, 2013 http://www.apfinance.gov.in/html/fin-min-speech-2009-middle.htm.

Gupta, I., & Chowdhury, S. (2014). "Public financing for health coverage in India: Who spends, who benefits and at what cost?." *Economic and Political Weekly* 49, No. 35 (August 30), 59–63.

Hooda, S.K. (2015). *Private Sector in Healthcare Delivery Market in India:Structure, Growth and Implications.* Working Paper 185. Institute for Studies in Industrial Development (December).

In Kakinada.com. (2009). *Aarogyasri Cancelled in 51 Hospitals.* 5 August. Accessed January 20, 2013. http://www.inkakinada.com/news/headline/arogyasri-cancelled-in-51-hospitals.

International Institute for Population Sciences, and Macro International. (2007). *National Family Health Survey (NFHS-3), 2005–06: India: Volume I.* Mumbai, IIPS.

Kameswari, S.V., & Vinjamuri. (2011). *Medical Ethics: A Case Study of Hysterectomy in Andhra Pradesh.* Life—HRG, Centre for World Solidarity and KICS.

Kumar, A. K. S., Chen, L.C., Choudhury, M., Ganju, S., Mahajan, V., Sinha, A, & Sen, A. "Financing healthcare for all: Challenges and opportunities." *The Lancet* 377, No. 9766 (January 11), 668–679.

Lal, B. S. (2017). Economic Analysis of the Rajiv Aarogysre (Healthcare) Scheme: An Emperical Study in Warangal District. Accessed Sept. 16, 2018. http:\\www.researchgate.net/publication/318493036_economic_analysis_of_the_Rajiv_Aarogyasri_Health_Care_Scheme_An_Emperical_Study_in_Warangal_District.

Mahapatra, P. 2001. *Estimating National Burden of Disease: The Burden of Disease in Andhra Pradesh in the 1990s.*. The Institute of Health Systems.

Mallikarjun, Y. (2009). Aarogyasri not in the pink of health. *The Hindu*, November 4. Accessed July 9, 2011. http://www.thehindu.com/2009/11/04/stories/2009110454540400.htm.

Mallipeddi, R., Pernefeldt, H., & Bergkvist, S. (2009). *Andhra Pradesh Health Sector Reform: A Narrative Case Study.* Technical Partner Paper 7. Access Health Initiative.

Mani, M. K. (2009). Letter from Chennai. *National Medical Journal of India, 22*(4), 207–208.

Ministry of Health and Family Welfare, Government of India. (2006). *Report by Working Group on Healthcare Financing Including Health Insurance for the Eleventh Five Year Plan* (October). Ministry of Health and Family Welfare.

Ministry of Health and Family Welfare, Government of India. (2015). *National Rural Health Mission: Report of the Task Force on Exploring New Health Financing Mechanisms.* October 18. Ministry of Health and Family Welfare.

National Commission on Macroeconomics and Health. Government of India. (2005). *Report of the National Commission on Macroeconomics and Health.* Ministry of Health and Family Welfare.

National Sample Survey Organisation. (2006). *Morbidity, Healthcare and the Condition of the Aged: NSS 60th Round, January–June 2004* (Report No 507 (60/25.0/1)). Ministry of Statistics and Programme Implementation, Government of India.

Patel, V., Parikh, R., Nandraj, S., Balasubramaniam, P., Narayan, K., Paul, V.K., Shiva Kumar, A.K., Chatterjee, M., Reddy, K.S. (2015). "Assuring health coverage for all in India." *The Lancet* 386, No. 10011 (December 12), 2422–35.

Planning Commission of India. (2011). *A Critical Assessment of Existing Health Insurance Models in India.* Research Study, Public Health Foundation of India. Accessed April 20, 2018. http://planningcommission.nic.in/reports/sereport/ser/ser_heal1305.pdf.

Pollock, M. A., Player, S., & Godden, S. (2001). "How private finance is moving primary care into corporate ownership." *British Medical Journal*, 332 (April 21), 960–963.

Prasad, N. P., & Raghavendra, P. (2012). "Healthcare Models in the Era of Medical Neo-Liberalism: A Study of Aarogyasri in Andhra Pradesh." *Economic and Political Weekly* 47, No. 43 (October 27), 118–126.

Qadeer, I., & Reddy, S. (2006). "Medical care in the shadow of public private partnership." *Social Scientist* 34, No. 9/10 (September-October), 4–20.

Qadeer, I., & Reddy, S. (2013). Medical tourism in India: Perceptions of physicians in tertiary care hospitals. *Philosophy, Ethics, and Humanities in Medicine, 8*, 20.

Qureshi Committee Report. (2001). High level committee for hospitals in Delhi. Enquiry Report. Government of National Capital Territory of Delhi, Health and Family Welfare Department.

Ram, F., Mohanty, S. K. & Ram, U. (2009). "Understanding the Distribution of BPL Cards: All-India and Selected States." *Economic and Political Weekly* 44, No. 7 (February 14–20): 66–71.

Rao, M., Kadam, S., Sathyanarayana, T.N., Shidhaye, R., Shukla, R., Ramachandra, S.S., Sitamma, M., & George, M.S.. 2012. "A Rapid Evaluation of the Rajiv Aarogyasri Community Health Insurance Scheme in Andhra Pradesh, India." *BMC Proceedings* 6, No. 1: O4. BioMed Central.

Reddy, D. (2013). "Andhra Pradesh has More Ration Card Holders than Households." *Business Standard.* July 4.

Reddy, S., & Qadeer, I. 2010. "Medical tourism in India: Progress or predicament." *Economic and Political Weekly* 45, No. 20 (May 15): 69–75.

Selvaraj, S., & Karan, A.K. (2012). "Why publicly—financed health insurance schemes are ineffective in providing financial risk protection." *Economic and Political Weekly* 47, No. 11 (March 17): 60–68.

Sen, K. (2001). "Health Reforms and Developing Countries—A Critique." In *Public Health and the Poverty of Reforms: The South Asian Predicament*, I. Qadeer, K. Sen, & K.R. Nayar (Eds.). Sage Publications Pvt. Ltd.

Shukla, R., Shatrugna, V., & Srivatsan, R. (2011). "Aarogyasri healthcare model: Advantage private sector." *Economic and Political Weekly* 46, No. 49 (December 3): 38–42.

Singh, P. V. (2009). "Arogyasri-Revolutionsing public Health through conviction and Innovative ICT Solution" http://ehealth.eletsonline.com/2009/07/11291. Accessed on September 28, 2018

Sood, N., Bendavid, E., Mukherji, A., Wagner, Nagpal, S., & Mullen, P. (2014). "Government health insurance for people below the poverty line in India: Quasi experimental evaluation of insurance and health outcome." *British Medical Journal* 349 (September).

Special Correspondent, *The Hindu.* (2008). "Aarogyasri Scheme Draws Flak." *The Hindu,* September 21. accessed August 28, 2017. http://www.hindi.com/2008/09/21/stories/2008092159510500.htm.

Venkatraman, A. (2014). "Private Sector and Public-Private Partnerships in Health Service Delivery in India." *India Infrastructure Report 2013/14: The Road to Universal Health Coverage.* IDFC Foundation. Hyderabad: Orient BlackSwan. 65–80.

Victoria, Y. F., Karan, A., & Mahal, A. (2012). *State Health Insurance and Out-of Pocket Health Expenditures in Andhra Pradesh, India.* Working Paper 298. June. Center for Global Development.

WHO. (1999). WHO Guidelines on Collaboration and Partnerships with Commercial Enterprises. Geneva, World Health Organisation. (Draft Discussion Document, June 24). In *Global Public—Private Partnerships: Part 1-A New Development in Health,* K. Buse & G. Walt. *Bulletin of the World Health Organisation*, 2000, 78 (4).

Chapter 11
Health Insurance to Achieve Health for All: A Critical Appraisal of Pradhan Mantri Jan Aarogya Yojana

Sourindra Mohan Ghosh and Imrana Qadeer

In the launch of Pradhan Mantri Jan Aarogya Yojana (PMJAY), the initiative was projected as a game changer in public-sector health care services for the poor[1]. It would give an insurance coverage for medical costs for hospitalization up to INR 500,000 per family in a year and it would benefit 100 million poor families, or over 500 million people. While giving it the tag of 'largest government-funded health care programme in the world' in its inauguration, it was pointed out that the 500 million beneficiaries under this scheme outstrip the populations of the US, Mexico and Canada taken together. But can India really implement the 'largest government-funded health care programme', while its government spending on health is one of the lowest in the world? According to the WHO data, India ranks 183rd in terms of government health expenditure as percent of GDP and 159th in terms of per capita government health expenditure in 2015, out of total 193 countries in the world[2]. Let us have a close look whether the budgetary allocations in this scheme is adequate to fulfil its promises.

Grossly Inadequate Budget

In this current 2020–21 fiscal year, INR 65 billion has been earmarked in the central government budget for expenditure towards health insurance scheme (which includes a small component towards Rashtriya Swasthya Bima Yojana [RSBY] along with PMJAY), which is basically the total premium paid by the central government to health insurance agencies (or trusts). Conservatively assuming there is no administrative costs or insurance overheads, health insurance agencies (or trusts) have only

S. M. Ghosh (✉)
Centre for Economic Studies and Planning, Jawaharlal Nehru University, New Delhi, India

I. Qadeer
Council for Social Development, New Delhi, India

I. Qadeer et al. (eds.), *Universalising Healthcare in India*,
https://doi.org/10.1007/978-981-16-5872-3_11

this INR 65 billion to pay the service providers for cashless hospitalization services they will provide to 10 crore beneficiary families. We have used the latest health survey data—National Sample Survey (NSS-2017–18)—to assess whether this fund is adequate to cover hospitalization costs. Table 11.1 shows total number of hospitalizations, out-patient department (OPD) treatments and their medical expenditures in the country in a year; we can have rough estimates for 100 million families from these aggregates. Calculating from that aggregated data, out of 100 million families there would be roughly 18.4 million hospitalizations in a year which means health insurance agencies have only INR 3532 to pay per hospitalization on average from INR 65 billion government funds. The average medical expenditure (excluding transport and other non-medical expenditures) per hospitalization works out to around INR 16,069. At these going rates, 100 million families under PMJAY with 18.4 million hospitalizations in a year will need INR 294.81 billion if they are to get cashless hospital services. These are 2017–18 expenditure estimates; even considering a minimal 5% annual inflation, it would be INR 358.3 billion in 2021–22 value. The actual financial requirements of PMJAY can be even higher if pre-hospitalization or post-discharge expenditures, some transportation costs etc. are to be provided and administrative cost or insurance overhead (which is always a substantial amount) is considered[3]. If hospitalization rates increase due to government's promotion of inpatient care through insurance coverage or, new individuals currently out-of-health coverage now seek access to hospitals, we will be looking at medical claims much higher than INR billion in a year under PMJAY.

The NITI Aayog has assured that eventually INR 100 billion will be allocated for the scheme[4]. That too is only a fraction of the amount required to give comprehensive coverage for in-patient care to 100 million targeted families. The assessment of budgetary requirements has clearly not been done in a scientific manner otherwise there would not be such a wide gap between allocation and requirement. In fact, no country has ever achieved such goals that PMJAY has set for itself with so little public spending. This scheme is expected to fail in living up to its promises. As the money for this scheme dries up and insurance agencies default on claims, service providers will start restricting the services/procedures available under PMJAY, charge money from patients or refuse services, as experience of other similar PFHI schemes in India suggests (Ghosh, 2014; Ghosh & Gupta, 2017).

Table 11.1 Estimated yearly hospitalizations and OPD treatments (incidence and costs)—all India aggregates, 2017–18

	Numbers (million)	Medical care OOPE (INR billion)
Total households	262	–
Hospitalizations	48	772.71
OPD treatments	2196	1331.01
Hosp + OPD	2244	2103.72

Source Authors' calculation, NSS 75th round unit data

Table 11.2 Major components of NRHM in Union Health Budget, 2016–17 to 2020–21 (INR billion, 2020–21 prices)

Service components	2016–17	2017–18	2018–19	2019–20	2020–21
	Actual	Actual	Actual	Revised	Budget
RCH flexible pool	73.68	85.34	57.96	59.21	57.03
Health system strengthening under NRHM	60.82	94.32	98.20	110.83	105.86
Flexible pool for communicable diseases	23.90	35.81	28.05	22.38	21.78
Flexible pool for non-communicable diseases, injury and trauma	5.89	10.31	5.84	7.35	7.17
Infrastructure maintenance	61.10	61.45	66.68	72.60	63.43
Ayushman Bharat Health and Wellness Centres	0.0	0.0	10.61	14.01	13.50
Others	4.43	5.19	5.02	2.55	1.62
NRHM total	229.82	292.40	272.36	288.94	270.39

Source Union Budget, various years

Inadequate Coverage and Containment of Out-of-Pocket Expenditure?

According to the Ministry of Health and Family Welfare, 12.6 million beneficiaries received free treatment since two years of its inception between September 2018 and September 2020[5]. This figure on an average will be half, i.e. 6.3 million, for a one year period. These 6.3 million beneficiaries who actually received free treatments in a year under this scheme is far less than the target when compared to the NSS 2017–18 data that shows 18.4 million hospitalisations among the targeted households in a year. Much has been made of the coverage provided by the PMJAY to COVID 19 patients during the pandemic as well. It is reported that according to the government sources 32,000 cases of COVID were treated under the scheme by September 2020[6] (HT). By September 21st 5,487,580 cases were reportedly diagnosed[7]; if it is conservatively assumed that 6 percent of this number were hospitalised (World Health Organisation [WHO, 2020] estimated that 13.8% diagnosed cases required hospitalisation), the number comes to 329,254 admissions. The 32,000 treated patients under PMJAY accounts for only 9.7% of this total admission for COVID which is far less than the expected coverage of the poor- which should be at least near 40%. Apart from these inadequate numbers covered, the claim of smooth cashless services is also problematic. This scheme offers coverage to pre-designated procedures and therapies. The package amount payable to the hospital by the government—is fixed based on predetermined criteria that do not factor in co-morbidities and duration of hospitalisation. At the time of billing therefore free service is only for procedures for which the hospital takes prior permission. This does not take into account comorbidities, and the duration of the stay. Both these increase patient's out-of-pocket expenditure

(OOPE), so the scheme is not necessarily free as projected. It is also well known that private tertiary care institutions charge heavily and often over investigate and treat. All this in fact adds to the patients financial burden, as highlighted during the pandemic (Thiagrajan Kamala, 2020). All of this revealed that the scheme has failed to lower OOPE (Garg et al., 2020). Also, there are reports of frauds by empanelled hospitals who charge patients, submit reimbursement documents for non-existent patients and indulge showing admissions of large numbers of COVID 19 cases difficult to verify given the in accessibility of COVID wards to investigators (Neetu, 2020).

An Inefficient Health Care Model

Over and above a grossly inadequate budget and inadequate coverage and cash free services under PMJAY is the issue whether India should at all push for a health care model that is essentially tertiary care based, techno-centric and hence expensive.

No Protection from OPD Expenditures

The majority of cases anywhere in the world are treated in the OPD and people spend more money in it rather than in hospitalizations. From Table 11.1, we see that yearly in India there are nearly 2200 million OPD cases (i.e. 97.9% of all cases) resulting in medical expenditure of INR 1,33,1.01 billion (i.e. 63% of medical expenditure). Hospitalizations account for only 2.1% of treated cases and PMJAY is restricted to only cover that much.

What India essentially need is a strong revamping of its primary health care system. In countries like the UK or Canada which provides Universal Health Care (UHC) to its citizens, such social health insurance model has been built on the back of a robust public primary and secondary health care (Macinko et al., 2003). Even when the first level care is typically provided by the private general practitioners within the primary/secondary care, their participation is strictly controlled by the rules and regulations of the state. All institutions participating in primary/secondary care are bound by these regulations. Role of tertiary care is to provide specialised treatment and intensive care for patients with diseases at an advanced stage (or when complications arise) and they are referred from the primary/secondary care. Over time in both these countries, hospitalization rate, per capita in-patient treatment/admission days etc. have gradually declined over time. One of the factors for this decline being the gradual strengthening of primary care as reflected in the OECD data over time[8]. India on the other hand could never develop a strong primary health care which has been its goal since independence and reiterated even in the latest National Health Policy, 2017 (GoI, 2017).

The Indian Government's effort to strengthen primary health care system must therefore be based on historical experience, clarity of vision and a sound financial policy. While efforts to rebuild the public infrastructure are critical, private practitioners—individual practicing doctors or small institutions—can be enrolled in a roster at a predetermined payment from government. The payments may be based on morbidity risk of the population they will serve for which they will provide cashless medical care services to all people in a designated area. Regulations such as, enrolled doctors can't accept any fee-for- service will be a necessary check against potential misuse of government funds. Such a predetermined payment directly to the service providers—instead of paying to insurance agencies—will cut-out the proverbial 'middle-man', will make the service-providers directly accountable to governments and will yet act as a social health insurance model.

A cursory look at Union Government Budget of last two fiscal years shows us how primary care in India is being neglected.

Undermining Primary Care

In the last several years, share of funds allocated to National Rural Health Mission (NRHM), which is the biggest component of rural primary health care infrastructure, has been rapidly falling, from 50.8% of total central health budget in 2016–17 to 40.3% in 2020–21. On the other hand, share of spending on the Pradhan Mantri Swasthya Suraksha Yojana (PMSSY) which aims to develop multi/super-specialty tertiary care institutions in States and PMJAY-RSBY increased sharply (Fig. 11.1). According to Rural Health Statistics 2016, there is 20% shortfall of health sub-centres, along with 22 and 30% shortage of primary health centres (PHC) and community health centres (CHC). The condition of primary care facilities have

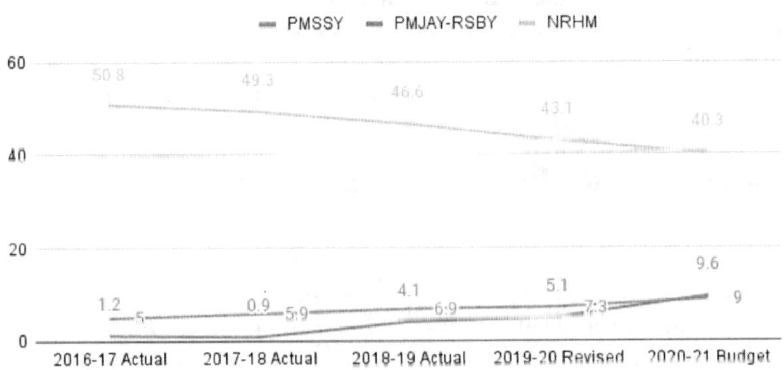

Fig. 11.1 Share (%) of centre's health spending on PMSSY, PMJAY-RSBY and NRHM. *Source* Union Budget, various years

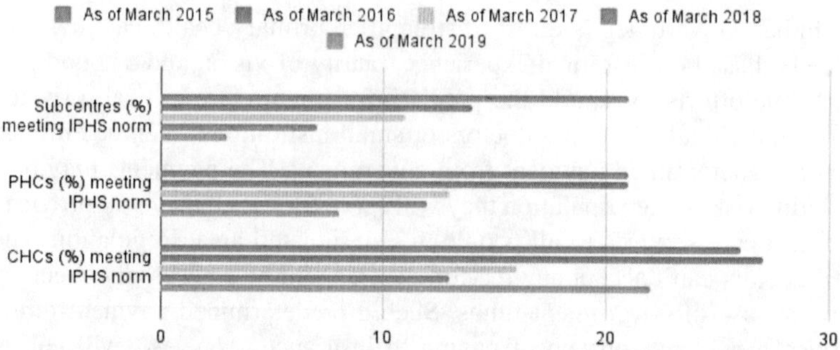

Fig. 11.2 Share (%) of primary healthcare facilities fulfiling Indian Public Health Standards (IPHS) Norm. *Source* Rural Health Statistics, various years

deteriorated as reflected in declining share of these facilities meeting Indian Public Health Standards (IPHS) norms in last five years (Fig.11.2).

Continuing neglect and deterioration of a primary health care that is already fragile cannot improve health of a population, even if a good coverage of tertiary care is provided. First of all, it undermines preventive care—which a comprehensive primary health care can provide—and focuses only on curative care (Keleher, 2001). Secondly, a weak primary care delays treatment, resulting in more complex and expensive medical interventions as well as deterioration of health if the patient is unable to get access. Along with investments in primary health care infrastructure, financial burden on the poor for tertiary care can be best handled by investing in building quality government hospitals rather than going through the insurance model which will end up fuelling corporate sector profits. The creation of National Health Authority (NHA), a stand-alone fully autonomous institution that implements PMJAY at the national level which has no integration with lower tier institutions, skews policy and further fragments health care delivery.

Within NRHM, allocations under reproductive and child health care (RCH flexible pool) and flexible pool for communicable diseases were cut significantly in real terms in last five years (Table 11.2).

Non-universal: A Faulty Application of Insurance Logic

For strengthening of primary care—through revamping public infrastructure and incorporating individual/small practitioners into the system for a social health insurance scheme—the government budgets need to increase many-fold. Direct taxation or compulsory contributory payments are two possible options for raising the funds. For that, universalizing would be the best bet for the following reason.

Any insurance works on the principle of hedging a financial risk with regular small payments over a period of time for the eventuality when that risk actualizes. We then don't need to spend a huge sum of money. Additionally, a universal social health insurance (financed by progressive taxation or contribution) distributes the risk of health expenditure in the eventuality of an illness across the rich—who can pay more—and the poor—who are less able to pay. By limiting any health insurance only for the poor, the government puts a limit on raising the money from richer population for strengthening its own institutions. Only if access is made universal, the substantial amount of OOPE that both the rich and the poor pay for medical care can be channelized efficiently through direct taxation or universal social insurance. This would certainly lead to a better outcome for both sections of the population over time.

Conclusion

Clearly PMJAY is a scheme which is not only insignificant in terms of its budgetary allocations and therefore inadequate to keep its promises or lower the out of pocket expenditures, but it is also not the right approach that the health care system in India needs today. Such an unbalanced promotion of tertiary care by the government might also increase health care costs. This can be disastrous for sections for whom the primary need is for comprehensive primary health care and where, any further aggravation of the imbalance of investment in the primary, secondary and tertiary health care can only add to their deprivation/burden. Any health policy aiming to further the prospect of UHC in India needs to take care of these issues and not ignore them any further.

Notes

1. This chapter has evolved out of a published paper in Social Change titled, "Pradhan Mantri Jan Arogya Yojana: A paper Tiger", Social Change, March 21, 2019.
2. Data can be accessed from http://apps.who.int/nha/database/Select/Indicators/en [accessed on 08.10.2018].
3. Estimates show that US has as high as 31% of health expenditures as overheads or administrative costs, while for Canada it is 16.7%.
4. https://www.thehindubusinessline.com/news/niti-aayog-seeks-world-banks-help-to-prevent-fraud-in-healthcare-insurance-programme/article23792632.ece [accessed 20.10.2018].
5. https://pib.gov.in/PressReleaseIframePage.aspx?PRID=1657981 accessed on 28.1.2021, Dr. Harsh Vardhan chairs Aarogya Manthan on 2nd Anniversary of Ayushman Bharat-Pradhan Mantri Jan Aarogya Yojana, "Free treatment to more than 1.26 crore beneficiaries since its launch in Sept 2018".
6. HT Correspondent 2020, "32,000 Covid patients treated under Ayushman Bharat: Centre". https://www.hindustantimes.com/india-news/32-000-covid-patients-treated-under-ayushman-bharat-centre/story-7kjhtzTPi06kmi7r2xb1dJ.html. Accessed 28.1.2021.

7. https://www.bloombergquint.com/coronavirus-outbreak/coronavirus-india-updates-new-cases-falls-to-lowest-in-nearly-six-months BQ Desk, 2020, Bloomberg Quint, Coronavirus India Updates: New Cases Fall To Lowest In Nearly Six Months, Dec 27.
8. Data can be accessed here https://stats.oecd.org/Index.aspx?DataSetCode=SHA# [accessed on 08.10.2018].

References

Garg, S., Bebarta, K. K., & Tripathi, N. (2020). Performance of India's national publicly funded health insurance scheme, Pradhan Mantri Jan Arogaya Yojana (PMJAY), in improving access and financial protection for hospital care: Findings from household surveys in Chhattisgarh state. *BMC Public Health, 20*, 949 (2020). https://bmcpublichealth.biomed-central.com/articles/. https://doi.org/10.1186/s12889-020-09107-4. Accessed January 31, 2021.

Ghosh, S. (2014). Publicly-financed health insurance for the poor understanding RSBY in Maharashtra. *Economic & Political Weekly, 49*(43–44), 93–99.

Ghosh, S., & Gupta, N. D. (2017). Targeting and effects of Rashtriya Swasthya Bima Yojana on access to care and financial protection. *Economic and Political Weekly, 52*, 61–70.

Government of India. (2017). *National Health Policy*. Ministry of Health and Family Health Care (New Delhi)

Kamala, T. (2020). Healthcare in India Covid-19 exposes the high cost of India's reliance on private healthcare. *British Medical Journal*, 2020; 370:m3506: published on 10 September 2020. www.bmj.com/content/370/bmj.m3506/rapid-responses. Accessed January 29, 2021.

Keleher, H. (2001). Why primary health care offers a more comprehensive approach to tackling health inequities than primary care. *Australian Journal of Primary Health, 7*(2), 57–61.

Macinko, J., Starfield, B., & Shi, L. (2003). The contribution of primary care systems to health outcomes within Organization for Economic Cooperation and Development (OECD) countries, 1970–1998. *Health Services Research, 38*(3), 831–865.

Neetu, S. (2020, September 8). Some hospitals under Ayushman Bharat may be attempting fraud over covid-19, *Live Mint*. https://livemint.com/news/india/some-hospitals-under-ayushman-bharat-may-be-attempting-fraud-over-covid-19-11599560408139.html. Accessed January 28, 2021.

Rythma, K. (2020). Only 6% cases need hospitalisation, over 40,000 have recovered: Govt. *Hindustan Times*. 21 May, www.hindustantimes.com/india-news/only-6-cases-need-hospitalisation-over-40-000-have-recovered-govt/story-4jTOt7S5TNhKpPzaBZ0YQI.html. Accessed on January 1, 2021.

WHO. (2020). *Report of the WHO–China Joint Mission on Coronavirus Disease 2019 (COVID-19)*. 28 February, viewed on 25 June. www.who.int/publications/i/item/report-of-thewho-china-joint-mission-on-coronavirus-disease-2019-(covid-19)

Part III
Drugs and Pharmaceuticals: Critique of Policies and Practices

Chapter 12
Developments in India's Domestic Pharmaceutical Sector and Implications for Universal Healthcare in India

Biswajit Dhar and Reji K. Joseph

Introduction

The economic reforms introduced in India in 1991 were a reversal of earlier policies which helped access to affordable medicines by the development of a strong generic pharmaceutical industry. Liberalisation of import restrictions, reduction of tariffs, removal of restrictions on foreign investment and introduction of product patents rights are all expected to have a profound impact on the industry. Cost of medicines being the most critical factor in the healthcare system in India, these reforms would have definite implications for the universal healthcare programme. This paper provides an analysis of the implications of reforms for the universal healthcare programme in the country.

Genesis of a Domestic Pharmaceutical Industry

The newly independent India was heavily dependent on imports for meeting its medicinal requirements. Indigenous production of drugs was worth only INR 100 million in 1947. The product patent regime 1911, which was in force at the time of independence, prevented Indian companies from producing patented drugs in India. Foreign companies which had the monopoly rights preferred neither producing the drugs in India nor supplying the drugs in India through imports. Keayla (1994) points out that in many cases drugs were not made available in India even after 15 years of their introduction in the international market. Besides, the drugs supplied by the foreign companies were exorbitantly priced. The report of the United States

B. Dhar (✉)
Centre for Economic Studies and Planning, Jawaharlal Nehru University, New Delhi, India

R. K. Joseph
Central University of Gujarat, Gandhinagar, India

I. Qadeer et al. (eds.), *Universalising Healthcare in India*,
https://doi.org/10.1007/978-981-16-5872-3_12

Senate states that "India which does grant patents on drugs provides an interesting case example. The prices in India for the broad spectrum antibiotics, Aureomycin and Achromycin are among the highest in the world. As a matter of fact, in drugs generally, India ranks among the highest priced nations of the world—a case of an inverse relationship between per capita income and the level of drug prices"(United States Senate, 1961: 112).

However, during the initial post-independence period, the policy of industrialisation by way of import substitution was not applicable to the pharmaceutical industry and foreign capital was encouraged. This was because, on the one hand there was no alternative available to the drug technology held by foreign companies (Narayana, 1984); and on the other the government expected that the foreign companies would help in building a strong industry within the new environment. The Industrial Policy Resolution of 1948 read that 'it should be recognised that participation of foreign capital and enterprise, particularly as regards industrial technique and knowledge, will be of value to the rapid industrialisation of the country' (Ministry of Industry and Supply, 1948: para 10). This liberal approach resulted in many foreign pharmaceutical companies opening their subsidiaries in India. Most of the foreign companies established themselves as mere trading concerns, importing finished drugs from abroad and selling them, without establishing manufacturing units in India (Ministry of Petroleum and Chemicals, 1975). The indigenous sector was also observed to be engaged mainly in the processing and formulation of medicines based on imported fine chemicals and bulk drugs, and the indigenous production of several new drugs had not commenced. The availability and prices of drugs continued to remain a major challenge for the policy makers. Realising the challenges in developing a vibrant pharmaceutical industry in the country with the help of foreign capital, the Government of India appointed four major committees to look into the matter and make recommendations. The Patents Enquiry Committee (1948–50) headed by Justice Bakshi Tek Chand was mandated to survey and report on the working of the patent system in India. Another committee headed by Justice N. Rajagopala Ayyangar was appointed in 1957 to examine the question of revision of the Patents Law and to advise the government in this regard (Ayyangar, 1959).

Alongside, the government gave due attention to the development of the pharmaceutical industry in the country. The Pharmaceutical Enquiry Committee headed by General Bhatia was appointed in 1953 with a detailed mandate to study the state of India's pharmaceutical industry and issues relating to the pricing of pharmaceutical products. The Committee was mandated to study the following: (i) working of the existing pharmaceutical manufacturing concerns in India; (ii) operations of foreign and/or Indian companies who import drugs and pack them in the country; (iii) extent of tie-up between the Indian concerns with foreign companies; (iv) recommend steps for encouraging the manufacture of important drugs, which are imported in the country; (v) distribution of pharmaceutical products, both imported or manufactured or packed in the country, the profit margins to Trade and Industry and the part played in this by purely Indian as well as foreign concerns (Kumar, 2004: 259).

The decade of the 1970s marked a turning point in the development of the Indian pharmaceutical industry as a result of three critical policy initiatives taken by the government: the Drugs Price Control Order (DPCO), which was adopted in 1970; adoption of the new Patents Act, which became effective in 1972; and adoption of a new drug policy in 1978. The framework for the new drug policy was provided in the Report of the Committee on Drugs and Pharmaceutical Industry commonly known as the Hathi Committee, Ministry of Petroleum and Chemicals 1975 (Government of India (GoI), 1975). Complementing these policy initiatives was yet another piece of legislation, the Foreign Exchange Regulation Act (FERA) of 1973, which aimed at reducing the share of foreign equity in enterprises registered in India to a maximum of 40%[1]. The above-mentioned policy initiatives were taken with two broad objectives in view: (i) to develop a strategy for the expansion of the domestic pharmaceutical industry by relying essentially on Indian enterprises, and (ii) to establish a structure for keeping the prices of drugs within affordable limits.

Possibly the most important policy reform which was instrumental in giving the Indian pharmaceutical industry global recognition was the Patents Act of 1970. The Act only provided for process patents in drugs and pharmaceuticals, the period of protection was reduced from 14 years to seven years (or five years from the date of sealing the patent, whichever is earlier) and the local production of patented subject matter was made compulsory. Indian pharmaceutical firms were able to produce patented drugs using alternate processes. An important outcome of this Act was that the gap period between the launch of a drug in the developed country markets and its launch in India got reduced considerably, to four to five years in contrast to much longer periods in the past (Keayla, 1994). Before the Patents Act, the Monopolies and Restrictive Trade Practices (MRTP) in 1969 came to curb the expansionist tendencies of big companies. The threshold limit for describing a unit as monopolistically large was fixed at INR 200 million. The prior approval of the central government became mandatory for the establishment of new undertakings, expansion of new undertakings, merger, amalgamation and takeovers and appointment of directors in certain cases.

The first step towards evolving a comprehensive policy regime for the Indian pharmaceutical industry was taken by the setting up of the Hathi Committee in 1974. The Committee, which presented its recommendations in 1975, had an exhaustive mandate that aimed at the realisation of the two broad objectives mentioned above. Following the recommendations made by the Hathi Committee, the government adopted the Drug Policy (DP) in 1978, which, till date, remains the most definitive statement justifying the establishment of the Indian pharmaceutical industry. Yet another step towards building an Indian pharmaceutical industry was taken by the 1978 DP. This policy stipulated that in order to promote small firms, the industrial licensing system must give preference to the small companies having Indian ownership, over companies belonging to the erstwhile monopoly houses and foreign-owned companies.

The new DP announced by the government in 1978 had the following five broad objectives: (i) to develop a strong Indian sector with the public sector playing a leading role; (ii) to channel the activities of the foreign firms in accordance with the national priorities and objectives; (iii) to deepen the production base of the domestic industry by ensuring that the production of drugs took place from as basic a stage as possible; (iv) to encourage research and development and improve the technological sinews of the industry; and (v) to provide drugs to consumers at reasonable prices.

The DP thus became an industrial policy instrument by linking up production, profitability to essentiality of medicine. In order to promote indigenous production from basic stages, the policy made mandatory for all firms producing formulations based on imported bulk drugs or bulk drugs manufactured from the penultimate stage, that they produce indigenously the bulk drug concerned from the basic stage within a period of two years. These firms were also required to supply 50% of the total production of bulk drugs to non-associate formulators. The policy also restricted the value of a firm's formulation production to five times the value of its total bulk drug production. All these measures amounted to a situation in which any significant increase in the production of formulations essentially depended on the increase in the indigenous production of bulk drugs. Companies were forced to engage in bulk drug production, which is the technology intensive phase in drug manufacturing. The practice of loan licensing, i.e. firms getting products manufactured by other firms and selling them under their own name, was also prohibited. The 1978 DP required the foreign firms operating in India with a turnover in drugs exceeding INR 50 million per year to have Research and Development (R&D) facilities in India. They were required to spend at least 4% of their turnover as recurring expenditure on R&D. The policy also liberalised licenses for the production meant for exports. A company could produce any amount for exports and had flexibility in the use of foreign exchange. The 1978 DP has been a milestone in the future development of the drug industry in India.

All these policy measures have had a profound impact on development of a strong indigenous pharmaceutical sector. The investment in the pharmaceutical industry increased from INR 240 million in 1952 to INR 2250 million in 1973 and further to INR 6000 million in 1982 (Hamied, 1988). The share of the domestic sector in total pharmaceutical production in India increased from 27% in 1975–76 to 52% in 1980–81 (Narayana, 1984). The indigenous production of drugs has grown from INR 100 million in 1947 to INR 1680 million in 1965–66 and to INR 82,200 million in 1993–94 (Ibid.). These measures also made a significant contribution towards self-reliance and self-sufficiency, using appropriate technology, based essentially on indigenous raw materials. In the production of bulk drugs, the share of the domestic sector had reached 82% in 1987 (Hamied, 1984). The drug prices in India had become one of the lowest in the world (Ghosh & Keayla, 1998) and the time lag for the introduction of a drug in India after its launch in the global market was reduced to less than 5 years (Keayla, 1994). The industry had transformed from a net importer to a net exporter. By the beginning of the 1990s, the Indian pharmaceutical industry was globally recognised as a powerhouse in reverse engineering. It contributes substantially to the facilitation of access to medicines in a number of countries other than India through its supply of drugs that are Good Manufacturing Practices (GMP) compliant at prices that are among the lowest in the world. This has earned the Indian pharmaceutical industry the epithet, 'the pharmacy of the world', coined by the global public health agency, Medecins Sans Frontiers (MSF).

In 1991, the Government of India liberalised its economic policies, which reversed many of the policies that had helped the development of the Indian pharmaceutical industry. The Industrial Licensing Policy Statement of July 1991 bears witness to this reversal in approach: it states that 'the role played by the government to be changed from that of exercising control to one of providing help and guidance by making essential procedures fully transparent and eliminating delays' (Ministry of Industry, 1991). The major features of this economic liberalisation were abolition of industrial licensing, abolition of FERA and introduction of automatic approval of Foreign Direct Investment (FDI), revision of the MRTP Act, and elimination of import restrictions and tariff liberalisation. All these reforms were introduced in the pharmaceutical sector in 1994 through the 'Modifications to the Drug Policy 1986'. The reforms in the pharmaceutical sector also eliminated the ratio parameter linking the production of bulk drugs and production of formulation, which was a crucial policy instrument in the development of the bulk drug industry in the country. The impact of this policy change was felt acutely by the two largest bulk drug producers in the country, the Indian Drugs and Pharmaceuticals Limited and the Hindustan Antibiotics Limited, both public sector undertakings. In the absence of support from the downstream producers, these firms were declared sick during the 1990s; an eloquent testimony to the problems that the market-oriented reforms had brought for the public sector enterprises.

Impact of Reforms on the Indian Pharmaceutical Industry

In the last two decades, the Indian pharmaceutical industry has become increasingly export-oriented. Exports as percentage of sales increased from 14% in 1994–95 to 44% in 2014–15[2]. With growing export orientation, the trade balance has also been growing positively, from US $287.3 million in 1994 to over US $10,000 million in 2013, before declining slightly (Table 12.1).

It has been primarily the domestic firms, including those taken over, which contributed to the exports. All the firms in the list of leading exporters in 2014–15 given in Table 12.2 are domestic firms.

Ranbaxy Laboratories and Mylan Laboratories (earlier Matrix Laboratories), two other leading exporters from India, do not figure in the list as their data for 2014–15 was not available in the Prowess database. For Ranbaxy and Mylan, exports had contributed to 53% and 79% of sales respectively in the previous year, i.e. 2013–14. Both these firms were taken over by foreign firms.[3]

As the pharmaceutical sector is increasingly becoming export-oriented, it is also becoming more formulation-oriented. Formulations are medicaments which are put into dosage forms and are ready for consumption. Share of formulations in exports has been on the rise in the last decade. It has increased from 70% in 2000 to 83% in 2014. And the positive trade balance has almost entirely been contributed by formulations.

Table 12.1 Export, import and balance of trade of different categories of pharmaceutical products (in US $ Million)

Years	Bulk drugs			Formulations			Total		
	Exp	Imp	BoT	Exp	Imp	BoT	Exp	Imp	BoT
1994	101.6	251	−149.4	484.2	47.5	436.7	585.8	298.5	287.3
1995	141.2	348.1	−206.9	582.9	56.9	526	724.2	405.1	319.1
1996	174.3	269.3	−95	639.7	37.4	602.3	814	306.7	507.3
1997	222.6	324.2	−101.6	724.6	64.6	660	947.2	388.9	558.3
1998	250.5	303.5	−53	683.2	80.7	602.5	933.7	384.3	549.4
1999	265.3	290.2	−24.9	802.9	82.6	720.3	1068.2	372.8	695.4
2000	341.8	281.1	60.7	805.1	92.8	712.3	1147	373.9	773.1
2001	363.3	303	60.3	959.1	97.6	861.5	1322.4	400.5	921.9
2002	451.7	404	47.7	1157.1	141.9	1015.2	1608.7	545.9	1062.8
2003	516.5	468.8	47.7	1455.4	141.2	1314.2	1971.9	609.9	1362
2004	482.5	493.9	−11.4	1789.1	186.4	1602.7	2271.6	680.3	1591.3
2005	543	662.4	−119.4	2218.8	275.3	1943.5	2761.8	937.8	1824
2006	644.5	789.3	−144.8	2771.6	392.2	2379.4	3416.1	1181.5	2234.6
2007	900.8	1101.2	−200.4	3576	515.1	3060.9	4476.7	1616.3	2860.4
2008	1015	1203.5	−188.5	4807.7	666	4141.7	5822.7	1869.6	3953.1
2009	1322.1	1312.4	9.7	4599.4	735.5	3863.9	5921.5	2047.9	3873.6
2010	1356.9	1598.5	−241.6	5767.2	835.9	4931.3	7124.1	2434.4	4689.7
2011	1828.6	1799.4	29.2	7674.1	935.7	6738.4	9502.6	2735	6767.6
2012	1871	1908.2	−37.2	8988.7	1161	7827.7	10,859.7	3069.2	7790.5
2013	2329.7	2042.3	287.4	10,844.70	1,019.00	9825.7	13,174.4	3061.3	10,113.1
2014	2242.9	2281.1	−38.2	10,692.40	907.3	9785.1	12,935.3	3188.4	9746.9

Source Compiled by authors based on DESA/UNSD, UN COMTRADE database (Rev.3)
Note This data is based on Standard International Trade Classification (SITC) Rev.3. SITC product group 541 refers to bulk drugs and 542 refers to formulations.

The changing pattern of exports has an impact on the production structure. As in the case of exports, growth in production too is focused on formulations. The Indian Drug Manufacturers' Association (IDMA) data on production that is available till 2014 shows that the growth dynamism of the production has changed in the post-1994 period, the year in which reforms were introduced into the pharmaceutical sector of India (Fig. 12.1).[4]

There has been a decline in the growth of bulk drugs production in the post-2000–01 to 2004–05 period, from around 20% during the 2000–01 to the 2004–05 period to less than 15% in 2005–06 to the 2009–10 period and further declined to around 10% during 2010–11 to 2013–14. The formulations segment which showed acceleration in production during the post-2004–05 period, exhibited a decline during the 2010–11 to 2013–14 period.

Table 12.2 Top 10 exporters in 2014–15

Company	Exp. ($Million)	%Sales
Dr. Reddy's Laboratories Ltd	1187.3	73.5
Aurobindo Pharma Ltd.	1001.0	75.7
Lupin Ltd.	936.5	59.5
Cipla Ltd.	758.4	46.3
Sun Pharmaceutical Inds. Ltd.	740.4	55.9
Glenmark Pharmaceuticals Ltd.	475.9	56.2
Cadila Healthcare Ltd.	449.6	56.5
Divi's Laboratories Ltd.	420.2	84.3
Ipca Laboratories Ltd.	266.2	53.0
Torrent Pharmaceuticals Ltd.	226.4	40.6

Source Compiled by authors from CMIE Prowess, Release 4.15

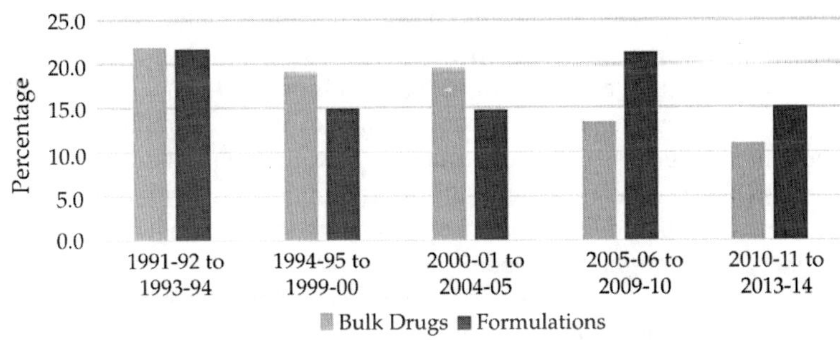

Fig. 12.1 Average annual growth production. *Source* Computed using data from IDMA Annual Publications. *Note* 2013–14 figures are estimated production

Expansion in the exports of formulations and decline in production of bulk drugs indicate more imports of bulk drugs. Firms are increasingly importing bulk drugs, their intermediates and fine chemicals as against relying on indigenous production as they used to do. It is seen in Table 12.1 that in bulk drugs, for most of the years, imports exceeds exports. Data from Prowess shows that the share of raw materials imported in sales turnover has grown from 9% in 1990–91 to 11% in 2000–01 to 12% in 2014–15[5]. There are different levels of value addition in bulk drugs manufacturing and the Indian bulk drug industry seems to focus particularly on the higher ends in the value chain. The abolition of the ratio parameter linking the production of formulations to indigenously produced bulk drugs from basic stages and reductions in import duty have eased the constraints on the imports of bulk drugs and other raw materials. Import duty on organic chemicals including bulk drugs has been reduced from 120% in 1990–91 to 7.5 in 2015–16. Another important factor contributing to decline in domestic production has been the implementation of Schedule M (concerning GMP) of the Drugs and Cosmetics Act since July 2005.

Consequently, a number of Small and Medium Enterprise (SME) bulk drug manufacturers had to shut down their operations. By January 2006, 70 firms were reported to have closed in the state of Andhra Pradesh alone due to implementation of GMP (Mahesh, 2006). Thousands of firms were reported to have shut down by the end of 2009 on account of their inability to comply with GMP standards (Mumbai Bureau, PHARMABIZ.com., 2006). Complying with GMP costs at least INR 20 lakhs for a SME firm, this was beyond the capacity of most SMEs. During our interaction with SME pharmaceutical representatives, it was established that not more than one percent of the SME pharmaceutical firms would be able to implement Schedule M. It was also reported that no new SME units came up during the three-year period ending in 2009, except in excise free zones. The SME sector has been a major producer of bulk drugs in India.

The bulk drugs segment is highly competitive with many players and hence the returns are very low. The Hathi Committee (Ministry of Petroleum and Chemicals, 1975) had worked out the capital invested-turnover ratio for bulk drugs and formulations manufacturing and estimated 1:1 for bulk drugs at its best and 1:2.6 for formulations on average, which in some cases would be as high as 1:7.2. Due to this, with the ratio parameter no more in force, firms in India tend to neglect the bulk drug segment and to concentrate on the production and export of formulations.

Though importing less costly bulk drugs and raw materials and exporting formulations which have higher investment-turnover ratio makes better business sense, the current pattern of import dependence causes concern from strategic as well as public health points of view. India has become dependent on one single country for half of its bulk drug imports. Since the turn of this decade, China has become the supplier of more than half of India's imports (Fig. 12.2).

The dependence on China shown above is for bulk drugs as a whole. In certain cases of bulk drugs the dependence is more substantial. The report of the Task Force on Strategy for Enhancing Exports of Pharmaceutical Products (Ministry of Commerce and Industry, 2008) has pointed out that in certain categories up to 70% of the requirements are met through imports from China. This very high import

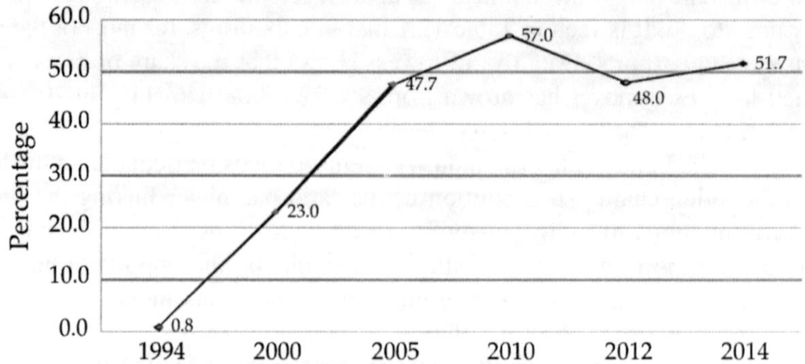

Fig. 12.2 Share of China in India's import of bulk drugs. *Source* Compiled by authors based on DESA/UNSD, UN COMTRADE database (Rev.3)

dependence on a single country can place India in trouble if the supply chains from China are cut. In fact, India has already experienced this risk once. The crackdown on the chemical industry in China in 2008 in order to enforce environmental legislation resulted in shortage of supply and subsequent hike in prices, affecting not only the bottom lines of Indian companies but even the very existence of many firms. Owing to shortage of raw materials and their rising prices, about 50 bulk drug manufacturing units were shut down while others cut down manufacturing of loss making drug categories (Dey, 2008). India's dependence on China is such that it does not have adequate domestic manufacturing capacity to meet the demand for intermediates and bulk drugs, if supplies from China are stopped for unforeseen reasons.

The cost advantage is the factor driving Indian manufacturers to shun indigenous production and engage in imports. For example, theophiline from China is 10% cheaper as compared to the cost of indigenous production. Chinese firms are able to sell bulk drugs at lower prices not only due to the subsidies, for example power subsidies, they enjoy but also due to better technologies. For example, in fermentation (an essential process for the production of bulk drugs) Indian firms still use sugar; whereas technology in China enables its firms to use cauliflower, which is much cheaper.[6] According to Y.K. Hamied, Chairman of Cipla, "if China decided one bright day to stop export to India, we would be finished."[7]

Excessive reliance on China for raw materials also raises challenges in ensuring quality of medicines. Recently, exports of certain medicines from India have been banned in the US on grounds of quality. Ensuring the quality of medicines is vitally important for the protection and promotion of public health.

Globalisation of the Indian Pharmaceutical Industry

The economic policy reforms paved the way for the 'globalisation' of the Indian pharmaceutical industry—which has now become part of the global production and development network of MNCs. A number of Indian (domestic) firms are in alliance with MNCs for contract manufacturing, joint marketing and contract research. Participation of Indian firms in the global network has become more of an income generation opportunity than a means for competence building. In 2010, the contract manufacturing market in India was estimated at US $ 2.3 billion (ICRA, 2011). It was expected to reach US $ 58.5 billion by 2015 (Shivakumar, 2012). Top global pharmaceutical firms like Pfizer, Merck, Glaxo Smith Kline (GSK), Sanofi-Aventis, Novartis, Teva, etc., largely depend on Indian firms for the supply of many of their Active Pharmaceutical Ingredients (APIs) and intermediates (FICCI, 2005).

Earlier, it was the smaller Indian firms which were into contract manufacturing, but lately larger firms like Dr. Reddy's are also into this business as part of much wider alliances, such as marketing and Research and Development (R&D) collaborations. The alliance between Dr. Reddy's and GSK provides that the latter would have exclusive access to Dr. Reddy's diverse portfolio and future pipeline of more than 100 formulations in therapeutic segments such as cardiovascular, diabetes, oncology, gastroenterology and pain management. The drugs will be manufactured by Dr. Reddy's and licensed and supplied by GSK in various developing countries in Africa, the Middle East, Asia Pacific and Latin America. In some markets, the drugs will be co-marketed by both companies (GSK, 2009). Revenues will be shared with Dr. Reddy's as per the agreement. Similar kinds of contract manufacturing alliances involving marketing tie-ups exist between Astra Zeneca and Torrent; Pfizer and Aurobindo; Pfizer and Biocon; and Boehringer Ingelheim and Cipla. The financial terms of these deals are often not disclosed and hence it is not possible to gauge the actual size of the contract manufacturing business as part of wider alliances.

In a similar way, a number of Indian firms are into various kinds of research collaborations ranging from contract research to collaborative research projects and in-licensing and out-licensing. The contract research business in India was estimated at $1.5 billion in 2010 (ICRA, 2011). It was expected to reach $31.5 billion by 2015 (Shivakumar, 2012). The contract research market in India is growing at a more rapid pace as compared to the global contract research market. Between 2007 and 2010 when the global contract research market grew at compound annual growth rate (CAGR) of 19% to reach US$25 billion in 2010, this market in India grew at CAGR 65% to reach $1.5 billion. The low cost of conducting research in India is an important factor for the outsourcing of research to India. R&D activities in India are estimated to be 60–65% cheaper as compared to the costs in the US. Labour cost in India is in the range of 10–15% of similar costs in the US. There is 25–50% reduction in the upfront capital requirements in setting up R&D projects in India due to locally fabricated equipment and high quality local technology/engineering skills (IBEF, 2011). The cost advantage of conducting clinical trials in India is more than 50% during phase I studies and more than 60% during the phase II and phase III studies (ICRA, 2011).

The liberalisation measures indeed had the objective that foreign investment and technology collaborations increasingly become important channels for competence building. In contract research, collaborative research projects, out-licensing and in-licensing partnerships, Indian firms have been partners of subordinate status who perform piecemeal projects in drug research and they are not exposed to the whole process of new drug development. In these collaborations, the scope for transfer of technology and joint ownership of technology is also very limited. The subordinate status of Indian firms in the long run may result in a dependency relationship of Indian firms with the MNCs. This can have harmful consequences for the country in many ways. Being trusted allies in the global strategy of MNCs, Indian companies may lose interest in those therapeutic areas which do not have a global presence (for example, neglected diseases). These allies might also withhold themselves from exercising compulsory licensing provisions, the Trade-Related Aspects of Intellectual Property Rights (TRIPS) instrument to counter abuse of patent monopoly rights as well as to address national health emergencies.

India has all rights under the TRIPS agreement to issue a compulsory license for making medicines more affordable for patients. The compulsory license over Bayer's Nexavar (anti-cancer drug) has reduced the cost for one month's course from INR 280,428 to INR 8800. But now India faces the challenge of no domestic firms coming forward to apply for compulsory licenses. Being part of the global networks of MNCs, it is quite expected that these firms would be unwilling to displease their global partners by applying for compulsory licenses. The lack of capacity of Indian firms in developing new drugs, both in terms of Science and Technology (S&T) skills and financial resources leave them with no other option but to collaborate with MNCs. In the earlier policy regime, the public sector companies and public sector laboratories had played a major role in augmenting the S&T skills of the private sector industry. Under the new policy regime, the public sector companies have been relegated and a few of them have already been closed down.

Implications for Universal Healthcare

Access to medicines at affordable prices is a critical factor for ensuring universal healthcare. The expenses on medicines constitute the single largest component of healthcare expenses both in in-patient and out-patient care. Expenditure on medicines alone constituted two-third (66.4%) of Out-of-Pocket Expenditure (OOPE) on healthcare in India in 2011–12 at the national level. It was 68.6% in rural areas and 62.9% in urban areas (Joseph, 2016). Given the fact that in India 69% of health expenditure is private spending and out of this two-third of spending is only on medicines, of medicines can be a strong determinant in patients accessing healthcare facilities. Various rounds of National Sample Survey (NSS) covering morbidity and healthcare shows that the cases of ailments not treated on account of financial problems are on the rise in the country (Table 12.3).

What emerges from the NSS data is that the financial problem is the most important constraint preventing people with ailments from getting treated[8]. With a very high share of out-of-pocket expenditure in healthcare, it is quite natural that poor people will find it difficult to seek healthcare services when they are ill. Given the significance of drug prices, any move to make drug prices more affordable alone will undoubtedly make more patients to seek healthcare services. It is worth noting in this context that within one year of the launch of the free medicines scheme in the state of Rajasthan[9], the out-patient visits rose by more than 50%[10] and in-patient admissions by 30% (Ebrahim, 2012).

The above discussion makes it clear that the policies adopted by the Government of India have resulted in the neglect of the bulk drug segment, the most crucial phase of drug manufacturing. Excessive reliance on one single country for the bulk drugs poses great risks to the universal healthcare programme as any disturbance in the supply from one country jeopardises the entire healthcare programme. Liberalisation has also led to globalisation of Indian pharmaceutical firms. Subsequently, most of the Indian firms are not keen to seek compulsory license options. Compulsory license

Table 12.3 Percentage of ailments not treated for their reasons during different rounds of NSS on morbidity and healthcare

Reasons for not treating Ailments	2004 (60th round) rural urban		1995–96 (52nd Round) rural urban		1986–87 (42nd round) rural urban	
No medical facilities available in the neighbourhood	12	1	9	1	3	0
Facilities available, but lack of faith	3	2	4	5	2	2
Long waiting	1	2	1	1	0	1
Financial problems	28	20	24	21	15	10
Ailment not considered serious	32	50	52	60	75	81
Others (including not reported)	24	25	10	12	5	6
	100	100	100	100	100	100

Source Compiled by authors from NSS data. Data from NSS 42nd and 52nd rounds have been accessed from NSSO (1998), and data from the 60th round from NSSO (2006)

also becomes a vital policy instrument in ensuring access to affordable medicines for universal healthcare.

Notes

1. The number of foreign subsidiaries in the pharmaceutical industry came down from 10 to two between 1973 and 1985 and the number of firms holding more than 50% equity declined from 21 to 14 during the same period (Pillai, 1984; Panikar et al., 1992).
2. Based on data from Prowess of CMIE. Information for 1994–95 is based on Prowess Release 4.13 and 2014–15 on Prowess Release 4.15.
3. Ranbaxy was taken over by Daiichi of Japan in 2008. The Sun Pharma of India bought Ranbaxy in 2015. The Matrix Laboratories was taken over by Mylan in 2006.
4. The Dept. of Pharmaceuticals data (available in its Annual Reports) on production is based on selected drugs and is available in terms of quantity only. IDMA Annual Publications provide the data on production of formulations and bulk drugs.
5. Based on data from Prowess of CMIE. Information for 1994–95 is based on Prowess Release 4.13 and 2014–15 on Prowess Release 4.15.
6. Informed by the Indian Drug Manufacturers' Association (IDMA) representative during the workshop on "Public Health and Pharma Industry", organised by

the Research and Information System for Developing Countries, on February 6, 2012, in New Delhi.

7. Hamied stated this during the stakeholders' meeting (civil society and Indian domestic pharmaceutical industry) held on November 24, 2013 in Mumbai, organised by Lawyers Collective.
8. 'Ailment not considered serious' is not a constraint.
9. The free medicines scheme launched in October 2011 began with free supply of 200 generic medicines in public hospitals. The Rajasthan Medical Services Corporation is the nodal agency implementing this scheme. For more details, see, Rajasthan Medical Service Corporation Limited. http://rmsc.health.rajasthan.gov.in/content/raj/medical/rajasthan-medical-services-corporation-ltd-/en/home.html#, http://rmsc.nic.in.
10. During the first anniversary of the launch of the scheme, the Chief Minister of Rajasthan is reported to have mentioned the increase in the number of patients visiting out-patient department. For details see (Special Correspondent, the Hindu, 2012)

References

Ayyangar, J. N. R. (1959). *Report on the Revision of the Patents Law*, Ministry of Commerce and Industry.

Dey, S. (2008). Sick Bulk Drug Cos May Get Life Support. *The Economic Times,* August 15, 2008.

Ebrahim, Z. (2012). India poised to supply free drugs to 1.2 billion people. *Inter Press Service News Agency,* November 8, 2012.

Federation of Indian Chambers of Commerce and Industry (FICCI). (2005). *Competitiveness of the Indian pharmaceutical industry in the new product patent regime* [FICCI Report for National Manufacturing Competitiveness Council (NMCC)]. FICCI.

Ghosh, A., & Keayla, B. K. (1998). *Report of people's commission on intellectual property rights.* National Working Group on Patent Laws.

Glaxo, Smith Kline plc. (GSK). (2009). *GSK announces a strategic alliance with Dr. Reddy's to further accelerate sales growth in emerging markets.* June 15, 2009. Accessed September 22, 2011. http://www.gsk.com/media/pressreleases/2009/2009_pressrelease_10064.htm

Hamied, Y. K. (1988). The Indian Patents Act 1970 and the Pharmaceutical Industry. *Conquest by Patent: On Patent Law and Policy.* National Working Group on Patent Laws.

Government of India. (1975). *Report of the committee on the drugs and pharmaceutical industry* (April 1975). Ministry of Petroleum and Chemicals.

IBEF (India Brand Equity Foundation). (2011). *Pharmaceuticals.* Accessed October 30, 2014. http://ukrexport.gov.ua/i/imgsupload/file/Pharma_sectoral.pdf

Information and Credit Rating Agency (ICRA). (2011). *CRAMS India: Overlook and outlook.* Accessed January 20, 2016. http://www.icra.in/Files/Articles/CRAMS%20Note,%20Overview%20and%20Outlook.pdf

Joseph, R. K. (2016). *Pharmaceutical industry and public policy in post-reform India.* Routledge.

Keayla, B. K. (1994). Patent protection and pharmaceutical industry. In K. R. G. Nair, & A. Kumar (Eds.), *Intellectual property rights.* Allied Publishers.

Kumar, V. (2004). *Committees and commissions in India Vol. 1: 1947–54.* Concept Publishing Co.

Mahesh, K. (2006). 70 Pharma Firms Shut Shop. *The Times of India,* January 24, 2006.

Ministry of Commerce and Industry, Government of India. (2008). *Strategy for increasing exports of pharmaceutical products.* Ministry of Commerce and Industry.

Ministry of Industry and Supply, Government of India. (1948). *Industrial policy statement*. Ministry of Industry and Supply.

Ministry of Industry, Government of India. (1991). *Statement on industrial policy.* Ministry of Industry.

Ministry of Petroleum and Chemicals, Government of India. (1975). *Report of the committee in drugs and pharmaceutical industry*. Ministry of Petroleum and Chemicals.

Mumbai Bureau, PHARMABIZ.com. (2009). *Empower SMEs while embracing GMP,* November 5, 2009. Accessed February 27, 2018. http://saffron.pharmabiz.com/article/detnews.asp?articleid=52445&sectionid=50

Narayana, P. L. (1984). *The Indian pharmaceutical industry: Problems and prospects.* National Council of Applied Economic Research.

NSSO (National Sample Survey Office). (1998). *Morbidity and treatment of ailments*, NSS 52nd Round, Report No. 441 (52/25.0/1). Ministry of Statistics and Programme Implementation, Government of India. Accessed November 14, 2014. http://mospi.nic.in/rept%20_%20pubn/441_final.pdf

NSSO (National Sample Survey Office). (2006). *Morbidity, healthcare and the condition of the aged*, NSS 60th Round, January–June 2004, Report No. 507 (60/25.0/1). Ministry of Statistics and Programme Implementation, Government of India. Accessed November 14, 2014. http://mospi.nic.in/rept%20_%20pubn/507_final.pdf

Panikar, P. G. K., Pillai, M. P., & Sundari, T. K. (1992). *International environment multinational corporations and drug policy*. Centre for Development Studies.

Pillai, P. M. (1984). *Multinationals and Indian pharmaceutical industry.* Kerala Sastra Sahitya Parishat.

Shivakumar, S. (2012). CRAMS in India. *Cutting edge* (March): 5–8. Special Correspondent, *The Hindu.* 2012. After Generic Medicine Supply, Rajasthan May Go for Free Diagnostic Tests. *The Hindu,* October 3.

United States Senate. (1961). *Study of administered prices in the drug industry (Report of the Committee on the Judiciary).* US Government Office.

Chapter 13
Vaccine Policy of the Government of India: Driven and Controlled by Vested Interests?

Jacob Puliyel

When trusted international organisations like the World Health Organisation (WHO) get co-opted, the onus falls on national governments to dispassionately evaluate vaccines for their people. The state cannot abdicate this responsibility. In this context the role of international philanthropic organisations influencing the functioning of national technical advisory groups on behalf of vaccine lobbies is deprecated.

Suppose it were ascertained that every child in the world could be rendered absolutely immune from all diseases during its entire life by taking half an ounce of radium to every pint of its milk. The world would be none the healthier, because not even a Crown Prince—no, not even the son of a Chicago Meat King, could afford the treatment. Yet it is doubtful whether doctors would refrain from prescribing it on that ground. The recklessness with which they now recommend wintering in Egypt or at Davos to people who cannot afford to go to Cornwall, and the orders given for champagne jelly and old port in households where such luxuries must obviously be acquired at the cost of stinting necessaries, often make one wonder whether it is possible for a man to go through a medical training and retain a spark of common sense (Shaw, 1906: Unpaged).

Vaccines need to be affordable before they can be useful. George Bernard Shaw believed that the medical fraternity was incapable of comprehending this basic truth. He attributed it to a lack of common sense. One century and a decade later, organisations like the World Health Organisation (WHO) and the Global Alliance for Vaccines and Immunisation (GAVI) are prescribing this champagne jelly to poor countries who cannot afford clean drinking water. Exorbitantly expensive vaccines against minor ailments are now being promoted and made mandatory for school admissions. The genius of vested interests lies in how they have co-opted these international agencies.

J. Puliyel (✉)
Paediatrics Department, St. Stephens Hospital, New Delhi, India

National Technical Advisory Group on Immunization (NTAGI), Government of India, New Delhi, India

I. Qadeer et al. (eds.), *Universalising Healthcare in India*,
https://doi.org/10.1007/978-981-16-5872-3_13

It has not always been like this. Most widely prescribed vaccines used to be inexpensive and a cost beneficial means of controlling disease. Immunisations against life threatening diseases like smallpox were a boon for public health. Early in the nineteenth century, India was at the forefront of this movement using vaccines for public health. Smallpox vaccine was discovered in 1798 and within 4 years in 1802, it was being used in India (Lahariya, 2014). The first plague vaccine was developed in India in 1897. The Haffkine Institute was set up in 1905 as the Plague Laboratory. The Pasture Institute was started in 1907 and it produced neural tissue anti-rabies vaccine (Ibid.). The Central Research Institute at Kasauli was set up in 1904 for research in immunology. India became smallpox free in 1977.

The Universal Immunisation Programme (UIP) started in 1985. Many consider protection with *Bacillus Calmette–Guérin* (BCG), Oral Polio Vaccine (OPV), Diphtheria, Pertussis and Tetanus (DPT) and measles vaccines are a part of the basic right of babies to healthcare. Full immunisation with all the UIP vaccines costs INR 20 (0.30 US $) (one US$ = approximately INR 60). However according to the District Level Household Survey-3 (DLHS) (2007–08) full immunisation with the Extended Programme on Immunisation (EPI) vaccination was achieved in only 53.8% of the population (Ministry of Health and Family Welfare (MoHFW), n.d.). The data from the DLHS 4 is even bleaker. In this context of the inability to provide basic, effective and inexpensive EPI vaccines to vast numbers of poor people living in remote areas in the country, newer and more expensive vaccines of doubtful utility are being sought to be introduced into the country's immunisation programme. These include vaccines against hepatitis B, H influenza B (Hib), rotavirus, pneumococcal and Human Papilloma Virus (HPV) vaccines. This paper examines the new scenario and the influences that bear on selection of vaccines for the national immunisation programme.

Introduction of New Vaccines: Role of WHO

In 1992, the World Health Assembly (WHA) passed resolution 45.17 that called on member states, '…to integrate cost-effective new vaccines, such as hepatitis B vaccine, into national immunisation programmes in countries where it is feasible…' (WHO, 2013a). Paradoxically, it was in the same year (that the WHA resolved that countries must integrate cost-effective vaccines), the WHO set a goal that all countries must integrate hepatitis B vaccination into EPI by 1997 (regardless of costs and benefits) (Ibid., WHO, 2002).

Hepatitis B

Hepatitis B can cause chronic hepatitis, liver cirrhosis and lead to hepatocellular carcinoma in susceptible persons. The risk of chronic infection is 90% in children infected under the age of one year and 2% for adults (Jensen & Balistreri, 2015).

The need for the Hepatitis B vaccination in India has been questioned because the incidence of hepatocellular carcinoma attributed to Hepatitis B in the country is very low. (Indian Council for Medical Research (ICMR) n.d.). Systematic review and meta-analysis done by Batham and colleagues using population-weights, estimated that the point-prevalence of hepatitis B was 3.70 (95% CI: 3.17–4.24) corresponding to a chronic carrier rate of 2.96% (Batham et al., 2009). The Indian Association for Study of the Liver (INSAL) estimates national average prevalence of Hepatitis B infection is 4.7% (INSAL, 2000). Assuming that 4% of the population are chronic carriers and extrapolating data from Taiwan, it was estimated that 184,000 to 250,000 persons die each year of hepatocellular carcinoma in India (Miller & McCann, 2000; Miller & Kane, 2000; Puliyel et al. 2001, 2004a, b; Tiwari et al., 2003). However, the Cancer Registry of the ICMR shows the incidence of Hepatocellular carcinoma (HCC) due to hepatitis B infection is only 5000 cases a year (Dhir & Mohandas, 1998). This is a mere 2% of the HCC load projected previously (Miller & McCann, 2000). Whatever the reason for the low HCC rate, immunising 25 million babies each year to prevent 5000 deaths from HCC and the corresponding number of deaths from cirrhosis liver, intuitively seems an uneconomic way to spend scarce health resources. The persuasions that caused the WHO to recommend universal immunisation are unclear.

Notwithstanding the concerns about the high costs and meagre benefits of the vaccine (ICMR, n.d.), Hepatitis B vaccine was introduced in the immunisation programme of the country starting with 10 states in 2007–8 (Lahariya et al., 2013). As a large proportion of births in India take place at home and are difficult to reach immediately after birth, a pragmatic schedule was adopted in India, vaccinating babies born in institutions at birth where possible and others were vaccinated starting at six weeks or later when they came for the DPT immunisation.

Evaluation of Benefits After Introduction of Hepatitis B

After the vaccine was introduced in India a serological survey of children aged five to 11 years in rural Andhra Pradesh was performed. Of those surveyed 2674 children had received hepatitis B immunisation and 2350 had not received the vaccine. Protective antibody (HBsAb) was seen in 18% of the unvaccinated children (33% in the unvaccinated at six years and 16% at ten years). The study also showed that the vaccine did not reduce the hepatitis B carrier rate. The frequency of chronic carriers (HBsAg positivity) was similar in the unvaccinated as in the vaccinated (0.17% and 0.15% respectively). The marker of hepatitis B infection in the past (HBcAb) was 1.79% in unvaccinated and 1.05% in the vaccinated (Aggarwal et al., 2014). These findings, demonstrating the futility of the vaccination, did not lead to any reassessment of the immunisation programme.

This was followed by a multi centre study in North India in children of the age group one to five years, funded by the ICMR (to be published). Forty percent of the unimmunized had protective levels of HBsAb (45% in the unvaccinated at one year and 29% at four years). The high levels of HBsAb seen among the unvaccinated in this study and that of Aggarwal point to passive transmission of natural immunity from mother to child, early in life (Ibid.). This natural immunity may be protecting babies from infection soon after birth, at the time when they are particularly vulnerable to develop chronic carrier status and HCC. This may be an explanation for the unexpectedly low levels of HCC seen in India. Universal immunisation will reduce this natural immunity and paradoxically it may increase the incidence of HCC in the country. The universal immunisation programme needs to be reevaluated given these findings.

H. Influenza B

The recommendation that all countries must include Hepatitis B vaccine in their immunisation programme (even if it were not needed) was followed by a similar recommendation for universal immunisation with Hib vaccine. This was mystifying initially. An editorial in the Bulletin of the WHO had questioned the need for Hib vaccine in Asia (Lau, 1999). In Asia the incidence of invasive Hib disease was considered to be very low even prior to the introduction of the vaccine. The Minz study found that the incidence of Hib meningitis in India was 7/100,000 children under five (Minz et al., 2008). At this rate if the birth cohort in India of 25 million is followed up over five years, there would be 1750 cases of Hib meningitis and 175 deaths (assuming mortality of 10%). The probe studies in Indonesia and Bangladesh found that the vaccine did not reduce pneumonia or meningitis (Baqui et al., 2007; Gessner et al., 2005). When the Bangladesh study showed no benefit from vaccination a misleading press release was issued by a number of organisations including the WHO, GAVI, United States Agency for International Development (USAID) and the Hib Initiative, a consortium of four organisations (Johns Hopkins Bloomberg School of Public Health, the London School of Hygiene and Tropical Medicine, the Centres for Disease Control and Prevention and the WHO) funded through a four-year, 37 million dollar grant from GAVI (GAVI, 2005). The press release stated deceptively that the Bangladesh probe study showed Hib vaccine protects children from significant burden of life-threatening pneumonia and meningitis (WHO, 2007). The involvement of international organisations in this deception was pointed out in articles published in the *British Medical Journal and the Indian Journal of Medical Research* (Puliyel, 2010; Puliyel et al., 2010).

It was around this time that the WHO suggested that, 'in view of their demonstrated safety and efficacy, conjugate Hib vaccines should be included in all routine infant immunisation programmes. Lack of local surveillance data should not delay the introduction of these vaccines, especially in countries where regional evidence indicates there is a high burden of disease.' (WHO, 2006).

In self-congratulatory articles, GAVI and the Hib initiative took credit for turning the tide against the Hib vaccine (GAVI, 2007; Levine et al. 2010). The article notes that given the controversies about whether there was a substantial burden of Hib disease, there was no strongly supportive WHO recommendation for vaccine use till the Hib initiative supported the revision of WHO Hib vaccine policy from a weak permissive statement (WHO, 2004) to a firm recommendation calling for universal vaccine introduction in all countries (WHO, 2006). This resulted in a rapid increase in application from GAVI countries for Hib conjugate vaccine. This highlights the influence GAVI and other vaccine-manufacturer-funded-organisations like the 'Hib Initiative' have on the WHO and how it impacts vaccine uptake internationally.

Accelerated Development and Introduction Plans (ADIP)

The Hib Initiative was only one of the accelerated development and introduction plans of GAVI (GAVI, 2007). Pneumo ADIP, located at the Johns Hopkins Bloomberg School of Public Health, is a small dedicated team supported by a 30 million dollar grant by GAVI[1]), working to accelerate the evaluation of and access to pneumococcal vaccines for the world's children. The WHO endorsed the pneumococcal vaccine for universal use (WHO, 2007) even when literature showed that vaccination reduced only 3.6 cases of pneumonia per 1000 child years (Madhi et al., 2008).

The Rota ADIP based in Seattle in the United States, was created to accelerate rotavirus vaccine introduction process and to make it available to children in developing countries as quickly as possible. It is a partnership with WHO and the CDC. Although the vaccine has only 50% efficacy in developing countries (Piple & Puliyel, 2015), this vaccine was recommended for universal use by the WHO (WHO, 2009).

Multivalent Pentavalent Vaccines and Adverse Events

Although adverse events are anticipated to occur more frequently after administration of a combination vaccine compared with administration of separate antigens at the same visit, Pentavalent vaccine (DPT, Hib HepB) was recommended by the CDC to improve vaccine coverage (Kroger et al., 2011). According to Madhavi and Raghuram, combination vaccines are a marketing trick invented to overcome poor penetration of the individual vaccines in the global market, as well as to overcome the expiry of their patents and establish eternal market monopolies (Madhavi & Raghuram, 2010). 'Every dubious new vaccine needs a piggyback ride on a diphtheria tetanus pertussis (DTP), measles or some other essential vaccine to get a back door entry into the UIP' (Madhavi, 2006). GAVI supports use of Pentavalent vaccine as a means of increasing uptake of Hib and Hepatitis B vaccines (GAVI, n.d.).

Rotavirus Vaccine

An 'Indian rotavirus vaccine' was introduced in the national programme recently. It illuminates the multifaceted ways in which international agencies and philanthropic organisations influence decision-making. Initially rotavirus was cultured from an asymptomatic neonate at the All India Institute of Medical Science (AIIMS). This was transferred to the USA and made into a vaccine (Bhan et al., 2014). The vaccine was patented by the Department of Health and Human Services USA. It was however misleadingly called an Indian vaccine and the Government of India was tasked to conduct clinical trials and license the vaccine. Ten years before clinical trials on the vaccine was undertaken an organisation called the Indo-US vaccine Action Programme selected Bharat Biotech to manufacture the vaccine and take all the profits. This company had no experience with vaccine manufacture and no licensed products at that time. Furthermore, government funds were used to build the manufacturing capacity of this private firm. The article by Bhan (Bhan et al., 2014) is co-authored by the owner of Bharat Biotech. It describes how, presumably because it would be illegal for the Department of Biotechnology of the Government of India to fund a private company, funds were given as grants to PATH (an organisation set up by the Bill Gates Foundation) which acted as a conduit to fund Bharat Biotech.

The vaccine was tested in a multicentre trial. Intussusceptiona are the dreaded adverse effect with the vaccine. The vaccine trial demonstrated that the incidence of intussusceptions was twenty times higher at the Vellore centre compared to Delhi. However without releasing the data on intussusceptions in Vellore the vaccine was licensed and introduced in the immunisation programme of the country. The Vellore data was not shared even with the National Technical Advisory Group on Immunisation (NTAGI). It is said that the government will monitor adverse events in the post-marketing surveillance within a small window period after vaccination but little reliance can be placed on such a study without reliable controls. A public interest litigation filed in the Delhi High Court asked for release of the data from the randomized trial in Vellore, but the government pleaded that "site specific data on safety is inappropriate for release as per protocol and its inappropriate interpretation or publication would lead to disinformation about the product (that has been) developed by government with great effort and expense, and will give unfair advantage to multinational products which were never tested in India, (and) yet (were) licensed." (Rathi, 2015: unpaged).

Ad Hoc Revision of the AEFI Classification: Downplaying Adverse Events

The introduction of the Pentavalent vaccine was associated with numerous deaths in different countries (Puliyel, 2013). The response of WHO to these deaths is educative. When there were 5 deaths in Sri Lanka with Quinvaxim (Pentavalent vaccine) a

WHO panel investigated the events and classified three deaths (cases D1, D3, and D6) as 'unlikely' to be related to vaccine after deleting the categories 'Probable' and 'Possible' from the standard Brighton classification (WHO, 2005).

Adverse Events Following Immunisation (AEFI) classification is best understood as an algorithm. All events that have a plausible temporal relation to vaccine administration are classified as either 'very likely/certain' or 'probable' or 'possible'. Adverse events are classified as unlikely or unrelated only if the timing makes a causal connection improbable or incompatible. The next level of the algorithm requires enquiry whether the adverse event can conclusively be attributable to other causes. If there are other possible explanations, the association with vaccine is classified as 'possible'. If another cause is not found, an adverse event after immunisation is 'probable'.

As mentioned above, while investigating the cluster of deaths in Sri Lanka the WHO panel deleted the categories 'probable' and 'possible' from the standard classification. All adverse events that could not be classified as 'very likely/certain' were classified as 'unlikely'.

Using the improvised classification (deleting 'probable' and 'possible'), three deaths that would have been classified as 'probable' related to immunisation were classified as 'unlikely' to be related to vaccine, although the authors note 'it could not be conclusively attributable to another cause'. The website of the WHO, published only the conclusions of the AEFI panel but not the methodology they employed (WHO, 2008a, b). It was possible to acquire the full report only after a petition was filed for a rational vaccination policy in India in 2010. It was then that the alteration of the categories was exposed through an article in the BMJ (Saxena et al., 2010).

The Official Revision of the AEFI Classification

The response of the WHO to this exposé was to officially change the way AEFI is classified in March 2013 (WHO, 2013b).The new algorithm for AEFI is reproduced in Fig. 13.1.

In the new scheme, causality is classified in 4 categories: 'Consistent causal association to immunisation', 'Indeterminate', 'Inconsistent causal association to immunisation' and 'Unclassifiable' Only events that occur after vaccine administration are eligible for AEFI causality assessment. 'Unclassifiable' are cases where the circumstances could not be investigated accurately.

Consistent Causal Association to Immunisation

A reaction can be classified as 'Consistent with causal association with immunisation' only if there is evidence in population-based studies that the vaccine has caused similar adverse events.

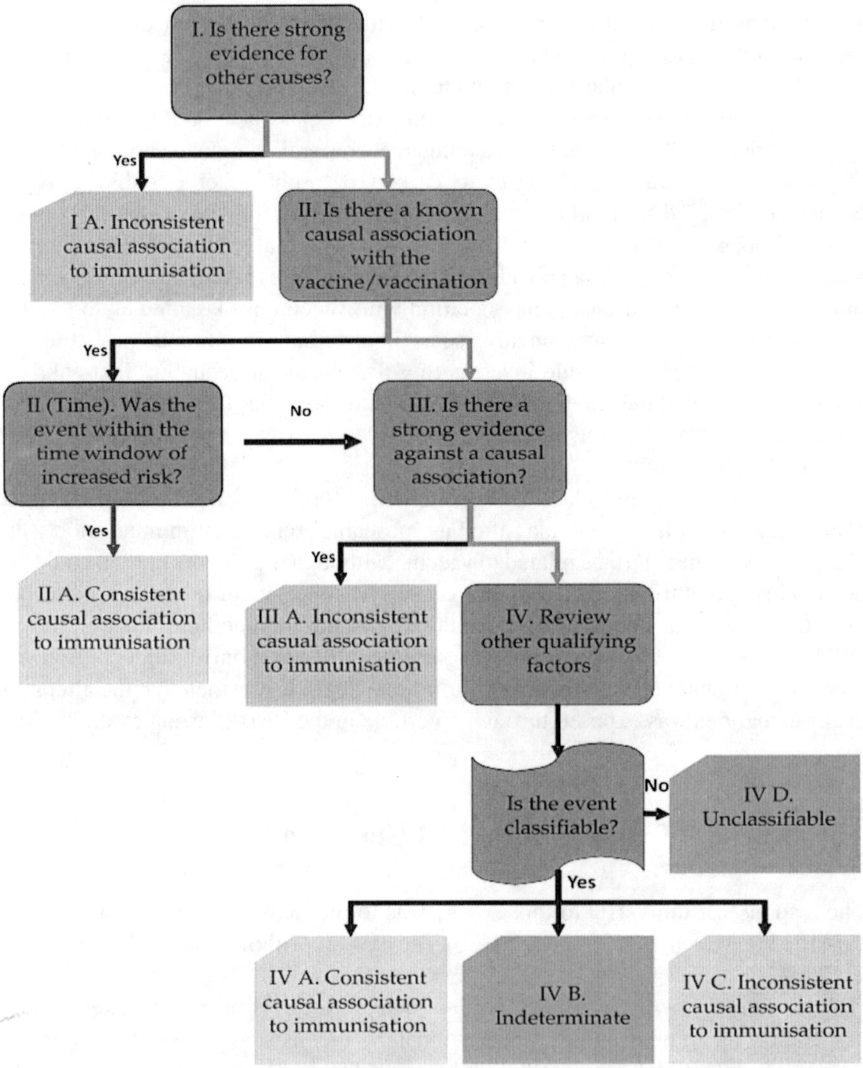

Fig. 13.1 The new algorithm for AEFI

No new association discovered in Phase 4 trials will qualify. On the other hand, if it is a known adverse reaction within an acceptable window period, causal association is accepted even where the events could have happened by coincidence. For example, just because intussusceptions are acknowledged as an adverse event following use of rotavirus vaccine, it does not follow that all intussusceptions in the critical window of increased susceptibility are necessarily caused by it. The residual uncertainty ensures that even if an adverse event is classified as 'Consistent with causal association with immunisation' 'coincidence' is still a possibility. Thus no reaction is classified as 'certainly' related to vaccination in the new scheme—not even if the reaction was duplicated on re-challenge.

Inconsistent Causal Association to Immunisation

At the bottom of the new causality classification hierarchy is 'Inconsistent causal association to immunisation'. Even reactions for which there is no alternate explanation will fall in this category, if causal association with immunisation has not been documented in prior epidemiological studies. In the revised scheme, this term is also used to suggest that there is no relation between the AEFI and immunisation. No matter how frequently the reaction categorised as 'Inconsistent with causal association' occurs, it would not be investigated as new signals of a causal association.

Indeterminate

Theoretically this group is reserved for reactions that could have been caused by immunisation, but for which causal association has not been documented in epidemiological studies previously. It is stated that information on AEFI that are classified as indeterminate will be pooled and analysed in order to understand if the AEFI represents a new signal of an unrecognised event. However a dictum introduced by the Council of International Organisation of Medical Sciences (CIOMS)/WHO ensures that reactions are not investigated as new signals.

CIOMS/WHO Report on Vaccine Pharmacovigilance

Forty experts (of whom 19 were industry representatives with possible conflicts of interest) helped to write this report on vaccine pharmacovigilance (CIOMS/WHO, 2012). It is acknowledged in the revised AEFI causality assessment document that the definitions and concepts of the CIOMS/WHO Pharmacovigilance report are used. The CIOMS/WHO document, under the heading 'Notes for Guidelines', states in small print:

> If there is adequate evidence that an event does not meet a case definition, such an event should be rejected and should be reported as 'Not a case of [AEFI]'. Such evidence is considered adequate, if an exclusion criteria is met, or an investigation reveals a negative finding of a necessary criterion (necessary condition) for diagnosis. Such an event should be rejected and classified as 'Not a case of [AEFI]'. (CIOMS, 2012: 170)

This passage implies that if the reported event does not meet an existing CIOMS/WHO case definition, even if they follow on after immunisation, it will be reported as 'Not an adverse event following immunisation [AEFI].' Besides being illogical and a contradiction in terms, this is at odds with the advice on page 11 of the CIOMS/WHO document which is that a case definition can be adopted from the standard literature or by the reviewers themselves; not necessarily 'an existing case definition'. After this CIOMS/WHO report, when they were called in to investigate 9 deaths in Vietnam with Quinvaxim (the vaccine used in Sri Lanka prior to the deaths there), the WHO presumably reclassified the AEFI they had previously reported in Sri Lanka as 'AEFI—Unlikely to be related to vaccination' changing it to 'Not a case of [AEFI]'. In the Vietnam report they then wrote 'Quinvaxem was prequalified by WHO in 2006…no fatal AEFI has ever been associated with this vaccine' (WHO, 2013c). One can see that each reaction is classified as 'Not a case of [AEFI]' and so none of them—no matter how frequently they recur—need to be assessed as a new signal.

The latest causality assessment of 132 reported serious AEFI cases, approved by the National AEFI Committee in India[2] has been uploaded on the Ministry of Health and Family Welfare website[3]. Of these AEFI reported between 2012 and 2016, 78 babies survived hospitalisation and 58 died. Among those who survived, the causality assessment suggests that 37 (47.4% of reactions) were vaccine product-related reactions classified as (A1). Among those that died 52 (96%) were classified as unclassifiable (D) or coincidental due to something other than vaccine. Not even one was classified as a vaccine product related reactions (A1) (Table 13.1).

Thus using the revised scheme of AEFI classification, a child who is admitted with intractable convulsions with onset after vaccination, the reaction could be classified as a vaccine product related if he survives, but if he dies during hospitalisation, it will be classified as coincidental death—underlying or emerging condition, or condition caused by something (anything) other than vaccine or (D)unclassifiable.

Table 13.1 Causality classification of 132 cases approved by the National AEFI Committee

Causality classification categories	Survived ($n = 78$)	Died ($n = 54$)
A1 Vaccine product related reaction	47. 4% (37)	0% (0)
A2 Vaccine quality related reaction	0% (0)	0% (0)
A3 Immunisation error related reaction	12.8% (10)	0% (0)
A4 Immunisation anxiety related reaction	2.6% (2)	0% (0)
B1 Temporal relationship but insufficient definitive evidence for vaccine causing event	1.3% (1)	1.9% (1)
B2 Conflicting trends of consistency and inconsistency with Causal Association	17.9% (14)	1.9% (1)
C Coincidental underlying or emerging condition, or condition caused by something other than vaccine	14.1% (11)	53.7% (29)
D Unclassifiable	2.6% (2)	42.6 (23)

TOKEN Study and Population Based Evidence of AEFI

Deaths are now classified as 'Not a case of [AEFI]', and all memory of numerous deaths from the Pentavlent vaccine have been erased on the ground that deaths have not been reported as AEFI in epidemiological studies involving the vaccine. However the TOKEN study contradicts the assertion that deaths have not been reported in population-based studies (Schlaud et al., n.d.).

The TOKEN study was done specifically to assess a possible causal relationship between vaccination and unexplained Sudden Unexpected Death (SUD) of children between their second and twenty-fourth month of life. von Kries et al. had previously found a statistically significant increase in the Standardized Mortality Ratio (SMR) within two days after vaccination with one of the two licensed hexavalent vaccines (Hexavac) (von Kries et al., 2005), and the TOKEN study was done to confirm or refute the association. The study was sponsored and supported by the Paul-Ehrlich-Institute (PEI) and the Federal Ministry of Health (Bundes ministerium für Gesundheit).

Temporal association of SUD to vaccination was examined in a Self- Controlled Case Series (SCCS) design. Parents of children who had died of SUD were requested to participate in the study. Total 254 cases (37.6% of all the eligible cases) could be included in the study. Parental participation was more than twice as high for children who had died within one week after vaccination (80%) as for children who had not been vaccinated within one week prior to their death. To account for this bias, inverse probability weighted analysis were conducted in addition to the pre-planned, unweighted analyses. The weight in this case was a method to compensate for the overrepresentation of parents of children who died soon after vaccination. The results obtained from these weighted analyses are regarded as more valid. The authors note that weighted analysis could only account for the selection bias among the exposed cases aged up to nine months and enrolled by the forensic institutes. Therefore, the results of the weighted analyses are likely to still overestimate the risk of SUD.

The weighted SCCS analysis, relative risk of SUD after pentavalent vaccination (first and second year of life) looking at risk period 0–3 days after vaccination versus control period 4–28/183 days showed Relative Risk (RR) of 8.11 ($p = 0.006$, 95% CI = 1.81–36.24; Table 41 in the TOKEN Report). The weighted SCCS analysis, relative risk of SUD after hexa or pentavalent vaccination (first and second year of life) looking at risk period 0–3 days versus control period 4–28/183 days showed RR 2.19 ($p = 0.031$, 95% CI = 1.08–4.45; Table 36 in the TOKEN Report) (Schlaud et al. n.d. :102).

It is clear from the above that there is reasonable evidence in epidemiological studies that SUDS can occur as AEFI following use of the Pentavalent vaccine and the deaths following the use of this vaccine should not be classified as 'Not a case of [AEFI]' using even the revised AEFI criteria.

Inflating Benefits to Match Cost

The role of the GAVI and WHO has been to try and find justifications for its use and recommend every vaccine that appears on the firmament. Chickenpox being a mild disease in the vast majority, prevention by vaccination was unlikely to match cost. Among children, varicella is usually a self-limited disease that lasts 4–5 days and is characterised by fever, malaise, and a generalised vesicular rash typically consisting of 250–500 lesions. Adolescents, adults, and immune-compromised persons usually have a more severe disease and are at higher risk for complications. When only direct medical costs were considered, the benefit–cost ratio was 0.90:1 (CDC, 1996). In Germany, vaccination at 15 months was not cost beneficial from the healthcare payer's point of view (Beutels et al., 1996). The wages of parents purportedly lost for looking after the sick child were added to make it appear cost-beneficial (Preblud et al., 1985).

Cost effectiveness of pneumococcal vaccine (Afonso et al., 2013), rotavirus vaccine (Patel et al., 2013; Rheingans et al., 2014), and the human papilloma virus vaccine (HPV) (de Kok et al. 2008; Isshiki, 2014; Kim & Goldie, 2008; Novaes et al., 2015; Sanders & Taira, 2003) have all been disputed.

WHO Cost-Effective Thresholds

Besides this, the WHO [Choosing Interventions that are Cost-Effective (WHO-CHOICE)] suggests that vaccination for Low- and Middle-Income Countries (LMICs) that cost one to three times the per capita income of the countries per disability-adjusted life-year saved should be considered cost-effective to help assist decision-makers. Newall and colleagues examined the results of reviews of cost-effectiveness analyses of human papillomavirus and rotavirus vaccination in LMICs, to assess whether the results of these studies were reflected in funding decisions for the vaccination programmes. They found that in many cases, programmes that were deemed cost-effective were not subsequently implemented given budgetary constraints (Newall et al., 2014).

Pandemic Flu: WHO-Vaccine Manufacturer Nexus

The discussion above is suggestive of a cosy relationship of WHO with vaccine manufacturers. However categorical evidence of this was provided in the declaration of the influenza pandemic in June 2009 that resulted in stockpiling of millions of dollars worth of flu vaccine and oseltamivir (Tamiflu) and zanamivir (Relenza). Investigations showed that WHO was advised by experts who had declarable financial and research ties with pharmaceutical companies producing antivirals and influenza vaccines. Scientists involved in WHO were funded by pharmaceutical firms that stood to gain from the guidance they were drafting. Initially the identity of these experts was kept a secret (Cohen & Carter, 2010).

National Technical Advisory Groups

Inevitably, the trust and faith in the WHO has eroded. It has become crucial for developing countries to evaluate vaccines and their costs and benefits for themselves. To take advantage of the prevailing mood of distrust the World Bank recommended that countries have their own NITAG (John, 2002). It was anticipated that national governments would more likely heed their own advisors than they would the WHO. Governments were then sought to be influenced through their NITAGs. On December 14, 2009, the Health Secretary in India chaired a meeting where it was pointed out that the NTAGI sub-committee that had recommended Hib vaccine had overlooked data from a multicentre study done specifically to advise policy on the Hib and Pneumococcal vaccines (Kant, 2009). The study had shown that the incidence of pneumonia was only a tiny fraction of what was being projected to recommend Hib vaccination (Lone & Puliyel, 2010).

Public Interest Litigation for Vaccine Policy

It was under these circumstances of distrust of the NTAGI, that a petition was filed in the Delhi High Court in the public interest seeking a direction to the government to formulate a rule-based rational vaccine policy by which vaccines are scientifically evaluated in a transparent manner before they become part of the country's UIP. For example, it pointed out that NTAGI, the government body responsible for conducting the relevant studies before recommending introduction of any vaccine, had recommended that a 10-valent pneumococcal vaccine be introduced from 2010 when the vaccine had not even been developed, let alone tested. Thus, NTAGI has recommended the introduction of a vaccine in the public health system without any trial (Delhi High Court, 2009).

Immunisation Policy for Namesake

After prodding from the High Court, a National Vaccine Policy was drafted (Ministry of Health & Family Welfare, 2011)[4]. The NTAGI directed two members to initially draft the policy[5]. The minutes were altered with the connivance of the Ministry of Health and Family Welfare[6] so the policy could be drafted by one person. The draft policy was vetted by international organisations before being presented as national policy. Various aspects of the final policy have been criticised by experts (Matharu, 2011).

Quoting from Houweling and colleagues (Houweling et al., 2010), Bhan has pointed out that vaccine introduction must be dependent on the burden of disease and seriousness of the disease, availability of vaccine to reduce the burden, with a good safety profile and which is cost-effective (Bhan, 2010). However the new vaccine policy states that 'industry must be provided a channel to voice opinion to be utilised in framing policy (MoHFW, 2011: 10).' The fact that this would invite conflicts of interest because of the tension between the profit motives of industry and the promotion of public health is ignored. Bending over backwards to oblige vaccine manufacturers the policy states that if industry has a 'genuine concern that a decision is made to its detriment' (Ibid.), there must be a speedy redressal by an independent mechanism (of government) (Puliyel, 2011).

Advance Market Commitments (AMC) are advocated. AMCs aimed at providing incentives for new vaccines through guaranteeing the market for the product even before it is tested—the government promising it will buy a certain amount of vaccines at a given price. It is to be binding even if the vaccine produced has poor efficacy or even if the market price of the vaccine is a fraction of the AMC price. AMC was first used for pneumococcal vaccine research. The money for the vaccine in the AMC must be deposited with the World Bank even before the delivery of vaccine, so the directors of the pharmaceutical do not have to lose sleep about marketing the drug or about withdrawal of orders on account of the low efficacy of the product. The policy drafters understand the government will not be able to foot the hefty bill. The draft, therefore, helpfully suggests 'innovative financing' to be able to make the money available to the World Bank upfront. The term 'innovative financing' is 'GAVI–speak' and must be understood as such. The Government of India is being urged to issue sovereign bonds in the capital markets so that investors and speculators can put up the money. This is a win–win situation for the pharmaceutical industry and the bond investors—for all, except perhaps the taxpayer (Puliyel, 2011; Sengupta, 2012).

Madhavi and Raghuram (2012) discuss the overarching emphasis on supply-side factors, Public Private Partnerships (PPP), innovative (read speculative) financing, global fund (read advance market commitments to further MNC pharma businesses), etc. It seems that the government has fallen for the same 'global' slogans of the World Bank that has pushed the world into recession and the aid politics of Gates Foundation, WHO, GAVI, multinational pharma industry, etc. They write that the vaccine policy is not designed to enhance national public capacities for public immunisation programmes, but to justify spending public money on privately produced vaccines in the name of protection from diseases, whose incidence figures and public health statistics are dubious and industry-manufactured (Madhavi & Raghuram, 2012). Our vaccine policy must attend to the health of the children in the country and it should not be overly concerned with the viability of the vaccine industry. This looks like a policy not to have a policy, but to use vaccines indiscriminately (Puliyel, 2011).

It will be clear to any objective observer that the order by the Delhi High Court asking the government to draft a clear policy on immunisation was not used by government to reevaluate its stand or for course correction. In fact, the court's intervention seems to have hardened the resolve of international organisations to control policy. NITAGs (called National Technical Advisory Group on Immunisation (NTAGI) in India) are supported by the *Supporting National Independent Immunisation and Vaccine Advisory Committees* (SIVAC Initiative) funded by Bill & Melinda Gates Foundation and GAVI. It was launched as an interactive platform involving all NITAGs worldwide in an active network and through the NITAG Resource Centre (NRC)[7]. The NRC offers NITAG members and secretariats technical reports and updates from partners. The SIVAC advocates all NITAG members be sworn to secrecy about the proceedings at the meetings. Even the confidentiality statement required to be signed by the NITAG in India is prescribed by the SIVAC[8] so the public are kept in the dark about how vaccine recommendations are made. This is in stark contrast to what happens in the USA where the meetings are open to the public (Smith, 2010). The NTAGI is appointed according to the whims of the ministry unlike in the USA where persons apply and are selected on merits by an independent body (Ibid.). The secretariat of the NTAGI in India used to be housed in the Public Health Foundation of India (PHFI)[9]. The Immunisation Technical Support Unit (ITSU) used to be funded by the Bill and Melinda Gates Foundation. The ITSU brings in the agenda for the NTAGI and records the minutes (PHFI n.d.). This abdication of responsibility by the MoHFW set an undemocratic and unwelcome precedent. Private philanthropic institutions are accountable only to their business-dominated boards of directors. Rosenthal (2015) has noted that philanthropic foundations pay little or no tax on their income, and most contributions are tax deductible. Even though foundation funds are subsidised by the public, the public has no say in how the money is spent. It is this money that is used to subvert health policies for private ambitions. It took a concerted drive by nationalistic organisations to move the NTAGI back to the MoHFW. Ironically soon after this news appeared, the Health Ministry denied it was severing links with the Gates Foundation (PTI, 2017). For all the efforts to develop an independent National Policy on Immunisation, it is clear that the interests of private players will be the controlling factor for a long time.

Way Forward: A NICE Solution Suggested Previously

The National Institute of Clinical Excellence (NICE) in the UK decides cost effectiveness of medical interventions for the UK National Health Services (Martin, 2001). NICE calls for registration of stakeholders before interventions are evaluated. It then assesses the clinical evidence and the economic data on benefits. Based on the evidence, draft guidelines are drawn up for assessment by the registered stakeholders. The guidelines are revised if more evidence is provided by the stakeholders. An 'independent-review-panel' then reviews the guidelines to decide if all stakeholder comments have been taken into account. The final guidelines are then issued and the government has clear and unbiased advice on which to base decisions. India could set up such a body to independently evaluate vaccines (Dhanasiri & Puliyel, 2007). Having said this, it must be noted that NICE has not evaluated cost benefit of any vaccine so far.

The Health Economics Model

The process of selection of vaccines for UIP must address and evaluate the following:

1. Does it have a good risk–benefit ratio?
2. Is it cost-effective compared to the other interventions already in place?
3. Is it capable of providing better returns than other uses of this resource?
4. Defining whether the intervention is affordable may help. A general guideline is that interventions that cost less than the per capita Gross National Product (GNP), per Quality Adjusted Life Year (QALY) saved are considered affordable
5. 'Optimal decision rule' involves ranking the incremental cost- utility ratios of different interventions and selecting those with the lowest ratio ('best value') till the budget is depleted.

A hypothetical example may be used to clarify this. Assume polio control costs INR 350 crores and saves 1 QALY per INR 10,000 spent, rotavirus control costs INR 200 crores and saves one QALY per INR 20,000 spent, and tuberculosis control costs INR 700 crores and saves one QALY per INR 5000 spent. Assume also a budgetary constraint of INR 1000 crores. The first programme to be accepted would be TB control as it provides the best utility (one QALY/INR 5000). Once this is accepted there is only INR 300 crores left in the budget. The next programme to be accepted must be polio control. Rota virus control costs only INR 200 crores which is less than the cost of polio control (INR 350 crores) but polio control takes precedence as it provides more utility (Dhanasiri & Puliyel, 2007).

Notes

1. See www.preventpneumo.org and www.gavi.org/Library/Documents/AMC/PneumoADIP/ accessed on 6.2.2012.
2. http://www.mohfw.nic.in/showfile.php?lid=4081.
3. http://www.mohfw.nic.in/index1.php?lang=1&level=4&sublinkid=3928&lid=2421.
4. http://jacob.puliyel.com/download.php?id=294.
5. http://jacob.puliyel.com/download.php?id=294.
6. http://jacob.puliyel.com/paper.php?id=293.
7. Accessible at http://www.nitag-resource.org.
8. http://www.nitag-resource.org/uploads/media/default/0001/02/bac6de3049176de187f9abbfeb7ca6ebe0172bf8.pdf.
9. In February 2017 the NTAGI was moved from ITSU-PHFI to the National Institute of Health and Family Welfare, under the Ministry of Health and Family

Welfare. The ITSU was to continue functioning till February 28, 2017 and its future functioning from PHFI and support from the Gates Foundation were being worked out (Ministry of Health and Family Welfare, 2017).

References

Afonso, E. T., Minamisava, R., Bierrenbach, A. L., Escalante, J. J., Alencar, A. P., Domingues, C. M., Morais-Neto, O. L., Toscano, C. M., & Andrade, A. L. (2013). Effect of 10-valent pneumococcal vaccine on pneumonia among children, Brazil. *Emerging Infectious Diseases, 19*(4), 589–597.

Aggarwal, R., Babu, J. J., Hemalatha, R., Reddy, A. V., Sharma, D., Kumar, T. (2014). Effect of inclusion of Hepatitis B vaccine in childhood immunisation programme in India: A retrospective cohort study. *Indian Pediatrics, 51*(6) (November), 875–879.

Bhan, A. (2010). Ethical considerations in developing a national vaccine policy. *Indian Journal of Medical Research, 132*(August), 226–227.

Bhan, M. K., Glass, R. I., Ella, K. M., Bhandari, N., Boslego, J., Greenberg, H. B., Mohan, K., Curlin, G., Rao, T. S. (2014). Team science and the creation of a novel rotavirus vaccine in India: A new framework for vaccine development. *Lancet, 383*(9935) (June 21), 2180–2183.

Baqui, A. H., El Arifeen, S., Saha, S. K., Persson, L., Zaman, K., Gessner, B. D., Moulton, L. H., Black, R. E., Santosham, M. (2007). Effectiveness of Haemophilus Influenzae type B conjugate vaccine on prevention of pneumonia and meningitis in Bangladesh children: A case control study. *Pediatric Infectious Diseases Journal, 26*(7) (July), 565–571.

Batham, A., Gupta, M. A., Rastogi, P., Garg, S., Sreenivas, V., & Puliyel, J. M. (2009). Calculating prevalence of Hepatitis B in India: Using population weights to look for publication bias in conventional meta-analysis. *Indian Journal of Pediatrics, 76*(December), 1247–1257.

Beutels, P., Clara, R., Tormans, G., Van Doorslaer, E., & Van Damme, P. (1996). Costs and benefits of routine Varicella vaccination in German children. *Journal of Infectious Diseases, 174* (Supplement 3), S335–S341.

CDC. (1996). Prevention of Varicella: Recommendations of the Advisory Committee on immunisation practices (ACIP). *MMWR Recommendations and Reports, 45*(RR–11), 1–36.

CIOMS/WHO. (2012). Definitions and application of terms for vaccine pharmacovigilance. *Report of CIOMS/WHO Working Group on Vaccine Pharmacovigilance.* Geneva CIOMS/WHO. Accessed January 25, 2016. http://www.who.int/vaccine_safety/initiative/tools/CIOMS_report_WG_vaccine.pdf

Cohen, D., & Carter, P. (2010). Conflicts of interest. WHO and the Pandemic Flu "Conspiracies." *BMJ.* June 3, 2010. 340, c2912.

de Kok, I. M., Habbema, J. D., Mourits, M. J., Coebergh, J. W., & Van Leeuwen, F. E. (2008). Insufficient basis for the inclusion of human Papillomavirus vaccination in the national immunisation programme in the Netherlands. *Ned Tijdschr Geneeskd, 152*(37) (September 3, 2008), 2001–2004.

Delhi High Court. (2009). Advocate: Prashant Bhushan Advocate, Petitioners: Saxena K.B., Mittal S.K., Banerji D., Imrana Qadeer, Kurien, N.J., Priya R., Mira Shiva, Puliyel J.M., Dabade G., Writ Petition (Civil) No. 13698 of 2009. Public Interest Litigation. http://delhihighcourt.nic.in/index.html2009

Dhanasiri, S. K., & Puliyel, J. M. (2007). Regulating vaccines: Can health-economics tools be used profitably? *Indian Pediatrics, 44*(1), 11–14.

Dhir, V., & Mohandas, K. M. (1998). Epidemiology of digestive tract cancers in India. III. Liver. *Indian Journal of Gastroenterology, 17*(3) (July–September), 100–103.

PTI. (2017). Health Mission: Government Denies Ending Ties with Gates Foundation. February 8, 2017. *DNA News.* Accessed February 27, 2017. http://www.dnaindia.com/health/report-health-mission-govt-denies-ending-ties-with-gates-foundation-2316347

GAVI. (2005). Hib Initiative—A new force in the fight against Hib Meningitis and Pneumonia. Accessed January 25, 2016. http://www.gavi.org/library/news/press-releases/2005/hib-initiative-a-new-force-in-the-fight-against-hib-meningitis-and-pneumonia/

GAVI. (2007). Evaluation of Gavi's efforts to introduce new vaccines via the accelerated development and introduction plans and the Hib initiative. Accessed January 25, 2016. http://www.gavi.org/results/evaluations/adips-and-hib-initiative/

GAVI. (n.d.). Pentavalent vaccine support. Accessed January 25, 2016. http://www.gavi.org/support/nvs/pentavalent/

Gessner, B. D., Sutanto, A., Linehan, M., Djelantik, I. G., Fletcher, T., Gerudug, I. K., Ingerani, D.M., Moniaga, V., Moulton, L. H., Moulton, L. H., Mulholland, K., Nelson, C., Soemohardjo, S., Steinhoff, M., Widjaya, A., Stoeckel, P., Maynard, J., & Arjoso, S. (2005). Incidences of vaccine-preventable Haemophilus Influenzae Type B Pneumonia and Meningitis in Indonesian children: Hamlet-Randomised vaccine-probe trial. *Lancet, 365*(9453) (January), 43–52.

Houweling, H., Verweij, M., & Ruitenberg, E. J. (2010). National immunisation programme review committee of the health council of the Netherlands: Criteria for inclusion of vaccinations in public programmes. *Vaccine, 28*, 2924–2931.

ICMR. (n.d.). Minutes of the Expert Group Meetings on Hepatitis B and Hib Vaccines. Accessed January 25, 2016. http://icmr.nic.in/minutes/Minutes%20Expert%20Group%20%20Hepatitis%20B%20and%20Hib%20vaccines.pdf

Indian Association for Study of the Liver (INSAL). (2000). Hepatitis B in India; Therapeutic options and prevention strategies-consensus statement. *Indian Journal of Gastroenterology, 19*(Suppl. 3) (December), C4–C66.

Isshiki, T. (2014). HPV vaccination for cervical cancer prevention is not cost-effective in Japan. *Asian Pacific Journal of Cancer Prevention, 15*(15), 6177–6180.

Jensen, M. K., & Balistreri, W. F. (2015). Viral Hepatitis. In R. M. Kliegman, B. Stanton, J. S. Geme, N. F. Schor, & R.E. Behrman (Eds.), *Nelson Textbook of Pediatrics* (Vol. 1, 20 ed.). Elsevier Science Health Science.

John, T. J. (2002). National technical advisory group on immunisation: A major step forward for child health. *Indian Pediatrics, 39*(4), 327–330.

Kant, L. (2009). NTAGI subcommittee recommendations on Haemophilus Influenzae Type B (Hib) vaccine introduction in India. *Indian Pediatrics, 46*(11), 945–954.

Kim, J. J., & Goldie, S. J. (2008). Health and economic implications of HPV vaccination in the United States. *The New England Journal of Medicine, 359*(8) (August), 821–832.

Kroger, A., Ciro, T., Sumaya, V., Pickering, L. K., & Atkinson, W. L. (2011). General recommendations on immunisation: Recommendations of the Advisory Committee on Immunisation Practices (ACIP). *60*(RR02), 1–60. Accessed January 17, 2016. http://www.cdc.gov/mmwr/preview/mmwrhtml/rr6002a1.htm?s_cid=rr6002a1_e

Lahariya, C. (2014). A brief history of vaccines and vaccination in India. *Indian Journal of Medical Research, 139*(4) (April), 491–511.

Lahariya, C., Subramanya, B. P., & Sosler, S. (2013). An assessment of Hepatitis B vaccine introduction in India: Lessons for roll out and scale up of new vaccines in immunisation programmes. *Indian Journal of Public Health, 57*(1) (January–March), 8–14.

Lau, Y. L. (1999). Haemophilus Influenzae Type B disease in Asia. *Bulletin of the World Health Organisation, 77*(11), 867–868.

Levine, O. S., Hajjeh, R., Wecker, J., Cherian, T., O'Brien, K. L., Knoll, M. D., Privor-Dumm, L., Kvist, H., Nanni, A., Bear, A. P., & Santosham, M. (2010). A policy framework for accelerating adoption of new vaccines. *Human Vaccines and Immunotherapics, 6*(12) (December 1, 2010), 1021–1024.

Lone, Z., & Puliyel, J. M. (2010). Introducing pentavalent vaccine in the EPI in India: A counsel for caution. *Indian Journal of Medical Research, 132*(July), 1–3.

Madhavi, Y. (2006). New combination vaccines: Backdoor entry into India's universal immunisation programme? *Current Science, 90*, 1465–1469.

Madhavi, Y., & Raghuraman, N. (2010). Pentavalent and other new combination vaccines: Solutions in search of problems. *Indian Journal of Medical Research, 132*(October), 456–457.

Madhavi, Y., & Raghuraman, N. (2012). National vaccine policy in the era of vaccines seeking diseases and governments seeking public private partnerships. *Current Science, 102*, 557–558.

Madhi, S. A., Levine, O. S., & Cherian, T. (2008). Incidence of pneumonia is not reduced by pneumococcal conjugate vaccine, author's reply. *Bulletin of the World Health Organisation, 86*(10) (October): Author's Reply A-C.

Martin, B. (2001). Implications of the appraisal function of the National Institute of Clinical Excellence. *Value Health, 4*(3) (May–June), 212–216.

Matharu, S. (2011). Experts contest new vaccine policy document. *Down to Earth*, September 15, 2011. Accessed January 29, 2016. www.downtoearth.org.in/news/experts-contest-new-vaccine-policy-document-34021

Miller, M. A., & McCann, L. (2000). Policy analysis of Hepatitis B, Haemophilus Influenza Type B-, Streptococcus Pneumoniae–conjugate and rotavirus vaccines in national immunisation schedule. *Health Economics, 9*(1) (January), 19–35.

Miller, M. A., & Kane, M. (2000). Routine Hepatitis B immunisation in India: Cost-effectiveness assessment. *Indian Journal of Pediatrics, 67*(4) (April), 299–300.

Ministry of Health and Family Welfare. Government of India. (2017). Press Note. Press Information Bureau. Accessed February 13, 2017. http://pib.nic.in/newsite/mbErel.aspx?relid=158277.

Ministry of Health and Family Welfare. Government of India. (2011). *National Vaccine Policy*. Accessed January 28, 2016. http://mohfw.nic.in/WriteReadData/l892s/1084811197NATIONAL%20VACCINE%20POLICY%20BOOK.pdf

Ministry of Health and Family Welfare. Government of India. (n.d.). *Universal immunisation programme*. Accessed January 25, 2016. http://mohfw.nic.in/WriteReadData/l892s/Immunisation_UIP.pdf

Minz, S., Balraj, V., Lalita, M. K., Murali, N., Cherian, T., Manoharan, G., Kadiravan, S., Joseph, A., & Steinhoff, M. C. (2008). Incidence of Haemophilus Influenzae Type B Meningitis in India. *Indian Journal of Medical Research, 128*(1) (July), 57–64.

Newall, A. T., Jit, M., & Hutubessy, R. (2014). Are current cost-effectiveness thresholds for low- and middle-income countries useful? Examples from the world of vaccines. *Pharmacoeconomics, 32*(6) (June), 525–531.

Novaes, H. M., de Soárez, P. C., Silva, G. A., Ayres, A., Itria, A., Rama, C. H., Sartori, A. M., Clark, A. D., & Resch, S. (2015). Cost-effectiveness analysis of introducing universal human papillomavirus vaccination of girls aged 11 years into the national immunisation programme in Brazil. *Vaccine, 33*(1), A135–A142.

Patel, H. D., Roberts, E. T., & Constenla, D. O. (2013). Cost-effectiveness of a new rotavirus vaccination programme in Pakistan: A decision tree model. *Vaccine, 31*(51) (December 9), 6072–6078.

Piple, J. K., & Puliyel, J. (2015). 116E rotavirus vaccine may have less impact in India than projected. *Vaccine, 33*(51) (December 16), 7142.

Preblud, S. R., Orenstein, W. A., Koplan, J. P., Bart, K. J., & Hinman, A. R. (1985). A benefit-cost analysis of a childhood Varicella vaccination programme. *Postgraduate Medical Journal, 61*(Suppl. 4), 17–22.

Public Health Foundation of India (PHFI). (n.d.). *Immunisation technical support unit*. Accessed February 28, 2018. https://www.phfi.org/news-and-events/key-projects/immunisation-technical-support-unit

Puliyel, J. M. (2004a). Policy analysis of the use of Hepatitis B, Haemophilius Influenzae Type B, Streptococcus Pneumonia-conjugate and rotavirus vaccines in the national immunisation schedules. *Health Economics, 13*(11) (November 9), 1147–1148.

Puliyel, J. M. (2004b). Plea to restore public funding for vaccine development. *The Lancet, 363* (February 21), 659.

Puliyel, J. M. (2010). GAVI and WHO: Demanding accountability. BMJ, *341* (August 4), 4081.

Puliyel, J. M. (2011). Vaccine policy and advance. Market Commitments. *Economic and Political Weekly, 46*(44–45) (November 5, 2011), pp. 18–19.

Puliyel, J. M. (2013). AEFI and the pentavalent vaccine: Looking for a composite picture. *Indian Journal of Medical Ethics, 10*(3) (July-September 2013), 142–146.

Puliyel, J. M., Mathew, J. L., & Priya, R. (2010). Incomplete reporting of research in press releases: Et Tu, WHO? *Indian Journal Medical Research, 131*(April), 588–589.

Puliyel, J. M., Taneja, V., Jindal, K., & Thomas, N. (2001). Hepatitis B leading to Hepatocellular Carcinoma: Calculating the risk. *Indian Journal of Gastroenterology, 20*, 251–252.

Rathi, N. (2015). *How Rotovac vaccine controversy questions the transparency of clinical trials. DNA*. September 22, 2015. http://www.dnaindia.com/analysis/column-how-rotovac-vaccine-controversy-questions-the-transparency-of-clinical-trials-2127424

Rheingans, R., Anderson, J. D., Anderson, B., Chakraborty, P., Atherly, D., & Pindolia, D. (2014). Estimated impact and cost-effectiveness of rotavirus vaccination in India: Effects of geographic and economic disparities. *Vaccine, 32*(1) (August), A140–A150.

Rosenthal, S. (2015, May). Philanthropy: The capitalist art of deception. *Socialist Review, 402*.

Sanders, G. D., & Taira, A. V. (2003). Cost-effectiveness of a potential vaccine for human papillomavirus. *Emerging Infectious Diseases, 9*(1) (January), 37–48.

Saxena, K. B., Banerji, D., Qadeer, I., Kurian, N. J., Priya, R., Shiva, M., Puliyel, J., Dabade, G. (2010). "Antivaccine Lobby" Replies to the BMJ. *BMJ, 341*, c4001.

Schlaud, M. M., Poethko-Müller, C., Kuhnert, R., Hecker, H., & Robert Koch Institute. (n.d.). *Study on deaths in young children (Second to Twenty-Fourth Month of Life)* (TOKEN Study). Accessed February 28, 2018. http://www.rki.de/DE/Content/Gesundheitsmonitoring/Studien/Weitere_Studien/TOKEN_Studie/Studyreport.pdf?__blob=publicationFile

Sengupta, A. (2012). (On Behalf of Jan Swasthya Abhiyan). Comments by Jan Swasthya Abhiyan on 'Draft National Vaccine Policy. Accessed January 29, 2016. http://phmindia.org/wp-content/uploads/2015/09/JSAssubmission-on-National-Vaccine-Policy.pdf

Shaw, G. B. (1906). Preface on Doctors. In G. B. Shaw (Eds.), *The Doctor's Dilemma*. Web edition. The University of Adelaide.

Smith, J. C. (2010). The structure, role, and procedures of the U.S. Advisory Committee on Immunisation Practices (ACIP). *Vaccine, 19*(28) (Suppl. 1) (April), A68–A75.

Tiwari, L., Varughese, R. M., & Puliyel, J. M. (2003). Computerised-Hepatitis B-model is subject to processing axiom: Garbage in, garbage out. *Journal of Hepatology, 39*(1) (July), 133–134.

vonKries, L. R, Toschke, A. M., Strassburger, K., Kundi, M., Kalies, H., Nennstiel, U., Jorch, G., Rosenbauer, J., & Giani, G. (2005). Sudden and unexpected deaths after the administration of hexavalent vaccines (Diphtheria, Tetanus, Pertussis, Poliomyelitis, Hepatitis B, Haemophilius Influenzae Type B): Is there a signal? *European Journal of Pedeatrics, 164*(2) (February), 61–69.

World Health Organisation. (2002). *Hepatitis B WHO/CDS/CSR/LYO/2002.2*. Accessed January 27, 2016. http://www.who.int/csr/disease/hepatitis/whocdscsrlyo20022/en/

World Health Organisation. (2004). Review panel on Haemophilus Influenzae Type B (Hib) disease burden in Bangladesh, Indonesia and other Asian Countries, Bangkok, January 28–29, 2004. *Weekly Epidemiological Record, 79*(18) (April 30), 173–174.

World Health Organisation. (2005). *Adverse Events Following Immunisation (AEFI): Causality assessment*. Accessed March 14, 2017.

World Health Organisation. (2006). WHO Position Paper on Haemophilus Influenzae Type B Conjugate Vaccines. (Replaces WHO Position Paper on Hib Vaccines Previously Published in the Weekly Epidemiological Record) *Weekly Epidemiological Record, 81*(47) (November 24), 445–452.

World Health Organisation. (2007a). Pneumococcal Conjugate Vaccine for Childhood Immunisation—WHO Position Paper. *Weekly Epidemiological Record, 82*(12) (March 23), 93–104.

World Health Organisation. (2007b). *Hib vaccine: A critical Ally in Asia's effort to reduce child deaths*. Accessed January 28, 2016. http://www.who.int/immunisation/newsroom/Hib_vaccine/en/

World Health Organisation. (2008a). *Investigation of adverse events following immunisation with liquid pentavalent vaccine in Sri Lanka.* Accessed March 16, 2017. www.who.int/immunisation_safety/aefi/investigation_pentavalent_Sri_Lanka/en/index1.html

World Health Organisation. (2008b). *Report of an Ad Hoc WHO Expert Panel to Review Reports of Serious AEFI following Administration of Pentavalent and Other Vaccines in Sri Lanka 2008.* http://jacob.puliyel.com/#paper_213

World Health Organisation. (2009). Rotavirus vaccines: An update. *Weekly Epidemiological Record, 84*(51/52) (December 18), 533–540.

World Health Organisation. (2013a). *Immunisation, vaccines and biological: Hepatitis B.* Accessed December 30, 2015. http://www.who.int/immunisation/diseases/hepatitisB/new_vaccine/en/index1.html

World Health Organisation. (2013b). *The causality assessment of adverse event following immunisation: User manual for the revised WHO classification WHO/HIS/EMP/QSS.* WHO, March 2013.

World Health Organisation. (2013c). *Safety of Quinvaxem (DTwP-HepB-Hib) pentavalent vaccine.* Accessed March 17, 2017. http://www.who.int/immunisation_standards/vaccine_quality/quinvaxem_pqnote_may2013/en/

Chapter 14
Availability and Access to Medicines: Some Issues in Pricing

S. Srinivasan and Malini Aisola

Introduction

In the context of Universal Access to Healthcare, issues related to medicine are very important. India's booming pharmaceutical sector has earned for itself the moniker of the 'pharmacy of the developing world', in the sense that most essential medicines including those for HIV/AIDS, for the Third World and for international procurement bodies, are sourced from India. But within India, the scenario is one of poor availability and access to medicines among plenty. Pricing of medicines is a key issue that determines the haves and have-nots in access to healthcare.[1]

There are several factors that affect the long-term sustainability of India's pharmaceutical sector. These include issues like: Foreign Direct Investment (FDI) in the pharma sector and takeover of Indian pharma companies by foreign entities; Trade-Related Aspects of Intellectual Property Rights (TRIPS) plus measures in Free Trade Agreements (FTA), trade and non-trade barriers by economic blocs that host the Big Pharma majors; lack of relevant Research and Development (R&D) within India; and competition from China from where a majority of the bulk drugs— Active Pharmaceutical Ingredients (APIs)—are being sourced for India's formulations. For more on some of these important issues, we refer the reader to other publications (Low Cost Standard Therapeutics (LOCOST) 2006; Phadke & Srinivasan, 2011; Srinivasan, 2011; 2012a, b; Srinivasan et al., 2013, 2014).

We discuss in this chapter the key features of India's pharma market and pricing of medicines, the price control of medicines through the Drug Prices Control Order 2013, and the attempts by certain states to provide free medicines. The chapter also talks of issues related to fixed dose combination and pricing of patented drugs, and concludes with a brief discussion on some current challenges in access to medicines.

S. Srinivasan (✉)
LOCOST (Low Cost Standard Therapeutics), Vadodara, India

S. Srinivasan · M. Aisola
All India Drug Action Network (AIDAN)., New Delhi, India

I. Qadeer et al. (eds.), *Universalising Healthcare in India*,
https://doi.org/10.1007/978-981-16-5872-3_14

A Brief Historical Context

The story of India's pharmaceutical industry is a success story by any standards. Even its worst critics concede that compared to the situation in 1970 and certainly compared to what it was at the time of independence in 1947, there has been a sea change. In 1947 most of the allopathic medicines used were imported. By 1970 the import content had come down but still most of the bulk drugs were made by foreign companies or were imported through their primary plants in the West, as most of the formulation industry in India was in the hands of Multinational Companies (MNCs).

The key event that changed this scenario of dependence on imports and led to the boom during the years 1971–2005 was the Patents Act 1970 passed in 1972. It did not allow 'product patents' in medicines; and as only process patents were valid in this period for medicines, any new patented medicine launched in the West would be made through reverse engineering in India within 3–4 years at a fraction of the price (say less than 10% of the innovator's price). By allowing only 'process patents' for medicines, the government opened the (doors?) for the boom in India's pharmaceutical sector. Using the process patent window, several groups and entrepreneurs within India also started making drug intermediates and APIs, as well as formulations. There was a period—especially from the late 1980s to 2005—when most of the bulk drugs India needed were made within India. Additionally the machinery and the technology for production were, and are, mostly indigenously available. (For some other milestones in the history of the developments of the pharmaceutical sector in India, see the chapter, "Developments in India's Domestic Pharmaceutical Sector and Implications for Universal Healthcare in India" by Dhar and Joseph in this book). India's pharmaceutical industry became, and continues to be, a place for low cost medicine production, especially in formulations. In December 2016, India's domestic sector formulations sales were worth INR 107,819 crores and about an equivalent amount for exports.[2]

The year 2005 was another critical milestone, when product patents were introduced. The product patents are valid for 20 years. By the mid-1980s, Big Pharma located in the West and think tanks funded by them, saw the impending threat to their hegemony, especially from China, India and Brazil. The ensuing discourse to clip the wings, as it were, of these emerging economies found expression by 1995 in institutions like the World Trade Organisation (WTO), and agreements like the Trade-Related Aspects of Intellectual Property Rights (TRIPS). Reverse engineering was made to look like a crime and 'intellectual' property right/product patents and associated instruments like data exclusivity were glorified as instruments of promoting innovation and creativity.

India's home grown pharmaceutical majors, with the aid of civil society activists and concerned politicians and intelligentsia, saw to it that acceding to the TRIPS/WTO framework by 2005, did not wreck India completely, even as the ground beneath their feet seemed to be slipping with the impending onset of product patents from 2005. The disadvantage post-2005 was minimised by the implementation of legal flexibilities wrought and won in the run up to the final TRIPS Agreement, and reiterated in the Doha Declaration of 2001, and in India's national laws. These flexibilities[3] include Section 3(d) of the Patents Act which prevents unwarranted extension of monopolies through the practice of 'ever greening'[4] and raised the standards of patentability. Novartis famously lost the case for a patent claim on its product Glivec (imatinibmesylate) in 2013 even as it sought to question the constitutionality of Section 3(d) of the Indian Patents Act.

The cartel of Big Pharma already had an experience of being pipped to the post in South Africa in the early 2000s, when Cipla challenged them and demonstrated its ability to make available an AIDS cocktail for less than a dollar a day (Muralidharan, 2001). The cartel did not want the experience repeated. So the narrative was fine-tuned: now even adhering to TRIPS/WTO is constructed as not good enough. Bilateral treaties with India are being drafted that try to side step TRIPS and seek to impose stricter Intellectual Property (IP) regimes. The 'stricter-IP-regime-is-good-for-your-country-and-your-people' narrative—see any business press report in the last 10 years—is unfortunately bought by India's own business press and sections of India's ruling and business elite. In spite of having complied with TRIPS requirements, India (at the time of writing) is deemed to not have a 'world class' IP regime: meaning India refuses to yield despite pressures from Western especially the US governments and, does not accede to TRIPS Plus[5]measures, such as longer patent periods, diluting Section 3(d) of the Indian Patents Act, adopting data exclusivity and patent linkage etc., none of which are required as per TRIPS. Part of the strategy of Big Pharma has been to create newer entry barriers for American and EU markets. However Indian companies have mostly overcome these entry barriers, defying local and global Cassandras. Attempts to create a scare about the quality and efficacy of Indian pharmaceutical products in the post-2005 era continue.

In the domestic context, some examples of big Indian pharmaceutical companies challenging foreign ones include: filing of pre- and post- grant oppositions contesting the patents granted to the Western companies, applications for compulsory license (CL) of some of the costly patented products (that have resulted in only one CL to date—sorafenib, brand Nexavar, useful in certain kinds of blood cancers), etc.[6]

But the tactics of the Western pharmaceutical lobbies seem to be paying and even major Indian pharmaceutical companies prefer to play along than resist and protect their autonomy. Companies like Cipla and Natco, which have been contesting the patentability of several products of Western pharmaceutical companies in Indian courts and with some success, have now thought it best to join hands with Western pharmaceutical companies. If you cannot beat them, join them—for instance, many have become willing partners in the so-called voluntary license agreement of Gilead for its costly Hepatitis C product Sovaldi (sofosvubir). Voluntary License (VL) is a misnomer: it has nothing voluntary to it, the terms are advantageous to the licensor and the hands of the licensee are tied in several ways including restricting the procurement of API from specific suppliers, etc. There is further discussion on VLs in the last section.

Medicine Pricing in India: Some Features

The pharmaceutical sector revolution of 1970–2005 in India led to a wide range of medicines being available in India, but access and affordability have continued to beset consumers and patients. The major reason for lack of access to medicines is of course overpricing of medicines and absence of assured access to free universal healthcare. Other endemic reasons are the predominance of irrational drugs and of irrational Fixed Dose Combinations (FDCs); irrational prescriptions by doctors; no prescription audit; poor or no adherence to Standard Treatment Guidelines; aggressive drug promotion by drug companies; and unethical drug promotion and a variety of inducements to doctors costs of the latter are passed on to consumers in the form of high prices (Table 14.1). Indeed certain undesirable features of the pharmaceutical market in India seem to be fairly well established:

- The same medicine is sold at a range of prices. (See Table 14.1 and picture on imatinib).
- Prescribers tend to advice patients to go in for the costlier versions. Patients are very vulnerable and there is little consumer resistance.
- As a result, costlier brands of the same medicine sell more with a few exceptions.
- It is up to patients to buy or not buy medicines from the retail pharmacy shops.
- The profit margins are anywhere between 100 and 4000%. (See column 6 in Table 14.2).
- As a result, competition seldom brings down the prices of the most sold brands.[7]
- In fact more players seem to result in a wider range of prices.
- Drug prices are fixed by the manufacturers as to what the perceived target market for the brand can take.

Table 14.1 Showing range of prices (in INR) to retailer (PTR) used for calculating simple average price

Name of drug with 1%	Lowest price market share	Highest Price with 1% market share	Simple average price (without 16% retailer markup)[a]
Acyclovir 200 mg tabs per 10	32.70	148.10	62.90
Atenolol 100 mg tabs per 10	3.00	42.30	32.10
Atorvastatin 5 mg tabs per 10	13.50	52.50	32.90
Azithromycin 500 mg tabs per 10	41.6	393.3	171.2
Losartan 50 mg tabs per 10	9.20	56	37.10

[a]Ceiling price is simple average price plus 16% retailer markup
Note The range of prices is from the simple average calculation sheets available at the NPPA Website for each drug. see http://www.nppaindia.nic.in/under 'What's New'. Many of these medicines are available at less than the lowest price indicated here. See Table 14.2 below

Table 14.2 Comparison of DPCO-2013 rates and RMSC/TNMSC rates (prices in INR)

No.	2	3	4	5	6
	Name of Drug, Strength and Use	Indication	Simple Avg ceiling price as per DPCO-2013 (valid as of August 2015)	Procurement rates of RMSC/TNMSC as of 2015–2016	DPCO-2013 ceiling price greater than RMSC/TNMSC rate (in percent)
1.	Imatinib Tab -400 mg, 10 tabs	Anti-cancer	2962.7	29.0	10,116
2.	Amlodipine Tab-5 mg, 10 tabs	Antihyper-tensive	31.3	1.0	3150
3.	Enalapril Maleate Tab-5 mg, 10 tabs	Antihyper-tensive	32.7	1.2	2739
4.	Atorvastatin Tab-10 mg, 10 tabs	Blood cholesterol lowering agent	67.4	2.5	2596
5.	Cetrizine Tab-10 mg, 10 tabs	Antiallergic	19.9	0.8	2522
6.	Atenolol 50 mg, 14 Tabs	Antihyper-tensive	31.92	1.6	1904
7.	Domperidone Tab-10 mg, 10 tabs	Antivomiting agent	24.9	1.3	1864
8.	Diclofenac Sodium Tab-50 mg, 10 tabs	Painkiller	21.5	1.3	1576
9.	Albendazole Tab-400 mg, 10 tabs	To treat worm infestation	103	7.3	1311
10	Fluoxetine hydro- chloride Cap 20 mg, 10 caps	Antidepressant	38.3	2.8	1251

*Rajasthan Medical Services Corporation (RMSC) & Tamil Nadu Medical Services Corporation (TNMC). Source of Prices: http://www.rmsc.nic.in; and www.tnmsc.com accessed on August 16, 2016, and DPCO-2013 ceiling prices as of August 2015. Rows 1 to 5 are from RMSC and 6 to 10 are from TNMSC

- Markets are distorted by unfair and unethical marketing practices of drug companies adding further to end consumer costs.

The resulting lack of access because of high prices of most prescribed brands is aggravated by the fact that if a patient goes to a public health facility, useful medicines are not stocked sufficiently, if at all, or the patient is asked to buy from a private retail pharmacy shop. The latter could mean a long trek for most rural patients.

What Can Be Done About Providing Medicines—To Those Who Need It—In the Public Health System?

The answer is: provide all essential medicines, and provide them free as it is eminently doable. The financial reasons are discussed later.

We need to make medicines available free in public health services for the following reasons:

- People seeking treatment in public health facilities will increase.
- There will be a decrease in patients going to private practitioners and retail drug shops.
- And patients will no more be exploited by the pharmaceutical industry-doctor nexus.
- There will be a decrease in related indebtedness and impoverishment since:
  - Healthcare expenditure is the second greatest cause of rural indebtedness in India today.
  - More than 70% (72% in the rural areas and 79% in the urban areas) of illness episodes were treated in the private sector of which around 70% was self-financed[8] (Government of India, 2015).
- Sixty-five percent of India's population lacks regular access to essential medicines (WHO, 2004:62).[9]
- Even if patients are able to receive a free check-up at a government clinic, they are often forced to pay out-of-pocket for the actual medicines prescribed for their illness.[10]
- At the local chemist's shop patients often pay a price 2 to 100 times higher than the cost offered by pharmaceutical companies to retailers, private hospitals, nursing homes and government agencies (See Table 14.2).

Feasibility of Public Provision: The Experience of Tamil Nadu and Rajasthan

Providing free generic medicines through the Public Health System is not as costly as assumed. But it needs careful management and fine tuning at several levels. It has been done most famously by the Tamil Nadu Government since 1995 (Tamil Nadu Medical Services Corporation (TNMSC), 2009); the experiment is being repeated in Kerala since 2007 and in Rajasthan since October 2011 (Lalita, 2008). In Tamil Nadu (population 7.2 crores) the medicine budget is of the order of INR 300 crores per year for medicines purchased by pooled procurement by the TNMC. If one extrapolates this to all-India population levels of say INR 130 crores, by assuming that like in Tamil Nadu, approximately a maximum of 40% of those who access healthcare services go to the public health facilities (which is more than most states of India), the cost of free medicines for all India will be around INR 5400 crores at TNMSC procurement prices.[11] For a general understanding of the price differentials of the TNMSC/RMSC procurement rates and the ceiling prices, (Table 14.2).

Drug Price Regulation

As most states in India still do not have a fully functioning public health system from primary to tertiary care, most patients tend to use the private sector.[12] Using the private sector often impoverishes the poor and the middle class alike and is often a cause of indebtedness. In addition, the decision regarding which medicine to buy is mostly made by doctors and drug companies. Consumers and their families often have to make these purchase decisions under distress and therefore there is no "choice" in the "free" market. In addition, given the market distortions by pharmaceutical companies in the form of unethical marketing, the pharmaceutical market is nowhere near the ideal of a free market and is by and large a case of market failure. Stiglitz (2009) and Akerlof (1970) have identified the existence of information asymmetries as a cause of market failure. The pharmaceutical market, the doctor-patient-pharmaceutical industry interface, is rife with asymmetries, leading to market failure.

State intervention and price regulation are therefore necessary when markets do not work in favour of the poor and vulnerable patients. Drug price regulation needs to cover at the minimum all essential and lifesaving drugs, must be based on a formula that does more than a tokenistic reduction of prices, discourages irrational Fixed Dose Combinations (FDCs), and addresses the high prices of patented drugs. The National Pharmaceutical Pricing Policy 2012 (NPPP, 2012) and the Drug Price Control Orders (DPCO 2013) must be seen mostly as not meeting these criteria, as we show below.

The current price control regime, the DPCO-2013, is a result of the National Pharmaceutical Pricing Policy (NPPP) 2012, and a byproduct of Supreme Court directives to the Government of India in a Public Interest Litigation (PIL)—Writ Petition (WP) (Civil) 423/2003, All-India Drug Action Network (AIDAN) and Ors. versus Union of India and Ors. The grounds for the PIL were, inter alia, the overpricing of most essential and lifesaving drugs in India and the need for their price regulation. The NPPP 2012 recommends price control only for the drugs in the National List of Essential Medicines (NLEM) 2011 (and its periodic revisions) and prescribes what is called a simple average formula to fix the ceiling prices. The simple average formula, in contrast to a cost- based formula (that is cost of all inputs plus margin), says the ceiling price will be the simple average of the brands, with one percent market share, of a drug formulation specified in the NLEM.

Limited Coverage of DPCO-2013: According to the government's affidavit filed in the Supreme Court during November 2013, only 18% (INR13,097 crores) of the then domestic market of INR71,246 crores was under price control (using Inter Continental Marketing Service (IMS) Transportation Security Administration (TSA) December 2012 Moving Annual Total (MAT) data). The actual decrease in prices was confined to less than 1.8% of the market (Public Health Foundation of India (PHFI)—Institute for Studies in Industrial Development (ISID), 2014).[13]

More recent unpublished estimates by authors (August 2015) show that the market under price control was around 13.4% of a total sale of INR84,017 crores (January 2015, PharmaTrac data).The breakdown of market excluded from price control per therapeutic category is as follows: anti-diabetes (93%), anti-malarials (75%), anti-infectives (69%), anti-neoplastics (80%), blood-related (86%), cardiac (80%), derma (95%), gastro intestinal (90%), hormones (65%), neuro/Central Nervous System (CNS) (89%), ophthal/otologicals (95%), pain/analgesics (93%), respiratory (96%), sex stimulants/ rejuvenators (100%), stomatologicals (100%), urology (96%), vaccines (71%), vitamins/minerals/nutrients (99%), others (99%).

This negligible impact is because the price control is applicable only to the specific strengths and presentations of the 348 drugs mentioned in the NLEM-2011; and because the ceiling price formula is market- based, rather than cost-based. We elaborate below.

The former meant that the following categories of drugs are excluded from price control:

- Those other than the specified strengths and presentations of the 348 essential drugs (eg. paracetamol 650 mg and 1000 mg tabs) are excluded from price control as only paracetamol 500 mg tab is specified in the NLEM-2011. Paracetamol 650 mg tab is included in NLEM-2015.)
- Chemical analogs are mostly excluded, e.g. atorvastatin is included because it is the only statin mentioned in the NLEM-2011 but all other statins like rosuvastatin, simvastatin, etc., are excluded. In NLEM-2015, ramipril has been included along with enalapril, but other Angiotensin-Converting-Enzyme (ACE) inhibitors will therefore continue to be excluded from price control.
- All existing combinations, of NLEM plus NLEM, NLEM plus non- NLEM, and non-NLEM plus non-NLEM medicines, are excluded from price control.

As per the so-called market-based formula, Ceiling Price, as we mentioned earlier, is decided by taking the simple average price of prices (to the retailer) of brands with more than 1% market share plus retailer's trade commission of 16%. This is contrasted to cost-based formula for the previous DPCO 1995 (that is cost of raw material plus conversion costs plus a 100% margin). The result of this is that if several brands of the same drug are priced at the higher end, the simple average and therefore the ceiling price tends to be high. In fact, in most cases because of the simple average formula, the DPCO-2013 prices are way high and therefore provide legitimacy to high prices of top-selling brands. These statements are illustrated in Tables 14.1, 14.2, 14.3.

Table 14.3 Conversion or manufacturing costs as percent of cost price; and cost price compared to DPCO-2013 ceiling price (in Rupees)

Name	Raw material price per kg	No of Tablets per kg of raw material	Cost of API per 10 tabs	Total raw material cost per 10[a] tabs	Conversion or Mfg costs per 10 tabs[b]	Total cost per 10 tabs	Conversion or Mfg cost as percent of total cost (8)	DPCO-2013 ceiling price as of Aug 2015 per 10 tabs
(1)	(2)	(3)	(4)	(5)	(6)	(7)	[6/7]	(9)
Albendazole tabs 400 mg	1337	2,500	5.35	5.99	2.91	**8.90**	33	**103**
Atorvastatin tabs 10 mg	16,887	89,000	1.90	2.07	1.22	**3.29**	37	**67.40**
Atenolol 50 mg tabs	1231	20,000	0.62	0.72	0. 82	**1.54**	53	**22.80**
Amlodipine 5 mg	3136	140, 000	0.22	0.36	0. 59	**0.95**	62	**31.30**
Cetrizine tablets 10 mg	3499	100,000	0.35	0.45	0.70	**1.15**	61	**19.90**

[a]Cost of API plus excipients. [b]Labour plus electricity plus packing material, etc. *Note* In the case of relatively low-priced material and with low strengths (like 5 mg, 10 mg) of medicines like cetrizine, amlodipine, etc., the cost of conversion is as almost as much as the Raw Material. In the case of amlodipine, the Raw Material cost is less than the conversion cost. Please compare the cost price (Col. 7) and DPCO-2013 ceiling price (Col.9) – both are in bold
Data Source: LOCOST 2015 and DPCO 2013 ceiling prices

Table 14.3 with data from LOCOST, the Vadodara-based not-for-profit generic manufacturer, compares by way of example, conversion costs and raw material costs of some tablets. It is seen that conversion costs as proportion of total cost of the tablets are 32% to 62%. Of worth comparing is Total Cost (Cost Price) in column 7 and the DPCO-2013 Ceiling Price as of August 2015 (Column 9). This illustrates the absurd nature of the overpricing legitimised by the Simple Average Formula and the so-called Market-based Pricing Mechanism.

Omission of Useful Life-Saving Drugs in the NLEM-2011 and NLEM-2015

As mentioned above, at the time of going to the press, a revised NLEM was announced in December 2015, hereafter NLEM-2015. Our comments below and elsewhere in the chapter are applicable to both NLEM lists unless indicated otherwise. Indeed the recommendations of the NLEM-2015 Selection Committee with respect to price control continue to be regressive: it leaves out, like NLEM-2011, all isomers, derivatives, chemical analogs, limits to specific dosages, etc. The problem is because the

NLEMs, either 2011 or 2015, were not made with price control as the major focus. In fact, there needs to be a separate expanded list of essential and lifesaving drugs that remedies the problems of relying on an NLEM for price control.

Highly expensive drugs like meropenem, imipenem, cilastatin, tigecycline, colistin, abciximab, tirofiban, eptifibatide, and many are out of the NLEM-2015 and hence out of price regulation. In addition, many useful drugs for asthma—for example monteleukast—are excluded from price control. For diabetes, only glibenclamide, metformin and insulin (of a certain kind only) were under price control as only these were mentioned in NLEM-2011. In the NLEM-2015, however glibenclamide has been replaced by the more useful glimepiride but other overpriced and useful diabetics like acarbose or gliptins continue to be excluded. (We should clarify that some anti-diabetics not mentioned in NLEM-2011, like glimepiride, gliclazide, migitol, repaglinide, pioglitazone, sitagliptin, voglibose and acarbose, were sought to be brought under price control on July 10, 2014, by the NPPA by special notification under Para 19 of DPCO-2013. Paragraph 19 empowers the National Pharmaceutical Pricing Authority (NPPA) to fix/revise the ceiling price or retail price of any drug which it deems necessary for the interest of the public in case of any extraordinary circumstances. But many leading manufacturers took the government to court, and obtained a stay on the ceiling prices to be further notified under Para 19. The stay has since been lifted in the Bombay High Court during September 2016 and an appeal by drug companies in the Supreme Court against the stay through a Special Leave Petition (SLP) was denied in October 2016. The legitimacy of price control using powers under Para 19 stands restored at the time of writing.

Case of Anti-Diabetics as Illustration of the Ineffective Price Control Policy

As mentioned earlier above, 93% of anti-diabetics are out of price control when many are costly. India has the largest burden of diabetics in the world, with an estimated 67 million patients with diabetes. Like tuberculosis, untreated diabetes is a killer disease and all anti-diabetics should be considered as life-saving medicines especially in view of the fact that diabetes runs a more pernicious course in Indian patients. However, most oral hypo-glycemics were not part of the NLEM-2011. The situation is true of NLEM-2015 too. Only two oral hypoglycemic medicines were included inNLEM-2011—metformin and glibenclamide—apart from certain types of injectable insulin. In NLEM- 2015, glibenclamide has been replaced by glimepiride. There is, however, a need to include the following groups of oral anti-diabetics too so that they all can be put under price regulation:

- Thiazolidinediones (e.g. pioglitazone)
- Dipeptidyl peptidase-IV (DPP-IV) Inhibitors (e.g. vidagliptin, sitagliptin),
- Alpha-glucosidase inhibitors (acarbose, miglitol),
- Megltinides (e.g. repaglinide, nateglinide, etc.)

Insulins: Insulins are life-saving injectable anti-diabetic medicines. If patients who need insulin are deprived of insulin they would undergo rapid worsening of diabetes leading to death. The NLEM-2013 covers regular and NPH insulins but does not mention most of their combinations. A combination of the two insulins is very commonly needed in patients with diabetes. Secondly, newer insulin analogs like glargine, detemir are also needed in many patients. They are very expensive and are not in neither NLEM-2011 nor NLEM-2015. These are lifesaving medicines and many patients in India need insulin- substitutes. As these are expensive and under patent, compulsory licenses must be thought of as a policy to make these medicines affordable.

Tables 14.4 and 14.5 below show that the majority of oral anti- diabetic medicines are out of price control. They show that before the July 10, 2014 notifications,[14] 4.7% (INR 228 crores) of the anti- diabetics market (without insulin) was under price control.

After July 10, 2014, the figure under price control was 25% (INR 1224 crores). But the July 2014 notifications giving ceiling prices of other non-NLEM anti-diabetics were indifferently, if at all, complied with pharmaceutical majors. During September 2016, the challenge to these notifications was dismissed.

Table 14.4 Details of anti-diabetics market

	Sales for 12 months ending January 2015 (in INR cr.)	Percentage
Fixed dose combinations	3266	51.1
Single ingredient	1694	26.4
Insulin	1448	22.6
Total	6408	100

Source Calculated from PharmaTrac January 2015

Table 14.5 Percent of anti-diabetics market (without Insulin) under price control

	Sales for 12 months ending January 2015 (INR cr.)	Percentage of total anti-diabetics market (without insulin)	Sales of market under price control related to NLEM 2011 medicines (INR cr.)	Sales of market under price control related to para 19 notifications (INR cr.)[a]
Fixed dose combinations	3266	65.8%	Nil	Nil
Single ingredient	1694	34.2%	228	996
Total	4860	100%	228	996
			(4.7%)	(20.5%)

[a]Sales figures correspond to a period of about 6 months before July 10, 2014 price notifications and 6 months after the notifications

Source Calculated from PharmaTrac January 2015

Fixed Dose Combinations and Price Control

The above figures for anti-diabetic combinations underlie a related malaise, namely of prevalence of unnecessary fixed dose combinations (FDCs) that also add to the problem of pricing. FDCs are acceptable as rational only when the individual dosage forms, when combined, ensures better compliance, or when the combination has a proven advantage, or synergy, in terms of better safety and efficacy, when taken simultaneously. Most fixed dose combinations are out of price control because they are not in the NLEM-2011 (and neither in the NLEM-2015). Many of them also happen to be irrational and deserve to be weeded out. They also have a problem of having been licensed for manufacture by the state licensing authorities without having marketing approval from the Drugs Controller General of India (DCGI) (If a formulation is new, its efficacy and safety data need to be first submitted to the DCGI for marketing approval. A drug is 'new' for 4 years after its introduction in the market). FDCs account for roughly about 42% of the domestic market that is about INR 37,800 crores of the INR 84,017 crores market[15] and not more than 50% of this figure is rational. (Estimates done for a Representation to the Government and Supreme Court, August 2015 by authors in the Public Interest Litigation All India Drung Action Network AIDAN and Ors. Versus Union of India and Others, Writ Petition (Civil) 423/2003). Much of the expenditure of patients goes for fixed Drug Combination (FDCs), many of which are overpriced, unscientific and unnecessary.

Table 14.6 below shows the anomalous situation of paracetamol (Brand: Crocin, Calpol, etc.), where the sales of the rational formulation paracetamol 500 mg is a fraction of other formulations involving the painkiller.

Under price control, those that are mentioned in NLEM-2011, are: 500 mg tablets, 150 mg/ml injections, 125 mg/5 ml syrup and suppositories 80 mg and 170 mg. Sales of these presentations under price control are INR 181.6 crores (30% of single

Table 14.6 Market for single ingredient versus Combinations of Paracetamol

	Sales for 12 months ending January 2015 (in INR crore)	As percent of total paracetamol market of INR 3285.5 crore (%)
Single ingredient formulations in price control	181.6	5.5
Single ingredient formulations not in price control Fixed Dose Combinations	427.5	13
(not in price control)	2676.4	81.5
Total	3285.5	100

Source Calculated from PharmaTrac January 2015 data. See Note 13

*Likely to be under price control after NLEM-2015 is taken as the basis for price control. Market Out of Price Control: Market for Paracetamol Combinations + Other Strengths of Paracetamol = INR 3285.5 crores. Out of this, 94.5% is out of price control. Total single ingredient paracetmol formulations is INR 609.1 crores out of which only 30% (INR 181.6 crores) is under price control.

ingredient paracetamol market and only 5% of the total paracetamol related formulations market, for 12 months ending January 2015. (Under NLEM-2015, as already mentioned above, paracetamol 650 mg tabs have been included although gh this is irrational. So it can be expected to be under price control in 2016).

The sale of fixed dose combinations of paracetamol (non-NLEM- 2011 medicines) at INR 2,676.4 crores is almost 14 times that of single ingredient paracetamol (NLEM-2011 medicine) sales (INR 181 crores). Even sales of non-NLEM single ingredient formulations of paracetamol at INR 427.5 crores are almost double (2.35 times) that of the sales of single ingredient paracetamol formulations under NLEM (Tables 14.6 and 14.7).

Over the last 10 years there have been sporadic efforts by the DCGI's office to clean up the situation regarding FDCs. On January 15, 2013, the DCGI again wrote a letter requesting the State Licensing Authorities (SLAs) to ask the manufacturers of such formulations to submit, to the office of DCGI within 18 months, the data on safety and efficacy of FDCs permitted by the SLAs but not approved by DCGI before October 1, 2012. In response, the Office of DCGI received more than 6,000 applications. A committee under the chairmanship of Prof. C.K. Kokate was constituted for examination of the 6000 plus applications in a timely manner.

The Kokate Committee gave its Report in March 2016. The committee recommended the ban of 344 FDCs—totalling about 1080 applications as several brands had the same FDC. Some top-selling brands that were recommended for ban included

Table 14.7 Breakup of single ingredient formulations of Paracetamol

Strength	Sales in INR cr. for 12 months ending January 2015	Under price control?
120 mg/5 ml (syrups)	23.4	No
120 mg/5 ml (syrups)	23.4	No
125 mg/5 ml (syrups)	46.8	**Yes**
150 mg injections	14.2	**Yes**
250 mg/5 ml (syrups)	117.2	No
300 mg tablets	1.6	No
325 mg tablets	0.3	No
500 mg tablets	120.4	**Yes**
80 mg and 170 mg suppositories	0.2	Yes
650 mg tablets	142.5	No
750 mg tablets	1.7	No
1000 mg tablets	7.7	No
Others	133.1	No
TotalCourt in its order Single Ingredient Sales	INR 609.1 cr	
With 70% of INR 609.1 cr out of price control		

Source Calculated from PharmaTrac January 2015 data

Corex, Phensedyl, Vicks Action 500, etc. The Delhi High Court stayed the ban during March–April 2016 as several aggrieved manufacturers approached it. The Court heard arguments for and against the ban during March- June 2016[16].On December 1, 2016, the Delhi High Court in its order quashed the ban on grounds that the Drug Technical Advisory Board (DTAB) was not consulted in the process leading up to the ban. The order is being appealed by the government in the Supreme Court. As and when the legal issues are finally settled, the Kokate Committee will pronounce on another 944 FDCs (corresponding to 1730 applications).

It is worth remembering that the FDCs considered for ban by the Kokate Committee are only those which were licensed for manufacture by the State Licensing Authorities without approval for safety and efficacy by the central government. There are another set of FDCs worthy of ban that are in the market because of approval by the central government but irrational. In the meanwhile, the government may consider bringing under price control, all FDCs in the market that contain one or more of the NLEM-2015 medicines. This will at least minimise the economic burden on patients. Weeding out many of these FDCs will lessen the burden on the patient by not having to consume irrational and unscientific FDCs. But the issue of high prices of those FDCs that remain in the market still needs to be addressed.

Pricing of Patented Drugs

Pricing of a patented drug has become a contentious issue as there is no clear agreement on what it costs to discover a drug. In a rather opaque study by the Tufts Center for the Study of Drug Development, a figure of US $2.6 billion was arrived at as the cost of discovery per drug for pharmaceutical companies.[17] There have also been recent incidents of other investment adventurism by some pharmaceutical companies in USA where prices of old drugs have been increased to new unimaginable and unaffordable levels. In the case of pyrimethamine, the 4,000% hike was defended by the company CEO as 'altruistic not greedy'.[18]

In India, post-2005, there are only three options to reduce the cost of high priced patented drugs sold in India:

(a) Use a standard formula that factors in the prices of the patented drug in the developed economies and per capita incomes in the respective developed countries.
(b) Negotiate with the patent holder companies for a lower price.
(c) Get the patented drug made by Indian drug manufacturers under CLor through government use of provisions of the Patents Act (Sections 84, 92, 100). These are TRIPS sanctioned flexibilities and therefore do not violate TRIPS obligations.

The first option: to date no formula that is acceptable and produces consistently acceptable results for all stakeholders has been evolved. The second option of price negotiations assumes that the government will have a base price to negotiate with the patent holder company. In the absence of transparency about what it costs to discover a drug, and because of considerable reluctance of pharmaceutical companies to share such data, it is next to impossible to arrive at a successful price negotiation of otherwise high price patented drugs. In both the above cases, in case the attempts to arrive at an agreed price for price control are successful but the resulting price arrived at is unacceptable to the consumers, options to renegotiate with the companies or use other policy options like a CL (see below) may be foreclosed. This is because if the matter goes to litigation, the government will not have a plausible argument to counter in the courts as it would have been a party to the formula/negotiation.

The third option of using a CL is more feasible. To hope that Indian drug companies will suo moto apply for CLs is not a steady option: one has to defence on a fortuitous chain of circumstances that includes filing of a CL by a private Indian company, and successful defence of its CL application at every stage of the inevitable opposition by the patent holder. This may take years and in case the courts overrule the CL application, then there would be no other route to lower prices but to wait out the expiry of the patent term.

Alternatively the government can use Section 92 of the Patents Act (notification by the government that a CL needs to be issued for public non-commercial use, national emergency or extreme urgency) for a broad class of diseases, and/or Section 100 (for government use). But here the major obstacle is the government itself and its various ministries. A government that is keen on cultivating a 'strategic' relationship with Western powers, especially the USA, will be hesitant to go in for CLs or government use as option for fear of stoking further the disinformation that India has an unfavourable IPR climate and a less- than-world class IP regime. No amount of comparisons with Thailand and no amount of if-Thailand-can-do-it-why-not-us arguments would appear to persuade the Government of India for government use CLs (Wibulpolprasert et al., 2011).

A fourth option that is being advocated as an option is something we mentioned in the earlier part of the paper, namely, VL: where the patent holder allows Indian drug companies to manufacture under a license with certain terms and conditions—conditions that may bind the Indian licensee to the price it can sell and the markets it can sell plus of course a royalty, even in cases where no patent has been granted for the medicine. A recent instance of VL is the case of sofosvubir for treatment in hepatitis C, and the VLs issued to eight Indian drug companies by Gilead. Gilead's price was/is 1000 dollars per 400 mg pill in the USA working out to USD$ 84,000 for the full 12-week course of treatment. As a result, the sales of sofosbuvir (brand Sovaldi) by Gilead were slightly over US $10 billion in 2014.[19] The voluntary license awarded to Indian companies was partly to ward off the criticism. The Indian companies under VL are selling at less than $480 for a 12-week course. Researchers from Liverpool University find that 'even assuming a 50% profit margin for the manufacturer to cover capital investment and return to shareholders, it would now be possible to sell a 12-week course of the drug for $178.'[20] Our point is that only manufacture under CL by several manufacturers in India will enable one to discover the equitable price of sofosvubir that is affordable for India's citizens.

"For example, if a doctor has to treat a patient with blood cancer, he may advise the salt imatinib by various brand names. If he has prescribed brand Glivec a month's course will cost INR114,400 to the patient. Whereas, the same anti-cancer drug, but with a different brand name Veenat costs just INR11,400. Cipla supplies the generic equivalent of this drug imatinib at INR8000 only, also Glennmark supplies it for INR5720. All these brands contain the same salt imatinib, in the same quantity, conform to the same quality standards and are equally effective" (RMSC website: unpaged).

Likewise imatinib mesylate tablets of 400 mg are now available at less than INR 100 for 10 tablets (Fig. 14.1). The RMSC procurement price is INR 29 for 10 (see row 1, Table 14.2). The same medicine as branded Glivec was being priced at around INR 4000 for 10 (or famously INR 1.2 lakh for a month's course at 13,700% more) before Novartis lost the case in the Supreme Court in April 2013. No amount of price negotiations or formulaic exercises would have been able to achieve such a drop in prices. The case for local manufacture and competition of many costly patented drugs seems to be strong. (The DPCO-2013 ceiling price fixed at INR 2,962.70 for 10 tablets, 100 times higher than the RMSC procurement price, only shows the ineffectiveness of the simple average mechanism of the DPCO-2013, as against the cost plus method of ceiling price fixation).

Patents are a form of monopoly. Patent holders will be reluctant to shed this monopoly unless compelled to do so in public interest by mechanisms like the compulsory license and government use provisions. In addition, countries like India need to be careful not to sign treaties like the Trans Pacific Partnership Agreement (TPPA) that can force adoption of TRIPS-plus provisions such as patent linkage, data exclusivity, patent terms extensions, arbitration outside the scope of India's legal system or undermine the carefully crafted public health safeguards in the Indian IPR regime.

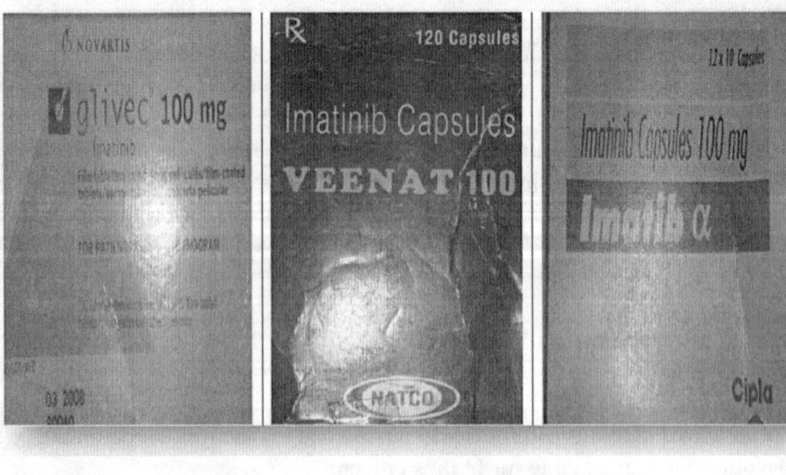

Fig. 14.1 Same drug: different prices. *Source* RMSC website, accessed January 9, 2016

Conclusion

Medicines are for promoting health and human welfare therefore, they cannot be left to the markets. Their prices need to be regulated as much as their quality. The DPCO-2013 while attempting to cap prices does so ineffectively. It has in many cases legitimised the already prevalent overpricing in the Indian market. We need a modified and improved pharmaceutical pricing policy that enlarges the scope to an enlarged list of essential and useful life-saving drugs and all formulations involving them. In addition, there is an urgent need to weed out irrational drugs and unscientific fixed dose combinations. Price control of patented drugs cannot be done effectively except by resorting liberally to use of compulsory license provisions by the government.[21] For the realisation of these reforms, we need a government with political will and which prioritises people's health above all.

A well organised procurement policy and free medicine scheme in all public health facilities on the lines of the Tamil Nadu and Rajasthan governments is an achievable goal for all state governments in India and it costs very little. Such a free medicine scheme needs to be a part of a larger comprehensive rational drug policy as was planned by the Delhi State Government in 1994.[22] It also needs to be part of a comprehensive understanding of the role of Intellectual Property Rights and patents in limiting access, availability and affordability to medicines, and the role of strategic use of TRIPS flexibilities so that India's pharmaceutical industry can be not only the pharmacy of the developing world but also a pharmacy to India's own poor and disadvantaged.

Notes

1. Parts of this chapter draw from the authors' previous works.
2. Source: Pharma Trac MAT for 12 months ending December 2016 and India Brand Equity Foundation, https://www.ibef.org/industry/ pharmaceutical-india.aspx, accessed March 30, 2017.
3. These flexibilities included among other things:

   - Section 3 (d) of the Patents Act was amended to exclude patentability of new forms (including derivatives of old drugs or combinations of old drugs) of known substances unless there is significant enhancement of efficacy;
   - New use of an old drug, is not to be considered an invention and hence not patentable;
   - Pre-grant opposition to patents applications was retained;
   - Post-grant opposition to granted patents was introduced.

   In addition, definitions of 'invention', 'inventive step', etc. that is of terms related to patentability criteria were modified by the 2005 amendments. Other measures to safeguard against patent abuse were introduced through the 2005 amendments as well as earlier amendments of the 1970s law were reinforced: Compulsory license (license to generic companies to produce and market); government use (public non-commercial use) patents; Bolar exception (preparation for generic launch, i.e. production for marketing approval) and parallel importation.

4. Evergreening refers to the tendency of patent holders to extend the life of the patent by claiming patents for new use or minor changes when the patent period is about to expire. It is almost always an abuse of the patent system.
5. According the Finance Minister, India was not ready to engage with any one on 'TRIPS PLUS' issues which could lead to ever-greening of patents or blocking of compulsory licences affecting access to medicines. October 20, 2016. https://www.thehindubusinessline.com/economy/policy/india-to-us-will-not-tighten-ipr-rules-beyond-trips-mandate/article9,246,323.ece
6. For a commentary, see Srinivasan (2012c).
7. We (authors) would like to qualify this. Competition in the classical sense (of many producers entering the field resulting in reduced price of a drug) does not occur in the Indian pharmaceutical market most of the time. When a generic enters the market for the first time, there is competition and lowering of prices, of the API as much as the formulation, with respect to the price of the innovator—but after some time when several producers start making the same formulation, the generic formulation is sold at a wide range of prices, positioned as it were to the varying purchasing powers of its buyers. However because of lack of choice for the consumer, the bulk of the market is skewed towards the higher priced brands. Therefore at this stage the principle that 'many producers will bring down the price of the product' does not work. There is competition of sorts but it does not work in favour of the consumer for he/she is told by prescribers and competing drug companies that the lower the price, the less the efficacy of the medicine, a fiction that is by now well-entrenched despite evidence to the contrary.
8. …more than 70% (72% in the rural areas and 79% in the urban areas) spells of ailment were treated in the private sector (consisting of private doctors, nursing homes, private hospitals, charitable institutions, etc.).
   Quoted in Para 3.2.5 along with graphic "Percentage distribution of spells of ailment treated during last 15 days by level of care separately for each gender" in Government of India, 2015:20.
9. This figure is for 1999, almost 20-years old. But things have not vastly improved since and in some states it is probably worse.
10. "Expenditure on merely 6% hospitalised treatment in urban areas was reimbursed partly or fully, whereas the similar figure for rural areas was only a meagre 1%." About 80% of those seeking treatment do not/did not have health protection in the form of insurance and the treatment costs are mostly self-financed. See statements 3.12 and 3.13, and related narration in Government of India (2015: 28–29).
11. This figure of INR5400 crores approximately is after making provisions for 20% of the population who are currently not able to access any form of health services (Phadke & Srinivasan, 2011). See also Gupta et al. 2015.
12. "In the rural areas, 42% hospitalisation took place in public hospitals, and 58% in private hospitals. The corresponding percentages in urban India were 32% and 68% respectively." Government of India (2015: 22, Para 3.3.3).

13. The figure of 1.8% is from *An Independent Evaluation of the National Pharmaceutical Pricing Policy 2012 and DPCO-2013, PHFI-ISID Collaborative Research Programme*, March 2014.
14. These notifications used powers under Para 19 of the DPCO 2013 to put other drugs—not in the NLEM 2015 and therefore not under price control—to be put under price control. These notifications were challenged by sections of the pharma industry. The Bombay High Court in September 2016 upheld these notifications and subsequently also the Supreme Court.
15. These figures are from Pharmatrac for January 2015.
16. For details of the context of the ban and the legal issues therein, see: Srinivasan et al. (2016).
17. See: https://csdd.tufts.edu/files/uploads/cost-study-backgrounder.pdf. Accessed January 8, 2016.
    For a commentary, see: Jerry Avorn, M. D. The $2.6 Billion Pill—Methodologic and Policy Considerations. *N. Engl. J Med* 2015; 372:1877-1879.
18. See https://www.washingtonpost.com/news/to-your-health/wp/2015/09/22/turing-ceo-martin-shkreli-explains-that-4000-percent-drug-price-hike-is-altruistic-not-greedy/. Also "No Justification for High Drug Prices", *New York Times*, Editorial, December 19, 2015.
19. Quoted at https://www.nytimes.com/2015/02/04/business/sales-of-sovaldi-new-gilead-hepatitis-c-drug-soar-to-10-3-billion.html. Accessed January 8, 2016.
20. Quoted at http://www.aidsmap.com/page/3021833/. http://www.aidsmap.com/page/3021833/. Accessed January 8, 2016.
21. As we go to the press, an interesting review paper prepared for the *Annual Review of Economics* has been under discussion. The author Petra Moser of the paper 'Patents and Innovation in Economic History' on the basis of empirical and historical evidence suggests, 'that patents were not a necessary condition for innovation, and that the large majority of innovations occurred outside of the patent system. Policies that limit the scope of patents (such as compulsory licensing) have encouraged innovation, while policies that strengthen the monopoly power conveyed by patents (such as unregulated patent pools) have unambiguously discouraged innovation.' On compulsory license, the author says: ' Firms under threat of compulsory licensing today argue that it will weaken their incentives to invest in R&D. The historical records, however, suggests the opposite. Baten et al. (2015) collect and analyse firm-level data on German patents to examine invention by German firms that were differentially affected by compulsory licensing under the TWEA. This analysis indicates that compulsory licensing was associated with a 28% increase in patenting by German inventors.' http://ssrn.com/abstract=2712428. Accessed January 20, 2016.
22. See: http://www.delhi.gov.in/wps/wcm/connect/f00bd00042170222b808bf2ac334b5d9/Drug_Policy_of_the_State_of_Delhi%5B1%5D.pdf?MOD=AJPERES&CACHEID=f00bd00042170222b808bf2ac334b5d9. Accessed December 1, 2015.
    For a detailed account, see: Roy Chaudhury et al. (2005), Mathur (2006).

References

Akerlof, G. A. (1970, August) The market for 'lemons': Quality uncertainty and the market Mechanism. *Quarterly Journal of Economics, 84*(3), 488–500.

Government of India. (2015). *National Sample Survey (NSS) 71st round social consumption: Health.* National Sample Survey Organisation, Ministry of Statistics and Programme Implementation. Government of India.

Gupta, N., Priyanka, & Pachauli, C. (2015, . January 21–22). *Report of the national forum on universal access to free medicines and free diagnostics: Complexities and prospects.* Delhi/Jaipur, JSA/Oxfam India/Prayas.

Lalitha, N. (2008, January). Tamil Nadu Government intervention and prices of medicine. *Economic and Political Weekly, 43*(1), 66–71.

LOCOST (2006). *A lay person's guide to medicines. What is in them and what is behind them?* LOCOST (Low Cost Standard Therapeutics).

Mathur, V. S. (2006). Implementing rational drug use: A success story. *Indian Journal of Pharmocology,* 38(2) (April), 93–94.

Muralidharan, S. (2001). New drug wars. *Frontline,* 18(5) (March), 3–16.

Phadke, A., Srinivasan, S. (2011, July 4). *Draft recommendations of the subgroup on drug regulation.* Unpublished Discussion Paper for the Subgroup Convened by the Ministry of Health and Family Welfare, for inputs to the Twelfth Five Year Plan.

PHFI-ISID. (2014, March). *An independent evaluation of the national pharmaceutical pricing policy 2012 and DPCO-2013.* PHFI-ISID Collaborative Research Programme.

Roy Chaudhury, R.R., Parameswar, U., Gupta, S., Tekur, S. U., & Bapna, J. S. (2005, March). Quality medicines for the poor: Experience of the Delhi programme on rational use of drugs. *Health Policy and Planning, 20*(2), 124–136.

Srinivasan, S. (2011, June 11). 'Medicines for All', the pharmaceutical industry and the Indian State. *Economic and Political Weekly, 46*(24), 43–50.

Srinivasan, S. (2012a, February 25). Medicines for all: Unexceptionable recommendations. *Economic and Political Weekly, 47*(8), 58–61.

Srinivasan, S. (2012b, June 23). A stinging indictment of India's drug regulation authority. *Economic and Political Weekly, 47*(25), 10–13.

Srinivasan, S. (2012c, April 7). The compulsory licence for Nexavar: A landmark order. *Economic and Political Weekly, 47*(14), 10–13.

Srinivasan, S., Srikrishna, T., & Phadke, A. (2013, June 29). Drug price control order 2013: As good as a leaky bucket. *Economic and Political Weekly, 48*(14), 10–12.

Srinivasan, S., Srikrishna, T., & Aisola, M. (2014, August 23). Pharmaceutical price control policy: Unrealistic and unfair. *Economic and Political Weekly, 49*(34), 13–15.

Srinivasan, S., Shiva, M., & Aisola, M. (2016, April 2). Cleaning up the pharma industry: A landmark ban on irrational drugs. *Economic and Political Weekly, 51*(14), 21–23.

Stiglitz, J. (2009). Chapter 1: regulation and failure. In D. Moss & J. Cisternino (Eds.), *New Perspectives on Regulation.* The Tobin Project.

Tamil Nadu Medical Services Corporation Ltd (TNMSC). (2009). *About us.* Accessed February 14, 2017. http://www.tnmsc.com/tnmsc/new/html/aboutus.php

Wibulpolprasert, S., Chokevivat V., Oh, C., & Yamabhai, I. (2011). Government use licenses in Thailand: The power of evidence, civil movement and political leadership. *Globalisation and Health, 7*(32). World Health Organisation (WHO)/EDM. 2000. *The Use of Essential Drugs:*

World Health Organisation (WHO)/EDM. (2000). *The use of essential drugs: The ninth report of the WHO.* WHO.

World Health Organisation. (2004). *The world medicines situation.* WHO/EDM/PAR/2004.5. WHO. Accessed March 5, 2018 http://apps.who.int/medicinedocs/en/d/Js6160e/9.html#Js6160e.9

Chapter 15
Vaccines and Vaccine Policy for Universal Healthcare

Y. Madhavi

Introduction

Vaccines are among the cost-effective preventive tools of disease management in primary healthcare. Vaccines are useful for mass immunisation, especially against diseases that are spread uniformly in populations and when their use is balanced with other public health measures. One should not forget that other public health measures such as sanitation, hygiene, safe drinking water, good living conditions and nutrition brought down infectious diseases in Western societies, even before vaccines were introduced (Mackenbach et al. 2008; CDC 1999). Traditionally, vaccines are developed, produced and supplied by public funded organisations all over the world. However, recent trends indicate just the contrary; where vaccines are produced predominantly by the private sector. Currently, the global vaccine business is dominated by the private industry concentrated in a few multinational corporations. The world vaccine market is worth US $24 billion in 2016, and it is expected to grow US $61 billion by 2020 (Guzman, 2016). The Indian vaccine market was placed at around US $500 mn in 2012 (Bhadoria et al., 2012: 11), and expected to grow by 5–7% to reach US $550 to 570 million by 2020 (Ibid.: 25).

Vaccines have always constituted a small share of the global pharmaceutical industry. The vaccine market share that was around 0.3% of the pharmaceutical industry in the USA, and 0.1% in India in the pre-1990s (Anonymous, 1985) has grown to 2% of the world pharmaceutical industry (Srinivas, 2004: 27). Vaccines have become the growth drivers of the global pharmaceutical industry today and are indispensable owing to global and national immunisation policies. Trends in the last two decades in India show steep growth of the private vaccine sector whose growth is reflected in the availability of abundant expensive new vaccines and their combinations. This is the case when there is shortage for primary vaccines that are under the national immunisation programme (Madhavi, 2005; 2009b). The shortage of primary

Y. Madhavi (✉)
National Institute of Science, Technology and Development Studies, New Delhi, India

I. Qadeer et al. (eds.), *Universalising Healthcare in India*,
https://doi.org/10.1007/978-981-16-5872-3_15

vaccines is largely attributed to the closure of around 23 Public Sector Units (PSUs) in the last 10 years. As of February 2008, only four functional vaccine PSUs existed in India (Madhavi 2009b). The growth of the private sector in India did not contribute to the reduction of demand–supply gaps in primary vaccines, as the private sector is interested in profitable new expensive vaccines. In fact, the steep growth of the private sector and the declining role of the public sector due to liberalisation distorted national immunisation and vaccine policies in India (Madhavi, 2005, 2008; 2009a, 2009b). The rate at which vaccine markets are growing and the aggressive vaccine promotional trends through a number of factors such as: (a) industry- sponsored advocacy; (b) donations; (c) international alliances (the Global Alliance for Vaccines and Immunisation (GAVI), the International AIDS Vaccine Initiative (IAVI), Malaria Vaccine Initiative (MVI), etc.; (d) global organisations (the World Health Organisation (WHO), World Bank (WB), United Nations Development Programme (UNDP), etc.; (e) advance market commitments; and (f) Public Private Partnerships (PPPs) indicate that the 'supply push' factors have come to determine the use of vaccines in public health. The current vaccine promotional trends indicate that vaccines are increasingly becoming the ideology of public health as 'one vaccine fits all' for all populations alike though pathogen strain specificity, variability and suitability from which vaccines are made is an important determinant of the suitability of the vaccine to local populations. Indian experience in vaccines is a glaring example and it underscores the need for an evidence-based sustainable national vaccine policy (Madhavi et al., 2010) for appropriate use of vaccines that are needed for public health for universal healthcare. Given this background, the current chapter analyses the context and the place of vaccines under universal healthcare proposed in the Twelfth Five Year Plan (FYP), to achieve health for all and its implication for public health, disease management and national health security.

Vaccines Under Universal Healthcare

Vaccines received scant attention in the working group reports of the Planning Commission (PC) for the Twelfth FYP under the banner 'universal healthcare', where emphasis was laid on access to essential medicines. There is no separate chapter on vaccines either in the High Level Expert Group (HLEG) or Steering Committee reports of the PC, though the importance of vaccine use was acknowledged, and emphasis was laid on continuation of mass immunisation of all existing vaccines (TT, DT, DPT, Measles, BCG, OPV and hepatitis B under the Expanded Programme on Immunisation (EPI) which is also referred to as the Universal Immunisation Programme (UIP) or National Immunisation Programme (NIP). Selective immunisation of Japanese Encephalitis (JE) vaccine in endemic regions was also recommended.

The Working Group on Communicable Diseases for the Twelfth Five Year Plan (Government of India (GoI), 2011) documented the formation of a new technical centre for vaccine preventable diseases that was approved in the Eleventh FYP by the Cabinet Committee on Economic Affairs (CCEA) in 2010, as a part of the expansion of the National Centre for Disease Control (NCDC). The mandate of the Centre for Vaccine Preventable Diseases is to work strategies for Polio/Measles/MMR/Meningitis, Rabies, viral Hepatitis and newer vaccines vigilance and policies (Ibid.).

The Working Group of the Planning Commission in its pharmaceuticals chapter makes a passing mention of vaccines and sera under the Public Sector Units (PSU) section and it is non-committal on vaccine PSU capacity building. It completely ignores the ongoing heated debate on Indian vaccine PSUs and their significant contribution in the development and production of EPI vaccines at crucial times when the demand–supply gap was at its peak since the closure of three crucial PSUs in January 2008 (MoHFW 2011; Madhavi, 2008; 2009a; Parliamentary Standing Committee on Health Reports 2009a, b, 2010, 2011). Despite shortcomings, PSUs have always met immunisation needs in times of crisis. This is a reflection of the fact that they can play a pivotal role in the production of essential vaccines (based on the need backed by scientific evidence) to suit the Indian population. However, it is not clear whether this deliberate silence in the PC reports on vaccine PSUs is to let the private sector and large Multinational companies (MNCs) capture the PSU's captive universal vaccine market through combination vaccines (pentavalent vaccines) in the future. The public sector is clearly sidelined in the policy discourse as the PPP model becomes the favourite slogan. This is evident from the fact that the Union Health Ministry has allotted 594 crores for the upcoming new vaccine park spread over 100 acres in Chengalpattu in Tamil Nadu (Sinha, 2012) with the PPP model, while vaccine PSUs that are under the same ministry are struggling to become WHO–cGMP (current good manufacturing practices) compliant.

A review of PPPs to access vaccines that are needed, an analysis of local evidence to establish vaccine need, a national vaccine policy for a rational decision-making in the following sub-sections would put the entire vaccine debate in context and its relevance in universal healthcare.

PPPs and Distorted Vaccine Needs

According to the WHO, PPP is a 'means to bring together a set of actors for the common goal of improving the health of the population based on the mutually agreeable roles and principles' (Buse & Walt, 2000: 549). Though the concept of PPP is defined by various scholars (Balgescu & Young, 2005) and agencies (UNDP, 1998; World Bank (WB), 1998), the most commonly used definition in the health arena is the one proposed by Kent Buse and Gill Walt, London School of Hygiene and Tropical Medicine: 'A collaborative relationship, which transcends national boundaries and brings together at least three parties, among them a corporation (and/or industry association), and an inter- government organisation, so as to achieve a shared health-creating goal on the basis of a mutually agreed division of labour' (Buse, 2004: 226).

PPPs have evolved in the post-1990s as a means to solve all health- related problems. They are perceived as complementing each sector's strengths to meet a common goal, to achieve equity in health between rich and poor countries. The enthusiasm for a PPP approach to global health problems arose in response to convergence of a number of forces during the mid- and late-1990s. First was the growing scepticism directed at an entirely private sector-driven approach. Second was a growing pattern of collaboration in the US between the government, private universities and private pharmaceutical companies as initiated by the Bayh–Doyle Act. Third was the decision by the Rockefeller Foundation, the Bill and Melinda Gates Foundation, etc., to rely on the PPP model to address the growing worldwide crises of HIV/AIDS, malaria, tuberculosis and other major diseases (Donald, 2007).

Collaboration of academic institutions with industry to develop specific medical products and therapies has become a common trend in the 1990s (Blumenthal et al., 1996). Organisations such as the WB, UNDP, and WHO have actively encouraged constructive partnerships with the private sector under the theme of the comprehensive development programme. The growth of international Non-governmental Organisations (NGOs) and their new interaction with private firms and international organisations also increased in the 1990s. Private foundations in the United States (US) assumed an active role to support PPPs. Increased NGO advocacy (for example, MSF, France) and influence pushed public health problems into international health and international policy agenda (Reich, 2002: 1–19). The period post-1990s witnessed the formation of such global alliances as partnerships between international organisations, philanthropic groups, private firms, national governments, NGOs and public funded organisations. Though there are several Global Public Private Partnerships (GPPPs) that have emerged to achieve equity in all spheres of health (Table 15.1), the current article focuses on GPPPs (Table 15.2) and PPPs in vaccines (Table 15.3).

Out of four GPPPs listed in Table 15.2, except GAVI, all the PPPs are for product development and Programme for Appropriate Technology in the Health (PATH) is a common partner in all of them except in the International AIDS Vaccine Initiative (IAVI). PATH announced its recent partnership with IAVI in August 2012 for

Table 15.1 List of WHO public–private partnerships

European Partnership Project on Tobacco Dependence Global Alliance for TB Drug Development
Global Alliance to Eliminate Lymphatic Filariasis Global Alliance to Eliminate Leprosy
Global Alliance for Vaccines and Immunization Global Elimination of Blinding Trachoma Global Fire Fighting Partnership
Global Partnerships for Healthy Aging Global Polio Eradication Initiative Global School Health Initiative Multilateral Initiative on Malaria Medicines for Malaria Venture Partnership for Parasite Control
Roll Back Malaria Stop TB Initiative
UNAIDS/Industry Drug Access Initiative

Source: World Health Organization website (www.who.int) search on 'partnership' and 'global alliance'

Table 15.2 Global PPPs in vaccines

Vaccine	*PPP Objective*	*Public Partners*	*Role of Public Partner*	*Private Partner*	*Role of Private Partner*	*Outcome*
Men Afrivac against meningitis A	nonprofit PATH, of Seattle, and the WHO set up the Meningitis Vaccine Project (MVP) to introduce an affordable vaccine specific for Africa	WHONIH, Bethedsa and USFDA	The US Food & Drug Administration laboratories in Bethesda, Maryland, licensed a technology for conjugating vaccine components from NIH. The WHO approved MenAfriVac in June 2010.	PATH (NGO), Bill and Melinda Gates Foundation.Synco Bio Partners – a ontract manufacturing company Amsterdam Serum Institute of India (SII), Pune India	$70 million in seed funding from the Bill and Melinda Gates Foundation in Seattle. Amsterdam-based Synco Bio Partners provided the polysaccharide ingredient,SII contributed the tetanus toxoid and affordable manufacturing	Vaccine developed priced at $0.50 a dose. Development took less than a decade and cost less than one-tenth the $500 million usually required to bring a new vaccine to market. (*Nature Biotech, 29, 99 20111.*) Requires 2 doses for full immunisation Undergone pahse I, II and III trials in India and Africa and additional testing is done in different sites..
Global Alliance for Vaccines and Immunisations (GAVI)	GAVI's mission is to save children's lives and protect people's health by increasing access to immunisation in the world's poorest countries. It's mandate is to introduce new vaccines in poor countries	The United Nations Children's Fund (UNICEF), the World Bank Group, and the World Health Organization. National governments, the Research, technical and public health institutions.	Contributions from Norway, the Netherlands, the United Kingdom, and the United States, for a total fund of over a billion dollars.	Gates Children's Vaccine Program at PATH, The Rockefeller Foundation the International Federation of Pharmaceutical Manufacturers Associations (IFPMA) Civil society organisations	Bill & Melinda Gates Foundation committed US$ 750 for 5 yrs when GAVI was launched in the yr 2000	Claims that it prevented over 5.5 million future deaths caused by Haemophilus influenzae type b (Hib), hepatitis B, measles, pertussis, pneumococcal disease, polio, rotavirus diarrhoea and yellow fever; • supported the immunisation of more than 325 million children; • committed US$ 7.2 billion to new and under used vaccines in developing countries. However, GAVI's unsustainable financial model is being criticized recently by Oxfam-Msf report 2010.

(continued)

Table 15.2 (continued)

Malaria Vaccine Initiative (MVI)	The PATH malaria initiative is a global programme launched in 1999 to develop malaria vaccines and to ensure availability and access to developing countries. MVI announced a partnership in 2011 between Tulane University and Gennova biopharmaceuticals Ltd. India	African researchers from different countries Two African researchers Tulane University	To develop vaccine against malaria Developed RTS S vaccine To develop transmission blocking vaccine against malaria	Bill & Melinda Gates Foundation, United States agency for international development and Exxon Mobile foundation GSK Gennova Biopharmaceuticals Ltd India	MVI was established with initial funding from Bill Gates Foundation. Receives funding from other donors as well Production and testing To produce and perform pre-clinical testing of transmission blocking vaccine	Claims that there are around 63 vaccine candidate portfolio including 41 in pre-clinical and clinical stages RTS, S, Phase III clinical trials are undergoing in 7 African countries. (http://www.malariavaccine.org/malvac-state-of-vaccine-dev.php MVi.org)
AIDs vaccine Development	The International AIDS Vaccine Initiative (IAVI) and Imperial College of Science, Technology and Medicine, in part with grants from US medical technology firm BD (Becton, Dickinson and Company; NYSE: BDX),	Imperial College of Science, Technology and Medicine, London	Key to the laboratory's mission is to provide training for developing country scientists and access to the most modern equipment. Initially, the London facility will work with IAVI-sponsored vaccine development teams now or soon to be	US medical technology firm BD (Becton, Dickinson and Company; NYSE: BDX's laboratory is located in London, at St Stephen's Centre, Chelsea and Westminster Hospital	The laboratory has been outfitted with state-of-the-art vaccine testing tools, in part by grants to IAVI from BD. BD's commitment includes both a direct contribution of US$1 million and a donation of a BD. FACS Calibur (TM) Automated Cell Analysis System from BD Biosciences,	Offers online databases of all AiDS vaccine trials on website. and published a report in 2010 on 'Progress on the path toward an AIDS vaccine'. In its first 10 years, IAVI developed six new vaccine products, established major new clinical trial capacity in Africa and Asia, mobilised more than $460 million in new funding for vaccine research.

(continued)

Table 15.2 (continued)

	have opened a laboratory to serve as a clearinghouse for coordinating the evaluation of AIDS vaccine candidates as they complete human trials at sites worldwide.		testing AIDS vaccine candidates in Kenya, Uganda, South Africa, India and China, as well as in the US and UK.		a business segment of BD, valued at US$100,000. This represents the largest ever direct financial contribution from a private company to IAVI's global AIDS vaccine development program. In addition, BD Biosciences will collaborate with IAVI to help monitor immune responses to the vaccines under study.	
Global Alliance for Vaccines and Immunisations (GAVI)	GAVI's mission is to save children's lives and protect people's health by increasing access to immunisation in the world's poorest countries. It's mandate is to introduce new vaccines in poor countries	The United Nations Children's Fund (UNICEF), the World Bank Group, and the World Health Organization. National governments, the Research, technical and public health institutions.	Contributions from Norway, the Netherlands, the United Kingdom, and the United States, for a total fund of over a billion dollars.	Gates Children's Vaccine Program at PATH, The Rockefeller Foundation the International Federation of Pharmaceutical Manufacturers Associations (IFPMA) Civil society organisations	Bill & Melinda Gates Foundation committed US$ 750 for 5 yrs when GAVI was launched in the yr 2000	Claims that it prevented over 5.5 million future deaths caused by Haemophilus influenzae type b (Hib), hepatitis B, measles, pertussis, pneumococcal disease, polio, rotavirus diarrhoea and yellow fever; • supported the immunisation of more than 325 million children; • committed US$ 7.2 billion to new and under used vaccines in developing countries. However, GAVI's unsustainable financial model is being criticized recently by Oxfam-Msf report 2010.

(continued)

Table 15.2 (continued)

Global Alliance for Vaccines and Immunisations (GAVI)	GAVI's mission is to save children's lives and protect people's health by increasing access to immunisation in the world's poorest countries. It's mandate is to introduce new vaccines in poor countries	The United Nations Children's Fund (UNICEF), the World Bank Group, and the World Health Organization. National governments, the Research, technical and public health institutions.	Contributions from Norway, the Netherlands, the United Kingdom, and the United States, for a total fund of over a billion dollars.	Gates Children's Vaccine Program at PATH, The Rockefeller Foundation the International Federation of Pharmaceutical Manufacturers Associations (IFPMA) Civil society organisations	Bill & Melinda Gates Foundation committed US$ 750 for 5 yrs when GAVI was launched in the yr 2000	Claims that it prevented over 5.5 million future deaths caused by Haemophilus influenzae type b (Hib), hepatitis B, measles, pertussis, pneumococcal disease, polio, rotavirus diarrhoea and yellow fever; • supported the immunisation of more than 325 million children; • committed US$ 7.2 billion to new and under used vaccines in developing countries. However, GAVI's unsustainable financial model is being criticized recently by Oxfam-Msf report 2010.
Malaria Vaccine Initiative (MVI)	The PATH malaria initiative is a global programme launched in 1999 to develop malaria vaccines and to ensure availability and access to developing countries. MVI announced a partnership in 2011 between Tulane University and Gennova biopharmaceuticals Ltd. India	African researchers from different countries Two African researchers Tulane University	To develop vaccine against malaria Developed RTS S vaccine To develop transmission blocking vaccine against malaria	Bill & Melinda Gates Foundation, United States agency for international development and Exxon Mobile foundation GSK Gennova Biopharmaceuticals Ltd India	MVI was established with initial funding from Bill Gates Foundation. Receives funding from other donors as well Production and testing To produce and perform pre-clinical testing of transmission blocking vaccine	Claims that there are around 63 vaccine candidate portfolio including 41 in pre-clinical and clinical stages RTS, S, Phase III clinical trials are undergoing in 7 African countries. (http://www.malariavaccine.org/malvac-state-of-vaccine-dev.php MVi.org)

Source Compiled from various published resources

Table 15.3 Public private partnerships in human vaccines in India

Vaccine	*Purpose of PPP*	*Public partners*	*Role of public partner*	*Private Partner*	*Role of Private partner*	*outcome*
Hepatitis B (Recombinant) (total cost of the project 2526 lakh INR) (total cost of the project 1221 lakh INR)	To develop recombinant Hepatitis B vaccine	TDB of DST with an agreement that 10% of sales revenue would be paid back to the DST 2. TDB of DST with an agreement that 10% of sales revenue would be paid back to the DST	Financial support (8.5 crores INR) Financial support (3.25 crores INR)	Shantha biotech Ltd., Hyderabad Bharat biotech International Ltd., Hyderabad	indigenous technology development indigenous technology development	Product launched in Indian market in 1997 Product launched in Indian market in 2000
Hepatitis B-DTP	To develop a combination vaccine of hepatitis B and DTP	TDB of DST and Exim Bank, Delhi	Financial support TDB (9 crores) Exim Bank (20 crores INR)	Shantha biotech Ltd., Hyderabad	Indigenous technology development	Product launched in Indian market in 2005

(continued)

Table 15.3 (continued)

HIV/AIDS (tripartite agreement between **NACO** under **MOHFW, IAVI** and **ICMR**)	The project aims to develop a safe and effective HIV/AIDS vaccine—such development has been mandated by the Indian government—for India and other developing countries. The vaccine has now been developed by ICMR in collaboration with Therion and is undergoing clinical trials.	ICMR, New Delhi, India NACO & MOHFW India International AIDS Vaccine Initiative (IAVI), New York,.	1. Infrastructure support for manufacture and conducting trials 2. selection of suitable Indian HIV strain 3. provide technical expertice Provides facilities permissions and permits. selection of Indian manufacturers 1. provides funding and access to technology from private company. 2. Assistance for designing, developing and evaluation of candidate vaccines suitable for India 2. Advocacy for vaccine trials 3. capacity building4. transfer of technology for manufacture of vaccine in India Biologicals	Therion Bologicals, Cambridge, Mass	1. developed vaccine with ICMR. IPR and confidentiality agreement between ICMR and Therion	1. Developed DNA/MVA HIV prototype vaccine from 6 genes of Indian HIV strains 2. Phase I prime-boost trials are being planned All new IP generated will be jointly held by IAVI & ICMR 3. Technology transfer agreement between ICMR & IAVI 4. Co-exclusive licensing bet. GOI & IAVI. GOI shall have the exclusive IP rights on inventions arising out of the program to benefit India and its neighboring countries and IAVI shall have IP rights for rest of the world

(continued)

Table 15.3 (continued)

Human Papilloma Virus	ICMR Signed an agreement with Merck to conduct clinical trials in India to observe safety and efficacy of the vaccine. ICPO signed a MOU with Merck to develop vaccine against HPV	ICMR India The Institute of Cytology and Preventive Oncology (ICPO) NOIDA.	Will facilitate and assist conducting clinical trials. Identified clinical trial cites in Delhi, Ahmadabd, Mumbai, TN and Hyderabad National Coordinating Centre for Indian HPV Vaccine Initiative	Vaccine developed by USA's, MERCK & Co and Merck & Co' Ltd., of India (MSD) would conduct trials in India	Developed vaccine named Gardasil Supplies vaccine free of cost for trials	Phase II Trials being carried out MSD has committed to supply vaccine at affordable prices if it is successful after trials. All global alliances-GAVI, WHO, The alliance for cervical cancer Prevention (ACCP), The International agency for research on Cancer (IARC), Bill Gates foundation and PATH are ready to provide technical and financial assistance to developing countries to deliver the HPV vaccine.

(continued)

Table 15.3 (continued)

Rotavirus	a large public-private partnership to develop 116E, an oral Rotavirus vaccine..	AIIMS, Delhi and Department of Biotechnology, New Delhi US Centres for Disease Control and Prevention (CDC), Stanford University, US National Institutes of Health, National Institute of Allergy and Infectious Diseases (NIAID), Society for Applied Studies, India's National Institute of Immunology, Indo-US Vaccine Action Program(on for the last 7years)	Isolated candidate molecule and developed vaccine with the help of NIH Technical assistanceFinancial assistance The Phase I/II clinical trial study was conducted by the Society for Applied Studies in New Delhi. A total of 369 infants were enrolled for the study.	Bharat Biotech International Ltd., Hyderabad Bill & Melinda Gates Foundation, PATH,	Developed 116 E Oral vaccine for conducting clinical trials Finanacial assistance	Phase II clinical trials
Malaria Vaccine	To develop a vaccine and conduct clinical trials	CDC Atlanta, ICGEB Delhi	Technological support	Bharat Biotech International Ltd., Hyderabad Bill & Melinda Gates Fondation, PATH	Falvac-1A (multiepitope antigen againt Pfalcparum) is being developed in collaboration with CDC Financial assistance	Will soon conduct pre-clinical tials

(continued)

Table 15.3 (continued)

Avian influenza virus (H5N1)	To develop vaccine against H5N1	Department of Biotechnology, GOI, India	Coordinator between BBIL and Novavax	Novavax USA, & Bharat biotech international Ltd., Hyderabad, India	Provides technology for producing virus like particle vaccine Manufactures vaccine & Will fund 100% for conducting clinical trialsResponsible for sales in India & other Asian countries	Unrestricted Access to entire pre-clinical & clinical trials data. Double digital royalty on sales of the product by BBIL
Tuberculosis (TB)	To develop vaccines against TB	CDC Atlanta St. John's National Academy of Health Sciences in Bangalore,	$925,000 to conduct epidemiological studies in preparation for conducting clinical trials to develop and expand sites for Phase II and Phase III clinical trials in Palamaner Taluk, Andhra Pradesh,	Aeras Global TB Vaccine Foundation (Philanthropic organization)	$2.7 million Funding to Develop TB Vaccine Financial assistance for conducting trials	To complete six phase I trials of TB vaccine candidates by 2010 in south Africa Europe and Asia

Source Compiled from websites of companies, ICMR annual report 2005–2006, Satyanarayana (2007), Shankar (2008), http://dst.gov.in/statuatory_board.htm and http://www.america.gov/st/washfile-english/2004/September/20040920155159lcnirellep2.230471e-02.html

selecting malaria vaccine candidates that are developed through MVI. One Meningitis A vaccine that was developed specifically for Africa in October 2011 through PPP was a successful example of PPP in new product development; it has completed Phase 3 trials and is undergoing additional testing at present. However, once the product was launched in the market, how the real issues of proprietary rights were shared among partners would determine the strength and sustenance of PPPs. In contrast to the Meningitis vaccine initiative, AIDs vaccine development through IAVI yielded very low efficacy vaccine candidates in clinical trials. MVI is also one of PATH's initiatives to develop vaccines against malaria for developing countries. MVI typically partners with various stakeholders as and when required for product development (vaccines against malaria), though high protection efficacy vaccine has not yet been developed so far. The malaria causing pathogen is so complicated that it is a challenge to make an efficient vaccine against malaria. The success of a safe and effective vaccine development has direct relationship with the nature and epidemiology of disease causing pathogen. This is evident from the fact that it is difficult to make safe and immunogenic vaccines against malaria and AIDS, whereas vaccines against Smallpox, DPT, Hepatitis B, etc., were highly protective.

GAVI is one of the major GPPP involving several multiple partners, and it is unique in the sense that this GPPP was not meant for product (vaccine) development but for vaccine introduction in poor countries. To put emergence of GAVI in context, PPPs were conceived as a means to access drugs and vaccines and were actively promoted in the late 1990s (Harrison, 1999; Reich, 2000; Smith, 2000). Vaccines are seen as magic bullets that prevent diseases in one shot. The vaccines which were already under EPI were not expensive and were accessible to all countries. However, there was a concern that the improved and new vaccines that were available in the West were not available in developing and poor countries owing to their high price. The champions of vaccines felt that the means to access new vaccines was through tiered pricing and through PPPs.

Initially, GPPPs in vaccines were meant to develop new vaccines through the Child Vaccine Initiative (CVI) for the poor countries. However, this effort could not be sustained as evidenced by the death of CVI despite the efforts of prominent actors to forge PPPs for the development of new vaccines for the poor (Muraskin, 2002). Then the concept of access to vaccines in poor countries became the objective of GPPPs like GAVI, whose main objective is to 'introduce' new expensive vaccines in those countries where vaccines are not affordable and cannot be accessed. GAVI is interested in introducing only new vaccines and preferably in combinations. It calls these new vaccines 'underutilised' vaccines, though this term is contestable in the context of a need-based approach and its meaning varies in different country contexts. For instance, the Oral Polio Vaccine (OPV) has not worked in the polio endemic states of India. But can OPV be called an underutilised vaccine in this context? Often, the ineffectual results are blamed on the lack of OPV coverage in these areas without realising the obvious need for generating unequivocal evidence by conducting post-vaccination studies to test protection achieved after immunisation. Critiques point out that the techno-centric approach of Global Polio Eradication Initiative disregarded the epidemiological features of polio (Bajpai & Saraya, 2012b).

GAVI claims that so far it has helped the introduction of 10 vaccines in 73 countries and was able to avert 8 million future deaths in developing countries, since its inception in 2000. It claims that it has brought down deaths in the under five age group by 3.6%, i.e. child deaths fell from 76 to a projected 63 deaths per 1000 live births between 2010 and 2015 and helped GAVI supported countries to achieve millennium development goals. GAVI—claims that it helped countries to avert more than 4 million future deaths during the period 2011–2015, by exceeding its target of 3.9 million for the five-year period (GAVI 2016). It also monitors the global rate of coverage and access to new vaccines. In their eagerness to promote vaccine introduction in poor countries to achieve equity in accessing vaccines, GAVI missed the important point that all vaccines are not suitable to all populations in the same manner. This assumption that 'all vaccines are suitable to all population alike' (Madhavi, 2005) distorts the national vaccine choices and needs.

The concept of 'need' for a vaccine based on scientific evidence from local regions gets distorted and the use of vaccine in isolation undermines the power of other preventive and public health measures in overall disease management strategy. GAVI's tendency to push new vaccines in poor countries irrespective of their need, safety and efficacy based on local epidemiological evidence, was criticised by experts and feared that it would push countries into the debt trap by enforcing advance market commitments (Puliyel, 2011). GAVI's unsustainable financial model has also been criticised by an Oxfam–MSF report (Wilson & Jones, 2010).

Though GAVI presents itself as a consortium that provides service to the poor nations, it influences and interferes with national vaccine priorities and policies. The Bill and Melinda Gates Foundation being the major fund provider of GAVI also tend to influence local governments through GAVI. It has been pointed out that the Bill and Melinda Gates Foundation, the largest contributor to vaccination programmes of GAVI, has substantial business interests in at least nine pharmaceutical majors, whose representatives sit on the Board of the Global Fund to Fight AIDS, Tuberculosis and Malaria. That the Foundation exercises considerable influence over India's health policies is evident from the fact that it sponsored the Commission on Macroeconomics and Health which held the protection of intellectual property as crucial to investment in drug development and influenced the report prepared by the Indian Council for Research on International Economic Relations that recommended the setting up of world class schools of public health in India. The Public Health Foundation of India (PHFI), a PPP, was set up soon thereafter and the Gates Foundation has an intimate association with PHFI (Sathyamala, 2006).

It is believed that PPP would improve equity, efficiency, accountability, quality and accessibility of the entire health system. The way PPPs developed in the West is different from those in the developing countries. In India PPPs are being imposed as an economic reforms measure irrespective of its socio-economic reality, while it is acknowledged that success or a failure of a PPP for specific purpose varies from case to case. PPPs in vaccines in India show that they are predominantly for conducting clinical trials (14. 3). It is pointed out by critics that clinical trials are less expensive and much easier to conduct in India as compared to Western countries because India offers cheap manpower and Contract Research Organisations (CROs) with poor regulatory structure. Clinical trial participants are often reduced to guinea pigs with no law that provides any compensation or treatment in case of any mishap during the trials (Nundy & Gulhati, 2005). The controversy over HPV vaccine trials where four girls died during the trial raised similar ethical concerns on informed consent, trial injury compensation, follow-up and record-keeping on trail participants (Sarojini et al., 2010; Sengupta et al., 2011). This controversy brought many issues to the forefront, such as the causes of cervical cancer, inability of HPV vaccine to reduce all causes of cervical cancer, and the need for regular screening in spite of HPV vaccine, etc. HPV vaccine trials in India were a PPP between Merck and the Indian Council of Medical Research (ICMR) to conduct clinical trials and to test the feasibility of HPV vaccine introduction in the Indian population. This PPP certainly did not benefit the women on whom the trials were conducted (Sarojini et al., 2010) but brought awareness in the society by highlighting several contentious issues in academia as well as the popular media.

AIDS vaccine trials, which are another PPP between ICMR, IAVI and a private company, Targeted Genetics in India, also created a controversy and brought to fore ethical and regulatory issues and the fact that the safety of trial participants was not ensured. Critics pointed out that India conducted Phase II clinical trials of the tgAAC09 vaccine against AIDS without conducting Phase I trials. The Phase II trials in India were conducted just two weeks before the announcement by Targeted Genetics that the Phase I trials conducted in Belgium proved that the AIDS vaccine tgAAC09 did not elicit significant immune response in trial participants. Since Target Genetics was also involved in conducting clinical trials in India, it raised scepticism about the sharing of the Belgium trial results with the Indian partners. Questions were raised about whether the Indian partners studied any preliminary trial data of the Belgium trials before launching Phase II trials and why Phase I trials were not conducted in India in the first place. Critics felt that this apparent lack of communication raises questions on the nature of partnerships between Indian and overseas partners (Jesani & Coutinho, 2007).

Unlike the above examples, indigenous development of Hepatitis B and Hepatitis B-DTP vaccine was a successful PPP between Shantha Biotech Ltd and the Technology Development Board (TDB) of the Department of Science and Technology under the Ministry of Science and Technology, where TDB provided financial support to the private company (Frew et al. 2007) However, Shantha Biotechnics Ltd., the most pampered private company by the Indian government as a model for home-grown, government-supported private enterprise, has now been taken over by the French multinational company Institut Merieux and is being eyed by another MNC GlaxoSmithKline (Madhavi, 2009a), indicating that the private sector cannot be a reliable/dependable partner to meet national vaccine requirements for stable affordable vaccine supply.

The above examples of access to vaccines through PPP in India reveal that vaccine development and vaccine clinical trials cannot deliver public health benefits in isolation without addressing ethical, regulatory and governance issues. Moreover, before entering into any PPP, the feasibility and health benefits that may accrue to local populations should be assessed for a vaccine to be developed. For a vaccine to be tested the basis should decidedly be local epidemiological evidence and the exercise should be in relation to prevailing diseases in the country. It must be imperative that PPPs ensure safety and vaccine injury compensation to trial participants while conducting clinical trials.

The experience of vaccine PPPs in India illustrates that public money is being spent for private profiteering without addressing issues of 'need' and without ensuring vaccine benefits. Yet, the Union Health Ministry announced the construction of a vaccine park, on a PPP model in Chengalpattu, Tamil Nadu, at a time when three crucial vaccine PSUs were closed down in January 2008 as they were alleged to be a non- WHO–cGMP complaint at that time. Another PSU, HLL Biotech Ltd, a 100% of HLL Lifecare Ltd. (HLL is Hindustan Latex Ltd.), a Government of India enterprise under the Ministry of Health and Family Welfare, is in charge of the upcoming vaccine park by drawing inspiration from Ernst & Young analysis of vaccine business in India. The Government of India mandated HLL to establish a state of art vaccine manufacturing unit termed as "Integrated Vaccines Complex" (IVC) at Chengalpattu near Chennai to produce lifesaving and cost effective vaccines primarily to minimise the demand–supply gap and support the government in the Universal Immunisation programme. IVC came into existence further to the proposal by the Ministry of Health & Family Welfare (GOI) to the Cabinet Committee on Economic Affairs (CCEA) for establishment of a centralised vaccines manufacturing facility with international standards in the government sector at an estimated cost of INR 594.00 crores and was declared as a Project of National Importance. The vaccine complex will be the nodal centre for research, manufacture and supply of vaccines at affordable prices for the Universal Immunisation Programme (UIP) of the Government of India. The vaccines to be manufactured in IVC are Pentavalent combination (DPT + Hep B + Hib), BCG, Measles, Hepatitis B, Rabies, Hib and JE vaccine. The annual capacity of IVC is expected to be around 585 million doses.[1] Work on this IVC was reported to have commenced as part of the Make in India project of the current government, in October 2016, and was to be completed in seven years (TNN, 2016).

Despite criticism from the civil society organisations, the health ministry closed its own PSUs while, around the same time, allotting INR 150 crores for setting up the vaccine park. Such policy measures had led to acute shortage of EPI vaccines as the private sector, despite having been supported by the public exchequer, refused to meet the shortages without increasing vaccine prices (Madhavi, 2008; Ramachandran, 2008). It is also interesting to note that HLL Biotech Ltd is also planning to access technologies from the existing PSUs for primary vaccine production in the vaccine park, while new vaccine production is envisaged through PPPs. This has led to fears that this vaccine Park is meant for marketing and distributing new vaccines and their combinations produced by multinational companies after exercising the simple expedient of repackaging from the bulk. This vaccine park thus apppears to be a bottling unit (Ramachandran, 2008) and cocktail factory of vaccines, where DPT may be procured from vaccine PSUs while the private sector may add new vaccines to make pentavalent (DTP–Hepatitis B–Hib) and tetravalent vaccines (DTP–Hepatitis B).

Epidemiological Evidence from India for New Vaccines

When the scientific community is divided on the issue of need for a vaccine and its safety and efficacy in populations, it becomes difficult for the decision-maker to make a rational choice of vaccines for mass or selective immunisation. Pressure from various stakeholders distorts local vaccination needs of the public, unless it is backed by published scientific evidence. Some examples from India are a reflection of the need for an evidence-based policy. The protection efficacy of any vaccine against a disease in a population is dependent on the strain specificity of disease-causing pathogen, which varies from region to region. A vaccine effective in Philippines need not necessarily be effective in India. Therefore, pathogen strain specificity and vaccine suitability are important issues in bringing down mortality/morbidity against a disease in mass immunisation strategies. Two highly debated Indian examples are highlighted here.

Rotavirus Vaccine

There is no scientific evidence for need and suitability of rotavirus vaccine in India. Rotaviral strains in India are different from those in other countries/regions (Bajpai & Saraya, 2012a), and new strains are continually emerging through re-assortment between animal and human strains. Natural infection of rotavirus does not provide protection to subsequent infections because of local, continuously evolving strains. However, in Mexico, natural infection does cause protection against subsequent infections (Puliyel & Mathew, 2012). These regional differences are indicative of local strain variation and prove that one region/country's experience cannot be extrapolated to other countries. The WHO recommended rotavirus vaccine to its member countries based on studies from Malawi (one of the poorest countries), Nicaragua and in a few developed countries (Ibid.). Most often the recommendation is based on disease burden estimates rather than on the actual number of cases and deaths in India. It was pointed out that the estimated figures of death due to rotavirus diarrhoea in India presumes uniform mortality rate for all causes of diarrhoea and the estimated Figures (122,000–15,300 deaths) were arrived at by multiplying the mean rotavirus case detection rate with the case fatality rate of diarrhoea, which wrongly assumes that all diarrhoeal cases are rotaviral diarrhoea cases. No rotaviral efficacy studies were done in India. Bacterial diarrhoea may cause more mortality due to systemic complications and sepsis, whereas rotaviral diarrhoea can be managed with simple measures to reduce dehydration. Fifty-eight percent of rotavirus cases are co-infected with other pathogens and attributing all deaths due to rotavirus will be an overestimate (Ibid.).

Two studies estimated that rotavirus vaccine is cost-effective in India by putting the vaccine price at 0.15 and 7 US $, respectively, while the open market price in middle income countries is US $50. Apparently, Brazil negotiated a vaccine price for 7 US $. Both the studies, by using vaccine efficacy studies from the West have been extrapolated to India as being cost-effective (Ibid.).

Pentavalent Vaccine (DTP–Hepatitis B–Hib)

There has been much debate over the introduction of pentavalent (Hb–Hib–DTP) vaccine; and the Indian government has gone ahead with its introduction in UIP despite the adverse events associated with it, including deaths (Lone & Puliyel, 2010; Madhavi, 2006; Madhavi and Raghuram 2010a, b). In fact, the debate on the introduction of the pentavalent vaccine in UIP is a test case for the future; new and combination vaccine introduction in Indian UIP.

The published epidemiological evidence from the few studies in India indicates that the Hib incidence is very low in the Indian population, around 0.007% (IBIS 2002; Minz et al., 2008). Moreover, evidence from other countries shows that in Hib vaccinated populations, some highly virulent Hib mutant strains are reported to have replaced the native strains (Bruce et al. 2008; Lipstich 1999; Muhlemann et al., 1996). Scientific evidence from India indicates that Indian children develop immunity against Hib during infancy (Puliyel et al., 2001) and it raises doubts about whether the mass vaccination against Hib is warranted. However, proponents of pentavalent vaccine and Hib vaccine cite hospital-based studies to show that Hib is responsible for a significant proportion of cases of bacterial meningitis (Bajpai and Saraya 2012b; IBIS 2002) and pneumonia (Bajpai and Saraya 2012a) in children below five years. However, these hospital-based studies cannot be extrapolated to the general population. The National Technical Advisory Group on Immunisation (NTAGI) in India estimated that the Hib disease burden in India is around 2.4 million cases and 72,000 deaths in children less than five years of age, accounting for approximately 4% of all child deaths in India in the year 2000. A particular point of contention was that NTAGI ignored the results of a multi-centric study conducted by ICMR to establish the prevalence of the Hib invasive disease in India, from July 2005 to December 2006 (Dutta & Puliyel, 2010). Results of this study did not support NTAGI's recommendation of including pentavalent Hib vaccine in EPI. Importantly enough, this led to a review of NTAGI's recommendation (Bajpai & Saraya, 2012b). Contrary to NTAGI's position, the opponents of Hib vaccine have pointed out the results from probe studies done in Asia to show that the vaccine did not reduce the burden of disease appreciably compared to placebo (Lone & Puliyel, 2010). Reference has been made to the role of GAVI, WHO, USAID, John Hopkins and the Hib Initiative in misleading the people about the efficacy of the vaccine (Lone & Puliyel, 2010; Puliyel et al., 2010). There are no well planned efficacy or cost- effectiveness studies from India yet to support or refute the efficacy of the vaccine. Expert opinions to the effect that 'the lack of local surveillance data should not delay the introduction of the vaccine especially in countries where regional evidence indicates a high burden of disease, that is being handed down by WHO, have served as a *fait accompli* for advisory groups like NTAGI while making their own recommendations' (Bajpai & Saraya, 2012b).

There are three most contentious issues on combination vaccines (Madhavi, 2006) that have not been answered by any international agency or by companies that invented them. They need the attention of policy-makers and readers in the interest of national sovereignty and health security.

First, why is it that every combination vaccine is a product of a combination of a UIP vaccine and a non-UIP vaccine? Is it because lack of demand–pull for individual new vaccines (for example, Hepatitis B, Hib) is sought to be covered up by the UIP vaccines that enjoy higher legitimacy? Virtually all combinations are a means by which new vaccines are gaining a backdoor entry through the captive UIP market by riding piggyback on UIP vaccines such as DTP, measles, IPV, OPV, etc. If a new vaccine can stand on its own merits (especially epidemiological merit), why does it need a piggyback ride?

Second, if a combination vaccine is nothing more than a cocktail then why does the price multiply? Is pricing of a combination vaccine a method of value addition or a means of cost recovery? If there is a qualitative difference in the technology, one can consider the legitimacy of recovering a cost of delivering it. However, combination vaccines are basically cocktail vaccines that are mixed in a vial and its price is much higher than the individual counterparts while it is expected that it can save costs of packaging, distribution, logistics and marketing. In that case, combination vaccine should be cheaper than all the individual vaccines combined. However, its high price compared to the total price of all individual vaccines indicates that the combination is made for the value addition but not for the benefit of the public.

As the patents on individual vaccines expire, combination of vaccines becomes a means to acquire new Intellectual Property Rights (IPR) advantage. Are combination vaccines IPR gimmicks or marketing gimmicks that give no additional health benefits than their individual components? Are combination vaccines driven by the same motives as drug formulations? When two individual drugs expire as product patents, combining makes them a new formulation which gives its own IPR advantages. For example, both Ibuprofen and Paracetamol are anti-inflammatory. When both are combined, it becomes a new formulation known as Combiflam but sells at a much higher price than the individual components. It is well-known among pharma critics that formulations are driven by business motives, which is why the majority of irrational drugs are actually formulations. One would like to ask whether vaccines are also joining the ranks of irrational drug formulations.

Third, do benefits of combination vaccines add up? Or is it only in terms of the number of injections reduced? Scientific literature shows that, in general, the safety and efficacy aspects of combination vaccines are not proven beyond doubt (Beeching et al., 2004; Beri et al. 2012; Comenge & Girard, 2006; Girard, 2005; Klein et al., 2010; Vesikari et al, 1991; WHO 2012: 1–4), and it is reported that they are less protective when compared to their individual components (AAP 1999; Buttery et al., 2005; FDA 1997; Greenberg et al., 2000; Kalies et al., 2004; White et al., 1997). In pentavalent vaccine (DTP–HB–Hib), lower immunological responses to Hep-B and Hib were observed when compared to their separate administration (Bar-On et al., 2009; Edwards & Decker, 1997; Jones et al., 1998; Pichichero et al. 1997; WHO, 2005). Critical studies point out that the new imported vaccines may not be cost-effective and beneficial in the Indian population keeping in view the epidemiology of prevailing diseases such as Hepatits B, Hib, rotaviral diarrhoea, etc. (Arora & Puliyel, 2005; Madhavi, 2003, 2006; Phadke & Kale, 2000).

The Need for an Evidence-Based Policy

The situation analysis of vaccines in India indicates that market forces and international organisations are distorting national vaccine needs by extrapolating other country experiences, overstating disease burden for vaccine-preventable diseases and pushing new vaccine into UIP without cost–benefit analysis. Lack of reliable surveillance data benefits private companies. Consumers are confused and unaware of the merits and demerits of new vaccines. This underscores the need for an evidence-based national vaccine policy for optimum utilisation of vaccines in public health. Two Public Interest Litigations on vaccine PSUs and pentavalent vaccines by civil society compelled the Indian government to draft a national vaccine policy in 2011. However, this policy document was an eye-wash and it actually endorses the current illegitimate practices of vaccine promotion.

Critique of the Health Ministry's National Vaccine Policy

The current national vaccine policy (April 2011) uploaded in the Ministry of Health and Family Welfare (MoHFW) website in July 2011 completely ignored a draft document for evidence-based national vaccine policy that emerged in June 2009 through an interdisciplinary workshop (Co- organised by ICMR and NISTADS) of scientists, doctors, health professionals, lawyers and activists. This document was submitted to the government for consideration and was also published in the *Indian Journal of Medical Research* (Madhavi et al. 2010), which was well received with no evidence of any credible critique of it so far. Some points to be noted are:

1. The policy of MoHFW (2011) does not provide an uncompromising scientific basis on which a vaccine can be introduced in Indian UIP and does not commit itself only to need-based and evidence-based vaccination.
2. In its eagerness to push vaccines, this policy completely missed the very idea of selective immunisation and implies that all immunisation is universal.
3. The government policy pays lip service to several important issues such as criteria for new vaccine introduction into UIP, including the Grades of Recommendation Assessment, Development and Evaluation (GRADE) system,

strengthening the surveillance of Vaccine Preventable Diseases (VPD) and Adverse Events Following Immunisation (AEFI), operational efficiency, etc. But the fact that these criteria are not mandatory may not ensure objective decision-making.

4. It concentrates more on supply-side factors, PPPs, innovative (read speculative) financing, global fund (read advance market commitments to further MNC pharma businesses), etc. The MSF–Oxfam report (Wilson & Jones, 2010) points out that the global financing model of GAVI that funds vaccine introduction in countries is also unsustainable as it gets its funding from the International Finance Facility for Immunisation (IFFI) and is based on the promise of future funding from donor countries, raising money in the meantime by issuing bonds to international capital markets which themselves operate in ways no less speculative than the American banks that triggered off the world recession (Madhavi & Raghuram, 2010a, b). 'Such policies are not only out of tune with national health security needs, but are also out of sync with the times that we live in; the yearning for health reforms in the US is a pointer to the incongruity of this policy framework. Clearly, this vaccine policy is not designed to enhance national public capacity for public immunisation programmes but to justify spending public money on privately produced vaccines in the name of protection from diseases whose incidence figures and public health statistics are dubious and industry-manufactured' (Madhavi & Raghuram, 2012). Moreover, advance market commitments to global financing schemes directly impinge on our sovereignty in subsequent decisions.
5. The government policy justifies the introduction of dubious, new combination vaccines (Section 5.2 of MoHFW policy) (MoHFW, 2011) in terms of the number of injections reduced and savings on logistics, while conveniently ignoring the fact that the cost of the combination vaccine multiplies manifold with each vaccine added. Most combination vaccines are just expensive cocktails with no net health benefit than their individual components other than the patenting, pricing and marketing advantages they offer to the company that makes them.

Conclusion

It is clear from the above trends that the push for new vaccines is aggressive through various means: (a) advance market commitments;

(a) setting international agendas; (c) through PPPs; (d) through national governments; (e) through mass immunisation programmes; (f) through IPR regimes, especially in large countries like India, China and Brazil as economies of scale determines the vaccine price and profits. The pressure to introduce new vaccines into UIPs is with the purpose of creating everlasting markets for all new vaccines. Even the deliberate politics of language is selling a vaccine by the disease rather than by the pathogen against which the vaccine is designed. For instance, the pneumococcal vaccine is called anti-pneumonia, though pneumonia is also caused by Hib and other pathogens. Similarly, the anti-rotaviral vaccine is called the anti-diarrhoea vaccine, which it is not. In fact an anti-diarrhoeal vaccine should be the one that protects against all causes of diarrhoea that is prepared with all anti-diarrhoeal antigens on a single epitope. In other words, there is a rationality crisis for combination vaccines and therefore legitimacy crisis and it becomes contentious. The aggressive marketing of new vaccines is also a crisis of financial speculation as it was reported in the Oxfam–MSF report. One wonders why supply push is becoming so desperate.

The cost of pentavalent vaccines in the US can only be brought down if it is adopted in the UIP of large countries like India, China and Brazil. There is the industry compulsion of economies of scale and the tendency to treat expansion of biopharma business as the best escape route from the drug-discovery deadlock in curative and synthetic medicine (Table 15.4).

Since 2005, only 11 molecules under product patent were launched in the Indian market. Even loans and aid as marketing tools have to depend on advance market commitments by GAVI, government guarantees on vaccines, funding commitments from donors and speculative loans from capital markets adoption. Pentavalent vaccine is an illustration that commercial success of any new vaccine anywhere in the world depends on economies of scale which, in turn, depends on its universal adoption in large countries. That means even if the rest of the world adopts a particular vaccine, it is still not sufficient for the company unless it is pushed into economies of scale. This is a circular profit model where any break in this link would collapse the entire structure, that is, if GAVI's aid or the World Bank loans are the inducement for adopting such vaccines in the absence of epidemiological evidence and if GAVI's own funds depend on loans raised by IFFI which, in turn, depend on the policy commitment of large countries, there can be no break in this chain. This raises the critical question about whether vaccines are driving the speculative biopharma boom as the best insurance against synthetic pharma doom. The lack of evidence-based vaccine policy in most countries of the world driving the speculative biopharma boom seems to be the best escape route from the impending doom in synthetic drug discovery. The slogan—'prevention is better than cure'—is more true today for the pharma industry's own health than for the health of people and nations.

Table 15.4 New drug approvals

New Drug	*Year of approval*	*Developer*	*Therapeutic value*	*Approver*	*Reference*	*Remarks*
lorcaserin (Belviq)	June 2012	Arena Pharmaceuticals	Prescription weight loss drug (3%)	FDA	Nature, 18(8), Aug 2012	In 2010, FDA rejected because it induces cancer in rats. Later new data presented that it doesn't apply to humans. FDA recommends post-market surveillance studies
Qsymia	July 2012	Vivus	Weight loss drug (8.9%)	FDA	Nature, 18(8), Aug 2012	Causes serious side effects like increased heart rate and risk of birth defects
HEV 239	Oct 2012 in china	Xiamen Innovax Biotech, china	Against hepatitis E	Chinese stte FDA (SFDA)	http://www.scientificamerican.com/article.cfm?id=hepatitis-e-vaccine-debuts	
Florbetapir, Amylo-beta imaging agent for	July 2012	Eli Lilly of Indianapolis, and its subsidiary Avid Radiopharmaceuticals	A diagnostic agent for suspecting alzheimers	FDA	Nature Biotechnology, 30, 575, 2012.	
Elelyso (taliglucerase alfa)	June 2012	Israeli company Protalix BioTherapeutics of Carmiel	Treating Gouchers' disease	FDA	Natue Biotechnology 30, 47, 2012	This is the first plant-made drug approved by the regulators. Protalix and US partner Pfizer of New York are pricing Elelyso at a 25% discount from Genzyme's Cerezyme (imiglucerase), the market leader, a price they hope will persuade clinicians and patients to switch.

Source Compiled from secondary sources

References

American Academy of Pediatrics (AAP). (1999, May). Recommendations of the advisory committee on immunisation practices (ACIP). *Pediatrics, 103*(5), 1064–77.

Anonymous. (1985, August). Just beginning: A new era of vaccines. *Chemical Weekly, 137*(9), 58.

Arora, R., & Puliyel, J. M. (2005). Economic evaluation tailored to promote vaccine uptake: How third world consumers can respond. *Expert Review of Pharmacoeconomics and Outcomes Research, 5*(5), 515–516.

Bajpai, V., & Saraya, A. (2012a, January–March). Agenda setting in vaccine policy and social relevance of the emerging vaccine technologies from public health perspective. Part 2. *International Journal of Medicine and Public Health, 2*(1), 16–25.

Bajpai, V., & Saraya, A. (2012b, August 21). Understanding the syndrome of techno-centrism through the epidemiology of vaccines as preventive tools. *Indian Journal of Public Health, 56*(2), 133–139.

Balgescu, M., & Young, J. (2005). *Partnerships and accountability: current thinking and approaches among agencies supporting Civil Society organisations.* Overseas Development Institute.

Bar-On, E. S., Goldberg, E., Fraser, A., Vidal, L., Hellmann, S., & Leibovici, L. (2009, July 8). Combined DTP–HBV–HiB vaccine versus separately administered DTP–HBV and HIB vaccines for primary prevention of Diphtheria, Tetanus, Pertussis, Hepatitis B and Haemophilus Influenzae B (HIB). In Cochrane Acute Respiratory Infections Group (Ed.), *Cochrane Database of Systematic Reviews* (pp. 1–57). Wiley.

Beeching, N. J., Clarke, P. D., Kitchin, N., Pirmohamed, J., Veitch, K., & Weber, F. (2004, November 15). Comparison of two combined vaccines against Typhoid fever and Hepatitis A in healthy adults. *Vaccine, 23*(1), 29–35.

Beri, R. S., Ojha, & Kant, R. (2012, November 6). Is Hib vaccination required at all in India? *Indian Pediatrics, 39*(11), 1067–1068.

Bhadoria, V., Gobinath, A., Mitra, P., & Narayanan, M. (2012, September 15). Transforming India's vaccine market. Prepared by Mckinsey and Company for Organisation of Pharmaceutical Producers of India (OPPI), Mumbai, pp. 1–33.

Blumenthal, D., Causino, N., Campbell, E., & Louis, K. S. (1996, February 8). Relationships between academic institutions and industry in the life sciences: An industry survey. *New England Journal of Medicine, 334*(6), 368–373.

Bruce, M. G., Shelley, L., Tammy, Z., Navarro, C., Case, C., Hemsley, C., Hennessy, T., Corriveau, A., Larke, B., Sobel, I., Lovgren, M., DeByle, C., Tsang, R., Parkinson, J. A., and the International Circumpolar Surveillance Hib Working Group. (2008, January). Epidemiology of Haemophilus influenza Serotype A, North American Arctic, 2000–2005. *Emerging Infectious Diseases, 14*(1), 48–55.

Buse, K., & Walt, G. (2000, April). Global public–private partnerships part I: A new development in vaccines? *Bulletin of the World Health Organisation, 78*(4), 549–561.

Buse, K. (2004). Governing public-private infectious disease partnerships. *Brown Journal of World Affairs, X*(2), 225–242.

Buttery, J.P. FRACP; Riddell, A. MRCPCH; McVernon, J. (2005, April 13). Immunogenicity and safety of a combination pneumococcal-Meningococcal vaccine in infants: A randomised controlled study. *Journal of the American Medical Association, 293*(14), 1751–1758.

Center for Disease Control and Prevention. (1999, July 30). Achievements in public health, 1900s–1999: Control of infectious diseases. *Morbidity and Mortality Weekly Report (MMWR), 48*(29), 621–629.

Center for Disease Control and Prevention Press Release. (2004, September 20). CDC *Funds studies for Tuberculosis Vaccine trials, Aeras Foundation helps prepare for vaccine clinical trials in India, Distributed by the Bureau of International Information Program.* US Department of State. Accessed December 25, 2012. http://www.america.gov/st/washfile-english/2004/September/20040920155159lcnirellep2.230471e-02.html

Comenge, Y., & Girard, M. (2006, September 21). Multiple sclerosis and Hepatitis B vaccination: Adding the credibility of molecular biology to an unusual level of clinical and epidemiological evidence. *Medical Hypothesis, 66*(1), 84–86.

Donald, A. B. (2007, January). Ethics in public health research: A research protocol to evaluate the effectiveness of public-private partnerships as a means to improve health and welfare systems worldwide." *American Journal of Public Health, 97*(1), 19–25.

Dutta, P., & Puliyel, J. M. (2010, June). NTAGI Recommendations Overlooked Crucial ICMR Data. *Indian Pediatrics, 47*(6), 542–543.

Edwards, K.M., & Decker, M. D. (1997). Combination vaccines consisting of a cellular pertussis vaccines. *Pediatric Infectious Diseases Journal, 16*(Suppl. 4), S97–102.

Food and Drug Administration (FDA). (1997, April). *Guidance for industry for the evaluation of combination vaccines for preventable diseases: Production, testing and clinical studies*. Docket No. 97N-0029. US Department of Health and Human Services, Food and Drug Administration, Center for Biologics Evaluation and Research.

Frew, S. E., Rahim, R., Stephen, S. M., Monali, R., Abdallah, D. S., & Singer Peter, A. (2007). India's health biotech sector at a crossroads. *Nature Biotechnology, 25*(4), 403–417.

Gavi, The Vaccine Alliance. (2016). Keeping Children Healthy: The Vaccine Alliance Progress Report 2015." (1–100). Geneva: Gavi Publication. Accessed 6 March, 2018. http://gaviprogress report.org/2015/.

Girard, M. (2005, February). Auto-immune hazards of Hepatitis B vaccine. *Autoimmunity Reviews, 4*(2), 96–100.

Government of India (GoI). (2011). Report of the working group on disease burden for the twelfth five year plan. *WG 3(1): Communicable Diseases*. Planning Commission.

Guzman, T. A. (2016). Big pharma and big profits: The multibillion dollar vaccine market. *Silent Crow News, 26*, 2016.

Ministry of Health and Family Welfare (MoHFW), Government of India (GoI). (2011). *National Vaccine Policy*. MOHFW.

MoHFW. Javed Chowdhury Committee Report. (2010). *Final Report of the Committee Set up to Determine the Reasons for the Suspension of the Manufacturing License of CRI Kasauli, PII Coonoor, and BCGVL Guindy, and to Draw the Road-map for the Revival of the Three Units* (1–74).

Greenberg, P., Wong, V. K., Partridge, S. B., Chang Swei-Ju, J., Jing, B. J., Howe, & Ward, J. I. (2000). Immunogenecity of a *Hemophilus Influenza* Type B–Tetanus Toxoid Conjugate Vaccine when Mixed with Diphtheria– Tetanus–Acellular Pertussis–Hepatitis B Combination Vaccine. *Pediatric Infectious Disease Journal, 19*(12), 1135–1140.

Harrison, P. H. (1999). A new model for collaboration: The alliance for microbicide development. *International Journal of Gynecology and Obstetrics, 67*(Suppl. S2), S39–S53.

Invasive Bacterial Infections Surveillance (IBIS) Group of the International Clinical Epidemiology Network. (2002). Are Haemophilus influenzae infections a significant problem in India? A prospective study and review. *Clinical Infectious Diseases, 34*(7), 949–957.

Jesani, A., & Coutinho, L. (2007). AIDS vaccine trials in India: Ethical benchmarks and unanswered questions. *Indian Journal of Medical Ethics, 4*(1), 2–3.

Jones, I.G., Tyrrell, H., Hill, A., Horobin, J.M., & Taylor, B. (1998). Randomised control-led trial of combined diphtheria, Tetanus, whole-cell Pertussis vaccine administered in the same syringe and separately with Haemophilus Influenzae Type B vaccine at two, three and four months of age. *Vaccine, 16*(1), 109–113.

Kalies, H., Verstraeten, T., Grote, V., Meyer, N., Siedler, A., Schmitt, H., Breuer, T., Moulton, L. H., & von Kries, R. (2004). Four-and a half year follow up of the effectiveness of Diphtheria–Tetanus Toxoid–Acelluar Pertussis/Hemophiplus influenza type B and Diphtheria–Tetanus Toxoid– Acellular Pertussis–Inactivated Poliovirus/H Influenza Type B combination vaccine in Germany. *Pediatric Infectious Disease Journal, 23*(10), 944–950.

Klein, N. P., Fireman, B., Katherine Yih, W., Lewis, E., Kulldorff, M., Ray, P., Baxter, R., Hambidge, S., Nordin, J., Naleway, A., Belongia, E. A., Lieu, T., Baggs, J., & Weintraub, E. (2010). Measles-Mumps-Rubella-Varicella combination vaccine and the risk of Febrile Seizures. *Pediatrics, 126*(1), e1–e8.

Lipsitch, M. (1999). Bacterial vaccines and Serotype replacement: Lessons from Haemophilus Influenza and prospects for streptococcus pneumonia. *Emerging Infectious Diseases, 5*(3), 336–345.

Lone, Z., & Puliyel, J.M. (2010). Introducing Pentavalent vaccine in the EPI in India: A counsel for caution. *Indian Journal of Medical Research, 132*(1), 1–3.

Mackenbach, J. P., Stirbu, I., Roskam, A. J., Schaap, M. M., Menvielle, G., Leinsalu, M., & Kunst, A. E., European Union working group on socioeconomic inequalities in health 2008. European Union Working Group on Socioeconomic Inequalities in Health: Socioeconomic Inequalities in Health in 22 European Countries. *New England Journal of Medicine, 358*(23), 2468–2481.

Madhavi, Y. (2003). The manufacture of consent? Hepatitis B vaccination. *Economic and Political Weekly, 38*(24), 2417–2424.

Madhavi, Y. (2005). Vaccine policy in India. *PLOS Medicine Weekly, 2*(5), e127: 387–391.

Madhavi, Y. (2006). New combination vaccines: Backdoor entry into India's universal immunisation programme?." *Current Science, 90*(11), 1465–1469.

Madhavi, Y. (2008). Vaccine PSUs: Chronicle of an attenuation wilfully caused. *Medico Friends Circle Bulletin (MFC), 329*, 1–7.

Madhavi, Y. (2009a, September 23). Home-grown Vaccines are Crucial for Public Health. Opinions, *scidev.net*. Accessed December 25, 2012. http://www.scidev.net/en/opinions/home-grown-vaccines-are-crucial-for-public-health.html.

Madhavi, Y. (2009b, November). Meeting local Needs in Global Times: The Case of Universal Vaccines in India. *Journal of Health Studies II, No., 2*, 81–105.

Madhavi, Y., et al. (2010). Evidence-based national vaccine policy. *Indian Journal of Medical Research, 131*(5), 617–628.

Madhavi, Y., & Raghuram, N. (2010a, May 17). Crisis of Speculation: Donors Should Fund Only Locally Proven Vaccine Needs and Local Capacity Building. *British Medical Journal, 340*, c2576. Accessed March 6, 2018 http://www.bmj.com/content/340/bmj.c2576/rapid-responses

Madhavi, Y., & Raghuram, N. (2010b). Pentavalent and other new combination vaccines: Solutions in search of problems. *Indian Journal of Medical Research, 132*(4), 456–457.

Madhavi, Y., & Raghuram, N. (2012). National vaccine policy in the era of vaccines seeking diseases and governments seeking public private partnerships. *Current Science, 102*(4), 57–58.

Minz, S., Balraj, V., Lalitha, M.K., Murali, N., Cherian, T., Manoharan, G., Kadirvan, S., Joseph, A., & Steinhoff, M.C. (2008, July). Incidence of Haemophilus Influenzae Type B Meningitis in India. *Indian Journal of Medical Research, 128*(1), 57–64.

Muhlemann, K., Balz, M., Aebi, S., & Schopfer, K. (1996, March). Molecular characteristics of Haemophilus influenza causing invasive disease during the period of vaccination in Switzerland: Analysis of strains Isolated between 1986 and 1993. *Journal of Clinical Microbiology, 34*(3), 560–563.

Muraskin, W. (2002). The last years of the CVI and the birth of the GAVI. In Reich, M. R. (Ed.),*Public private partnerships for public health.* Series on Population and International Health Harvard Centre for Population and Development Studies.

Nundy, S., & Gulhati, C.M. (2005, April 21). A new colonialism? Conducting clinical trials in India. *The New England Journal of Medicine, 352*(16), 1633–1636.

Parliamentary Standing Committee on Health and Family Welfare. (2009). *34th Parliamentary Standing Committee on Health and Family Welfare*. New Delhi: Parliament of India, Rajya Sabha, Government of India.

Parliamentary Standing Committee on Health and Family Welfare. (2009b). *38th Parliamentary Standing Committee on Health and Family Welfare*. Parliament of India, Rajya Sabha, Government of India.

Parliamentary Standing Committee on Health and Family Welfare. (2010). *43rd Parliamentary Standing Committee on Health and Family Welfare*. Parliament of India, Rajya Sabha, Government of India.

Parliamentary Standing Committee on Health and Family Welfare. (2011). *52nd Parliamentary Standing Committee on Health and Family Welfare*. Parliament of India, Rajya Sabha, Government of India.

Phadke, A., and A. Kale. 2000. "Epidemiology and Ethics in the Hepatitis B Vaccine." *Indian Journal of Medical Ethics* 8, No. 2 (April-June) C7: 8–10.

Pichichero, M. E., Thomas, L., David, I.B., Philip, H., Edward, C., Emmanuel, V., Carlton, M., & Robert, S. D. (1997). vaccine Antigen Interactions after a Combination Diphtheria—Tetanus Toxoid Acellular Pertussis/Purified Capsular Polysaccharide of Hemophilus Influenzae type B Tetanus Toxoid Vaccine in Two, Four, and Six-Month-Old Infants. *Pediatric Infectious Diseases Journal, 16*(9), 863–870.

Puliyel, J. (2011). Vaccine policy and advance market commitment. *Economic and Political Weekly, 46*, 44–45.

Puliyel, J. M., Agarwal, K. S., & Abass, F. A. (2001). Natural immunity to Haemophilus influenzae in infancy in Indian children. *Vaccine, 19*(32), 4592–4594.

Puliyel, J. M., Mathew, J. L., & Priya, R. (2010). Incomplete Reporting of Research in Press Releases: et tu, WHO?. *Indian Journal of Medical Research, 131*(4), 588–589.

Puliyel, J. M., GAVI (Global Alliance for Vaccines and Immunisation), and WHO. (2010). Demanding accountability. *British Medical Journal, 341*(7767), c4081–4266.

Puliyel, J. M., & Mathew, J. L. (2012). Should India launch a national immunisation programme against Rotavirus Vaccine?. *BMJ , 345:*, e7832. Accessed December 3, 2012. http://www.bmj.com/content/345/bmj.e7832.pdfpercent2Bhtml

Ramachandran, R. (2008). Vaccine worries. *Frontline, 25*(7), 4–27.

Reich, M. R. (2000). The global drug gap. *Science, 287*(5460), 1979–1981.

Reich, M. R. (2002). Introduction: Public Private Partnerships for Public Health. In M. R. Reich (Ed.), *Public Private Partnerships for Public Health,*. Harvard Series on Population and International Health. Harvard Centre for Population and Development Studies.

Sarojini, N. B., Sandhya, S., Madhavi, Y., Srinivasan, S., & Anjali, S. (2010). The HPV vaccine: Science, ethics and regulation." *Economic and Political Weekly, 45*(48), 27–34.

Sathyamala, C. (2006). Public Health Foundation of India: Redefining Public Health? *Economic and Political Weekly, 41*(30), 3280–3284.

Sengupta, A., Anjali Shenoy, N.B. Sarojini, and Y. Madhavi. 2011. "Human Papilloma Vaccine Trials in India." *The Lancet, 377*, 719.

Sinha, K. (2012, February 11). Public investment board gives nod to set up vaccine park near Chennai. *The Times of India*. http://timesofindia.indiatimes.com/india/Public-Investment-Board-gives-nod-to-set-up-vaccine-park-near-Chennai/articleshow/11843445.cms?prtpage=1&TOI_browsernotification=true

Smith, R. (2000). Vaccines and medicines for the world's poorest: Public–private partnerships seem to be essential. *British Medical Journal, 320*, 952–953.

Srinivas, S. (2004). *Demand Policy Instruments for R&D: Procurement, Technical Standards and the Case of Indian Vaccines* (BCSIA Discussion Paper 2004–09), December. Kennedy School of Government, Harvard University.

Times News Network (TNN). (2016, October 6). City to Get Vaccine Making Medical Park. *The Times of India*. http://timesofindia.indiatimes.com/city/chennai/City-to-get-vaccine-making-medical-park/articleshow/54706464.cms

United Nations Development Programme (UNDP). (1998). *The Global Sustainable Development Facility* (Internal Document).UNDP.

Vesikari, T., Ohrling, A., Baer, M., Delem, A., Bogaerts, H., & Andre, F. E. (1991). Evaluation of Live Attenuated Varicella Vaccine (Oka-RIT Strain) and Combined Varicella and MMR Vaccination in 13–17 month-old Children. *Acta Paediatrica Scandinavica, 80*(11), 1051–1057.

White, J., Stinson, D., Staehle, B., Cho, I., Matthews, H., Ngai, A., Keller, P., Eiden, J., Kuter, B., The MMRV Vaccine Study Group. (1997, May). Measles, Mumps, Rubella, and Varicella Combination Vaccine: Safety and immunogenecity alone and in combination with other vaccines given to children. *Clinical Infectious Diseases, 24*(5), 925–931.

Wilson, P., & Jones, A. (2010, April). Giving developing countries the best shot. An Overview of Vaccine Access and R&D." *Oxfam–MSF Report*. Geneva, Switzerland.

World Bank. (1998, May 20). *Partnerships for development: Proposed actions for the World Bank* (Discussion Paper, Partnership Group). World Bank. Accessed March 7, 2018. http://documents.worldbank.org/curated/en/789141468153858137/pdf/516050WP0Dev0i10Box342046B01PUBLIC1.pdf

World Health Organisation (WHO). (1999, June 24). *WHO guidelines on collaboration and partnerships with commercial enterprises* (draft discussion document). World Health Organisation.

World Health Organisation (WHO). (2012, June). *Information sheet observed rate of vaccine reactions Varicella zoster Virus Vaccine*. June 2012. (Global Vaccine Safety, Immunisation, Vaccines and Biologicals). WHO. 1–4. Accessed May 2, 2013. http://www.who.int/vaccine_safety/initiative/tools/Varicella_Zoster_Vaccine_rates_information_sheet.pdf

WHO. (2005, January 28). Pertussis Vaccines, WHO Position Paper. *Weekly Epidemiological Record, 80*(4), 31–39. http://www.who.int/immunisation/topics/wer8004pertussis_Jan_2005.pdf

Chapter 16
Drugs and Vaccines in Healthcare: Problems and Possibilities

Pushpa M. Bhargava

Drugs

The problems with regard to the use of allopathic drugs in India range from quality and regulation to irrational use because of the nexus between pharmaceutical companies and the largely commercial healthcare establishments. Fake or sub-standard allopathic drugs may represent as much as 25% of our drugs (IMPACT, 2006)[1] though there are no reliable estimates.

When a few years ago, members of the staff of the Sambhavna Trust set up in Bhopal to take care of the Bhopal gas tragedy victims, raided the dispensaries of government hospitals whose primary objective was to take care of the gas tragedy victims, and sent randomly selected drugs for analysis, it was found that most of them were fake or sub-standard (Anonymous, 2006). This was reported extensively but no action was taken against the manufacturers, many of them located in Indore. Then there is also the question of expired drugs being sold to unsuspecting and ignorant customers. The tragedy is that even when it is established that the drugs are fake or sub-standard, or drugs that were sold had crossed the expiry date, no action is generally taken against the culprit.

Till recently, the drug costs in India were the lowest in the world. This was largely because, till 2005, we had no product patent and our outstanding chemists devised better and cheaper processes than the patented ones for making the drug (Greene, 2007). Now that we permit product patent under pressure from the US and major multinational drug producers in the West, the situation has changed dramatically to the detriment of the interests of a vast proportion of our countrymen, unless we have the courage to make use of certain enabling provisions of the Trade Related Aspects of Intellectual Property (TRIPS) agreement, such as its Articles 7, 8, 28.2,[2] and the one concerning compulsory licensing.[3]

P. M. Bhargava (✉)
Centre for Cellular and Molecular Biology, Hyderabad, India

I. Qadeer et al. (eds.), *Universalising Healthcare in India*,
https://doi.org/10.1007/978-981-16-5872-3_16

Fortunately, the 2005 Act amending our patent rules does not allow patenting of minor chemical modifications or analogues of existing patented drugs. It also does not allow the patenting of microorganisms and other living entities, including genes. Recently our courts disallowed the application of Novartis (a major foreign drug producer) for a patent on account of the above provision in the amendment of 2005 to the Indian Patents Act. In my opinion, there was really no legal case at all in favour of Novartis.

There is an unfortunate but very widely prevalent and effective nexus between drug companies, on the one hand, and commercial healthcare establishments and doctors (with a few but notable exceptions) on the other. This nexus involves not only direct payments by drug companies to doctors but also indirect support to them through expensive gifts or financing of travel to meetings in India or abroad (Matharu 2012; Sinha, 2012). This leads to a vast proportion of our doctors, particularly those who work in corporate hospitals and other commercial healthcare establishments, to prescribe expensive and/or branded drugs when cheaper generic drugs would have been just as good from the point of view of the patient. In fact, many medical shops attached to commercial healthcare establishments do not keep generic drugs. Then, there is often no bulk purchase by government hospitals which would ensure reduction in cost.

Our doctors are generally far too busy making money. After all, in most cases, they have paid INR one crore or more for getting into a medical college and they have to recover that. Further, more often than not, they do not ask the patient if he/she is taking any other drug so that they can ensure that there is no interaction between a drug that the patient is already taking and the newly prescribed drug. In fact, most doctors are unaware of drug-drug interaction which is not emphasised in the course leading to a medical degree. I personally had an unfortunate experience of having been prescribed Diacerin for an orthopaedic problem a few years ago. It was supposed to be a miracle drug but I had a severe reaction to it which may have taken my life. Being a scientist who has dealt with medical literature for six decades, I decided to look at what was known about Diacerin. The literature clearly said that it must not be taken by patients who were using any other drug that would modify any function of the gastrointestinal tract. I was taking three such drugs: Ganaton, Naturolax and Duphalac!

Often the instructions given to the patients by the doctors with regard to the use of the prescribed drug are insufficient or not clear to the patient, with the result that compliance is poor. One result of poor compliance has been the development of antibiotics resistance which, as it turns out, is now very common in the country. We thus have a fair number of cases of infection by Methicillin-Resistant Staphylococcus Aureus (MRSA), a strain of Staphylococcus aureus that is resistant to all antibiotics except Vancomycin, which can be used only under careful medical care. In fact, we now have emergence of MRSA which is resistant also to Vancomycin (Weinstein, 1998); if you are infected with this organism, the chances that you will survive are extremely slim. In the USA antibiotic-resistant infections and hospital infections are reported to be a major public health problem (Berens, 2002; Weiner et al., 2016).[4,5]

Given the realities, it is not only important to have the right drug but also to make sure that it has been stored properly at the prescribed temperature. Some drugs require storage at, say, 4 °C which is generally the temperature in a refrigerator. In many places, there are long power cuts when the temperature of the refrigerator in a drug store would go up substantially. Few drug stores in the country, if any, have a back-up generator. Not only that a large number of medical shops in the country function as general merchants and have no trained pharmacists as required by law. There is no system to review medical stores in the country.

The government hospitals are supposed to provide free drugs to patients. However, often there is no stock of the required drug, or the quality of the drug supplied is poor. This is a consequence of the public sector healthcare becoming poorer everyday in every respect.

Often, the major drug companies advertise that a particular drug which has been approved for a particular use is also useful for other ailments without the drug having been properly tested for such ailments. There is, thus, misleading marketing of drugs, and bribing of doctors to prescribe such drugs for conditions for which they have not been approved. This, in medical terminology, is called 'off–label use'. (An example in our country has been that of Latrazole.) Such unfair practices led to a fine of US $13 billion imposed on leading American pharma companies (Varma, 2012). However, the fact is that such a fine would not make much difference to the pharma company. Thus, Pfizer was fined US $2.3 billion in 2009 which was very small compared to its revenue of US $67.4 billion during the same year.

In India the Drug Controller General of India (DCGI) approves drugs for sale here, which have either not been approved in the country of origin or their trials have been inadequate. Even in the case of appropriately approved clinical trials, the manner in which the trials are conducted leaves much to be desired, not only from the legal but also the ethical point of view. For example, the consent forms are not adequate or appropriate, and Serious Adverse Events (SAEs) are not reported.

Very often, prescription of a drug by a doctor depends on the results of a diagnostic test. We have a system of accreditation of diagnostic laboratories under the National Accreditation Board for Laboratories (NABL) which was set up nearly ten years ago at the initiative of an organisation in Hyderabad called the Medically Aware and Responsible Citizens of Hyderabad (MARCH). However, there are less than 200 laboratories accredited under this system, whereas my city (Hyderabad) alone may have a few thousand diagnostic laboratories. We have strong reasons to believe that the results of many of these laboratories are totally unreliable. This can be easily tested by giving the same sample to a number of laboratories at the same time. If the diagnostic tests are not reliable, the diagnosis could be incorrect and the patient could be prescribed a wrong drug.

There is another source of wrong drugs being prescribed. When you go to a clinical (diagnostic) laboratory for the prescribed tests, your values are given on the left while on the right are given the reference ranges for the parameter tested. As it turns out, there is a great deal of evidence that the reference ranges or standards we are using are derived from the West and may not be applicable to Indians. In fact, on account of the huge human biodiversity in India, we may not have just one set of reference standards for all Indians. At the initiative of the MARCH, the Indian Council of Medical Research (ICMR) set up a high-power committee to work out Indian reference standards,[6] but after spending nearly INR one crore on very useful meetings and plenty of ground work, the project was put into cold storage.

It is often said that drug prices are high because the cost of putting a new drug in the market today may be anywhere between US $ 1 and 1.5 billion. Apart from that, the number of new drugs (new chemical entities) appearing in the market is decreasing rapidly as years pass by, so that last year, probably, not more than 15 new drugs were put in the market. The solution is to screen the repertoire of traditional plant-based drug formulations, of which we have over 40,000, using 8000 to 10,000 plants (Bhargava & Chakrabarti, 2003). Even if 4000 of them were found to be valid using the stringent modern system of validation, in the next hundred years, India would become a world leader in healthcare.

The argument that the cost of a new drug is high because of the expenditure on research and development is not valid for India as drug companies spending say, INR 100 on Research and Development (R&D), get a tax rebate of at least INR 150!

If India wants to provide cheaper and reliable drugs to our people, we must not allow foreign companies to take over our companies in the pharma sector. In addition, we should not forget that a substantial part of the vibrancy in our pharma sector has been on account of the now defunct Indian Drugs and Pharmaceuticals Limited (IDPL). The lesson is that we must revive public sector investment in the drug sector.

Vaccines

While India has successfully deployed vaccines to eradicate diseases such as smallpox, there are serious issues with vaccine trials, especially in the context of the absence of a system for independent monitoring of quality and relevance to the population. We have tried vaccines in the country which were irrelevant. For example, the Indian component of the International Aids Vaccine Initiative (IAVI) funded by the Bill and Melinda Gates Foundation did a Phase-I trial of a vaccine even though it had failed in such trials in Europe and Africa. The reasons given for conducting the trial in India were totally unsatisfactory. We try out and use unnecessary and unproven vaccines; on poor unsuspecting patients without proper informed consent. We also do not recognise that any immunisation schedule for children would need to be culture-specific and country-specific.

We succumb to sacrificing our interests to satisfy foreign interests. We thus decided to close our vaccine manufacturing facilities in the public sector instead of improving them so that we can import foreign vaccine (fortunately, this decision was, reversed).

Shantha Biotech had to overcome a plethora of obstacles to manufacture and market its Hepatitis B Vaccine which is genetically engineered and brought its price down 50-fold. In fact, most of the funding for the above vaccine, the first genetically engineered product in India, came from Oman and not from India.

We make a wrong choice of vaccines when better alternatives are available. An example would be our choosing Sabin's Oral Polio Vaccine (OPV) to be given in more than a dozen doses as against the Salk's Injectable Polio Vaccine (IPV), which gives one hundred percent immunity with two injections. This was in spite of the fact that initially we had decided in favour of the Salk vaccine and even set up a company—Indian Vaccine Corporation Limited (IVCOL)—in 1989 in Gurgaon (where the National Brain Research Centre is currently located). This company had an outlay of INR 90 crores with Institut Merieux (one of the world's premier and ethical vaccine manufacturers) putting in INR 50 crores and the Department of Biotechnology (DBT) and Indian Petrochemicals Corporation Limited (IPCL) putting in INR 20 crores each. This company was wound up subsequently, after spending a substantial amount of money. This happened because in spite of the well-documented fact that OPV had problems in developing countries such as India, WHO had decided that the developing countries like India should shift to OPV. The reasons were clear. The developed countries had decided to move to IPV from OPV. Therefore, a market had to be found for the manufacturers of OPV in the Western world. The consequence was that several Secretaries and Joint Secretaries of the Department of Health of the Government of India, Directors of Medical and Health Services of the Government of India, and at least one Director-General of ICMR were given cushy jobs with the WHO (Bhargava, 1999, 2008).

Notes

1. IMPACT 2006 quotes Indian pharmaceutical companies as having suggested that in India's major cities, one in five strips of medicines sold is fake. The industry also estimates that spurious drugs have grown from 10 to 20% of the total market.
2. Article 7, Objectives: The protection and enforcement of intellectual property rights should contribute to the promotion of technological innovation and to the transfer and dissemination of technology, to the mutual advantage of producers and users of technological knowledge and in a manner conducive to social and economic welfare, and to a balance of rights and obligations.
   Article 8, Principles: (1) Members may, in formulating or amending their laws and regulations, adopt measures necessary to protect public health and nutrition, and to promote the public interest in sectors of vital importance to their socio-economic and technological development, provided that such measures are consistent with the provisions of this Agreement. (2) Appropriate measures, provided that they are consistent with the provisions of this Agreement, may be needed to prevent the abuse of intellectual property rights by right holders or the resort to practices which unreasonably restrain trade or adversely affect the international transfer of technology.
   Article 28.2, Rights Conferred: Patent owners shall also have the right to assign, or transfer by succession, the patent and to conclude licensing contracts.
3. Compulsory licensing is when the law of a member government authorises the use of a patented product without the agreement of the right holder under

the following conditions laid out in Article 31 of Trade-Related Aspects of Intellectual Property Rights (TRIPS): (a) authorisation of such use shall be considered on its individual merits; (b) such use may only be permitted if, prior to such use, the proposed user has made efforts to obtain authorisation from the right holder on reasonable commercial terms and conditions and that such efforts have not been successful within a reasonable period of time. This requirement may be waived by a member in the case of a national emergency or other circumstances of extreme urgency or in cases of public non-commercial use. In situations of national emergency or other circumstances of extreme urgency, the right holder shall, nevertheless, be notified as soon as reasonably practicable. In the case of public non-commercial use, where the government or contractor, without making a patent search, knows or has demonstrable grounds to know that a valid patent is or will be used by or for the government, the right holder shall be informed promptly; (c) the scope and duration of such use shall be limited to the purpose for which it was authorized, and in the case of semi-conductor technology shall only be for public non-commercial use or to remedy a practice determined after judicial or administrative process to be anti- competitive; (d) such use shall be non-exclusive; (e) such use shall be non-assignable, except with that part of the enterprise or goodwill which enjoys such use; (f) any such use shall be authorised predominantly for the supply of the domestic market of the Member authorising such use; (g) authorisation for such use shall be liable, subject to adequate protection of the legitimate interests of the persons so authorised, to be terminated if and when the circumstances which led to it cease to exist and are unlikely to recur. The competent authority shall have the authority to review, upon motivated request, the continued existence of these circumstances;(h) the right holder shall be paid adequate remuneration in the circumstances of each case, taking into account the economic value of the authorisation; (i) the legal validity of any decision relating to the authorisation of such use shall be subject to judicial review or other independent review by a distinct higher authority in that Member; (j) any decision relating to the remuneration provided in respect of such use shall be subject to judicial review or other independent review by a distinct higher authority in that Member; (k) Members are not obliged to apply the conditions set forth in subparagraphs (b) and (f) where such use is permitted to remedy a practice determined after judicial or administrative process to be anti-competitive. The need to correct anti- competitive practices may be taken into account in determining the amount of remuneration in such cases. Competent authorities shall have the authority to refuse termination of authorisation if and when the conditions which led to such authorisation are likely to recur; (l) where such use is authorised to permit the exploitation of a patent ('the second patent') which cannot be exploited without infringing another patent ('the first patent'), the following additional conditions shall apply:(i) the invention claimed in the second patent shall involve an important technical advance of considerable economic significance in relation to the invention claimed in the first patent; (ii) the owner of the first patent shall be entitled to a cross-licence on reasonable terms to use the invention claimed in the second patent; and (iii) the use authorised in respect of the first patent shall be non-assignable except with the assignment of the second patent.

4. In the USA the nosocomial infection rate was approximately five to six hospital-acquired infections per 100 admissions; however, because of progressively shorter inpatient stays, the rate of nosocomial infections per 1,000 patient days had actually increased 36%—from 7.2 in 1975 to 9.8 in 1995 (Weinstein, 1998).
5. *The Chicago Tribune* puts the death rate at 103,000 deaths linked to hospital infections in 2000. *The Chicago Tribune* examined hospital records, court records, and federal and state agency data pertaining to 5810 hospitals to reach its estimate (Berens, 2002).
6. Periodically there have been recommendations for establishing an Indian Medical Devices Regulatory Authority for certifying and regulating quality and marketing of medical devices in the country (Government of India, 2005: 10; 2014). In February 2017 the government notified the Medical Devices Rules, which will come into effect from January 2018 (Government of India, 2017).

References

Anonymous. (2006, December 14). Bhopal gas victims get spurious drugs, say activists. *IANS*. Accessed January 20, 2016. http://www.safemedicines.org/2006/12/bhopal-gas-victims-get-spurious-drugs-say-activists.html

Berens, M. J. (2002, July 21). Infection epidemic carves deathly path. *Chicago Tribune*. Accessed February 18, 2017. http://www.chicagotribune.com/news/chi-0207210272jul21-story.html

Bhargava, P. M. (1999, December 12). Fighting the polio virus. *The Hindu* (1999)

Bhargava, P. M. (2008, June 11). The politics of polio. *The Hindu*.

Bhargava, P. M., & Chakrabarti, C. (2003). *The Saga of Indian Science since independence: In a nutshell*. University Press (India) Private Ltd.

Government of India. (2005). *Report of the National Commission on Macroeconomics and Health*. Ministry of Health and Family Welfare.

Government of India. (2014, September 19 and 20). *Report on medical devices and diagnostics innovation parthership workshop*. Indian Council of Medical Research and Ministry of Human Resource Development. Accessed February 18, 2017. http://www.icmr.nic.in/final/Medical%20Technology%20and%20Innovation%20Partnership%20Workshop%20%20Report.pdf

Government of India. (2017). *Health ministry notifies medical device rules*. Press Information Bureau, Ministry of Health and Family Welfare. 2 February. Accessed February 18, 2017. http://pib.nic.in/newsite/PrintRelease.aspx?relid=157955

Greene, W. (2007, May). *The emergence of India's pharmaceutical industry and implications for the US generic drug market*. US International Trade Commission.

International Medical Products Anti-Counterfeiting Taskforce (IMPACT). (2006). *Counterfeit medicines: An update on estimates*. WHO.

Matharu, S. (2012, July 27). 15 doctors went on foreign Jaunt sponsored by Pharma Company, says Lok Sabha Member. *Down to Earth*.

Sinha, K. (2012, October 15). Medical council of India bans 25 doctors posing as fake faculty. *The Times of India*.

Varma, S. (2012, July 16). Unfair practices: Pharma companies fined $13bn in 4 years. *The Times of India*.

Weiner, L. M., Fridkin, S. K., & Aponte-Torres, Z. (2016, March 11). Vital signs: Preventing antibiotic-resistant infections in hospitals—United States, 2014. *Morbidity Mortality Weekly Report, 65*(9), 235–241. Accessed March 7, 2018 http://doi.org/10.15585/mmwr.mm6509e1

Weinstein, R. A. (1998, July–September). Nosocomial infection update. *Emerging Infectious Diseases, 4*(3), 416–420.

Part IV
Missing Links in the Debate

Chapter 17
The Elusive Development: Poverty, Inequality and Vulnerability

K. B. Saxena

Social Development in India has been characterised by marked inequities in the health services. Gaps in access to health services since the colonial period have not been bridged or significantly narrowed despite more than six decades of development and even faster rate of economic growth in the last decade. Rather, there is increasing evidence that inequities have worsened. The Committee on Social Determinants of Health set up by the World Health Organisation (WHO), attributed the persistence of inequities the world over to "unequal distribution of power, income, goods and services, globally and nationally, the consequent unfairness in the immediate visible circumstances of people's lives—their access to healthcare, schools and education, their conditions of work and leisure, their homes, communities, towns or cities and their chances of leading a flourishing life" (WHO, 2008: 1). This is not in any sense a natural phenomenon but the outcome of a 'toxic combination of poor social policies and programmes, unfair economic arrangements, and bad politics' (Ibid.). This chapter will examine whether the Economy and Development Policies in India have eliminated this toxic combination and bridged or significantly reduced these wide ranging inequities.

Two distinct watersheds can be seen in the evolution of the political economy in India. The first was the onset of colonial rule and the second was independence from it. The colonial rule was the most significant watershed in terms of the sharp change of direction and content of economy. The changes it ushered in should be seen with reference to the pre-colonial situation. The pre-colonial economy was, by available accounts, a vibrant subsistence economy characterised by high productivity, a large and expanding commercialised sector catering to a wide range of manufactured goods and marketable crops for the domestic and international market. This had generated a fair degree of integration of agricultural producers and rural manufacturers serviced by a market responsive credit structure (Raychaudhuri, 2005). The population was small with plenty of land for cultivation and the economy provided

K. B. Saxena (✉)
Council for Social Development, New Delhi, India

I. Qadeer et al. (eds.), *Universalising Healthcare in India*,
https://doi.org/10.1007/978-981-16-5872-3_17

sufficient elasticity for absorption of labour. As this economy had stabilised over centuries, no large-scale impoverishment or vulnerability of people was likely to emerge. The miserable position of Dalits, however, who were denied ownership of land and mobility in occupation and were tied to work as labourers on land of higher castes with a wage level barely sufficient for reproduction would have remained unaffected by the economy. Adivasis, in any case, were by and large outside the fold of state formation.

The colonial period registered a marked departure in this situation as its economic policies were geared to protect the British interests and their narrow ambit focused on tax collection and defence. These development policies catered to building of infrastructure—railways, ports, roads to transport raw material from rural areas for shipment to England and opening up the Indian market for British goods. No attention was paid to development of Indian agriculture, growth of industry or creation of social infrastructure. In fact, the colonial state was responsible for decline and even destruction of traditional industry with its large imports. The economy virtually stagnated with growth of aggregate output at less than two percent a year and per capita output at 0.5% a year (Vaidyanathan, 2005). There was stagnation in per capita income despite 0.4% rate of growth of population between 1871 and 1921. The economy remained agriculture-centric with low productivity, supporting 85% of the population, food grain per capita output growth at 1.14% per year and minimal increase in crop yields. The traditional industry employed less than 10% of the labour force. It is not surprising that there was marked food insecurity along with recurrent famines which killed thirty million people (Chandra, 1982). The extremely low level of social development was reflected in 84% illiteracy with 60% of children (6–11 years) out of school, high incidence of communicable diseases, average life expectancy of 32 years, absence of public health facilities and sanitation particularly in the rural areas (Vaidyanathan, 2005). The most negative of its contribution lay in introducing a regressive agrarian structure of intermediaries on peasant proprietors, resulting in sub-infeudation, tenancy and sharecropping, rack renting, high revenue demand and usury, which impoverished the cultivators, pushed them into the clutches of moneylenders for sheer survival and left no resources for investment and improvement in production. "Throughout the colonial period most Indians lived on the verge of starvation" (Chandra, 1982: 13). At the time of independence, per capita availability of cereals and pulses was at 349.9 g a day and of cloth at 10 m a year, the death rate of 27.4% per 1000 persons and infant mortality rate between 175 and 190 per 1000 live births, Malaria affecting one-fourth of the population and the under nourishment affecting one-fourth to 1.3 of the population (Bhatia as quoted in Kumar, 2013: 53).

The maladies of the economy and the plight of the people widely featured in the public discourse of national leaders. The development goals of the state were therefore settled in the preparatory work accomplished during the National Movement itself. The Directive Principles of state policy also laid down the objectives of the socio-economic policy which should be pursued by the state. There was consensus that the state would be the dominant player in the economy and planning would be its instrument of giving direction and content to it. The market was not perceived to harmonise the ends of social justice with need for modernisation and industrialisation (Nayyar, 2006). The very First Five Year Plan declared raising of living standards and provision of full employment at an adequate wage and reduction in inequalities in income and wealth as the goals of development. The attainment of a higher rate of economic growth was conceived as the strategy of realising these objectives.

The attainment of higher growth rate was sought to be realised by rapid industrialisation, particularly of basic and heavy industries. The transformation of social and economic life in rural areas was pursued through a variety of programmes, ranging from the community development programme to elimination of poverty with creation of employment opportunities from the Third Plan onwards and satisfaction of minimum needs from the Fifth Plan. These programmes were introduced as it was realised by the end of the 1950s that growth alone would not be instrumental in realising the development goals of poverty reduction with adequate employment and reduced inequalities. The subsequent plans, by and large, continued the programmes with revisions and refinements.

Multi-prolonged approaches were adopted to reduce poverty. The early period (1950–1960) was marked by emphasis on redistribution of land through a package of land reforms, including abolition of intermediaries, tenancy reforms aimed at giving land to the tiller and imposition of ceilings on large agricultural holdings and distribution of surplus land to the landless. The second phase starting from the late 1960s focused on creation of employment opportunities and distribution of renewable assets supplemented by food subsidies. In the third phase beginning in the mid-1970s, social development through provision of basic services, i.e. education, health, drinking water and shelter acquired primacy in this strategy. This phase also added two programmes for development of environmentally stressed regions (drought-prone and desert) and a programme for flood-prone areas. This phase also witnessed the maximum thrust on designing poverty alleviation programmes of asset distribution, development of skills, wage employment and housing. This was accompanied by nationalization of banks to smoothen the flow of credit to the poor. The fourth phase from the 1990s is characterised by four Rights Based legal entitlements i.e. (a) guaranteeing 100 days of unskilled work in rural areas; (b) giving legal recognition to rights in forest to tribals and other forest dwellers; (c) recently enacted food security legislation; and (d) providing full and compulsory education. This period has also seen introduction of an urban version of Poverty Alleviation Programme (PAP) focused on self-employment, wage employment and housing along with basic minimum services. It also added provision of social security, which included pension for the elderly, widows, disabled and maternity benefits and family benefits in case of the death of the breadwinner, health insurance and a package of services to unorganised workers. The latest additions to this package of affirmative action are programmes for women which provide credit and training for employment in addition to the PAPs which cover them, provision of nutrition to children and midday meals to school children. These programmes are funded from tax collections with their redistributive assumptions.

Economic Growth

Growth has been relied upon as the chief instrument to achieve the three goals of development—raising standards of living, provision of full employment at an adequate wage and reducing inequalities in income and wealth. Poverty alleviation programmes were only supplemental efforts to fill gaps in the trickledown effect of growth. Has this strategy succeeded? This would be examined with reference to the outcome of growth over the last sixty years. These 6 decades can be divided into two broad phases of Indian economy, conforming to the global political economy: (1) from the 1950s to 1980s when the economy was state-controlled (2) from 1990 onwards when it was changed to a market economy. The post-independence economy did witness a structural break with the colonial period, generating higher Gross Domestic Product (GDP) and per-capita income. In the period 1950–1980, GDP grew at 3.5% per annum—3 times the growth in the colonial period. But the income improvement per capita was between one percent and 1.95% which was a slow pace (Sengupta, 1998) and therefore insufficient to make a visible impact on poverty (Nayyar, 2006), which hovered around 50% (Ahluwalia, 1998). Documents of the Planning Commission themselves conceded that poverty and inequality were virtually unchanged over the years (Chandra, 1982). This was due to higher level of population growth and inability to generate sufficient employment to absorb the growing labour force. The decadal growth rate of GDP increased to 5.6% accompanying a sharp increase in per capita income to 3.24% in the 1980s facilitated by reduction in population growth. While it had a relatively favourable impact on reducing poverty, the deceleration in employment in agriculture limited this effect and therefore failed to register significant improvement in the standard of living. The decadal growth rate rose further to 5.8% during 1990–2000 along with per-capita income to 3.65%, and further up to 5.99% (2004–2005) with per capita income to 4.29% (1999–2000 prices) during the same period (Sengupta et al., 2008). The GDP growth during 2005–2006 to 2009–2010 averaged 8.4% per annum (at 2004–2005 prices) with a per-capita income growth which averaged 6.5% (GoI, 2012). The GDP growth rates have progressively declined from 8.6% in 2016 to 5.02% in 2019. But these high growth rates did not lead to transformation in the living conditions of the poor largely due to low rate of employment growth, increasing casualisation of employment, low status of human development and rising inequalities. Growth by virtue of its cumulative effect leads to acceleration in income growth. According to Nayyar (2006) income doubling in 20 years with a growth of 3.5% per annum, in 14 years with a growth rate of 5% per annum, in 10 years with a growth rate 7.0% and in 7 years with a growth of 10% per annum.

But higher growth by itself would not improve living standards unless it is accompanied by growth of secure employment with increase in real wages and social security. This is crucial for breaking the structural roots of income poverty (Dev & Ravi, 2007). The higher growth in output in the later part of the past decade was not achieved with higher level of formal employment and increase in real wages. This happened due to deceleration in employment, 'virtual jobless growth' (Kannan & Raveendran,

2009) resulting from loss of organised employment in the public sector not compensated by its growth in the private sector and capital intensification. The casualisation of labour in the informal and even formal sector and ruthless self-exploitation of self-employed workers were responsible for lack of growth in real wages. Besides, economic growth even with improved income and employment is not sufficient for reduction in poverty and improvement in the living standard unless it also leads to enhancement of human capital as reflected in the Human Development Index (HDI). The latter is a function of social development expenditure the increase of which the higher GDP growth should facilitate. The period of higher growth, however, has not seen much improvement in social sector spending as a percentage of GDP (Joshi, 2006) in the reform period even compared to the 1980s, notwithstanding some increase in overall per capita expenditure (Dev & Mooij, 2004). The status of Human Development of the vast majority of population is low when compared to some of the neighbouring countries like Sri Lanka, China, etc.; not to mention the norms laid down by the United Nations Development Programme (UNDP) (Kannan, 2012). Further, to be equitable in its outcome the growth process must reduce deeply entrenched inequalities which constrain participation of traditionally underprivileged sections of population and lead to denial of equal social opportunities. The growth has been most negative on this score. There is overwhelming evidence of in-equalising nature of growth in the post-reform period which has affected the pace of poverty reduction as well. (National Commission for Enterprises in the Unorganised Sector (NCEUS) 2007; Dubey & Thorat, 2012; Bhaduri, 2008; Dev & Ravi, 2007; Hirway, 2012; Kannan, 2012).

Creation of Employment

The impact of growth on poverty reduction and improving the living standard is realised foremost when adequate regular employment with decent wages is available. Generation of adequate employment has been the Achilles heel of Indian planning. Conceptually, it was viewed as integral to the process of development and not needing special treatment. The Second Five Year Plan estimated a backlog of 5 million unemployed with an addition of 2 million new entrants to the labour force. The economy with an average growth rate of 3.5% registered an employment growth of over 2% per annum in the 1960s and 1970s which, however, was lower than the addition to the labour force of around 2.5% per annum. This resulted in a backlog of unemployment of 11 million by 1977–1978 (Pappola, 2014). In the farm sector too, the Green Revolution technology failed to generate levels of employment matching output. In the circumstances, the process of growth was supplemented by programmes of self-employment and wage employment on public works to meet the deficit. But the higher rate of economic growth per annum during the 1980s and continuation of special employment programmes failed to generate adequate employment to absorb the labour force.

Employment status is measured by the National Sample Survey Organisation (NSSO) in terms of four different statuses, Usual Status, further divided into Usual Principal Status (UPS) and the Usual Principal Subsidiary Status (UPSS). UPSS captures chronic unemployment. UPS provides a picture of open unemployment. Current Weekly Status (CWS) indicates open unemployment in the reference week and Current Daily Status (CDS) represents utilisation of labour force, i.e. person days of employment. CDS is able to estimate unemployment as well as visible under employment. Growth employment (UPSS) has been at the rate of 2.4% per annum during 1972–1973 to 1983, 2.02% during 1983 to 1993–1994, 1.84% during 1993–1994 to 2004–2005 and 0.45% during 2004–2005 to 2012 which shows a declining trend from one decade to another the sharpest being during 2004–2005 to 2011–2012 (Institute of Human Development (IHD), 2014). The rate of employment growth was less than the rate of growth of the labour force. Employment Elasticity has also been consistently declining from 0.52 to 0.41 to 0.29 and finally to 0.04 respectively during the above periods. The notable feature in this trend is the asymmetry between the economy and employment growth, i.e. the declining employment growth with increasing GDP growth highlighting the lowering of employment content in the latter. The agriculture sector which employs the largest workforce witnessed the least employment growth from 1.7% in 1972–1973 to 1983, to 1.35% during 1983 to 1993–1994, to 0.67% in 1993–1994 to 2004–2005 and—1.98 in 2004–2005 to 2011–2012 (Ibid.). This has lowered worker productivity in agriculture and increased disparity with non-agriculture from 1.36% in 1950 to 1.6% at present with an obvious adverse impact on wages and incomes of those employed in agriculture.

Unemployment data does not present a realistic picture as its level is underestimated due to its coexistence with under-employment and disguised employment. Unemployment rates between 1972–1973 and 2011–2012, on UPS basis, fluctuated between 3.6 and 2.7%, between 1.61 and 2.20% in terms of UPSS and between 8.34 and 5.6% as per CDS. The difference between UPS and CDS rates connotes the level of under employment which was much higher at 5% in the first three NSS rounds and is now at 3%. The two taken together present a realistic picture of unemployment, i.e. lack of adequate work with reasonable income. The rates of open and chronic unemployment for rural areas are lower but are higher for urban areas. This data clearly highlights the long term visible unemployment in urban areas and low income self-employment in rural areas, both of which contribute to income poverty.

In the subsequent period, ILO's estimate of unemployment rate for 2013–14 is 3.4%, 4.9% for female and 2.9% for male (ILO, 2016). For subsequent period, as per Labour Bureau (2015–2016) unemployment rate on usual principal status basis was 5.0% for persons 15 years and above who were available for work but could not get it. It was 5.1% for rural areas and 4.9% for urban areas. Female rate of employment was 8.7% while for male it was 4.0% (GOI, 2016). The findings of Periodic Labour Force Survey which substituted National Sample Survey Organisation's Employment and Unemployment surveys of the renamed National Statistical Office based on data from July 2017 to June 2018 shows that unemployment rate in rural and urban areas was highest ever with 6.1% in according to usual status and 8.9% according to weekly status. Unemployment rate in urban areas are higher than those in rural areas

(Jeetendra, 2019). This is corroborated by study of Mehrotra and Parida which finds an unprecedented trend of falling total employment from 2011–2012 to 2017–2018 with massive loss of jobs. The growth process during the period has been 'termed as 'Job loss growth different from Jobless growth earlier (Kannan and Ravindran, 2019). The slowing down of economy from 2017, resulting from demonetization and faulty GST (Goods and Services Act) implementation, resulted in huge loss of employment, leading to reverse migration to villages and closure of small businesses (Manmohan Singh cited in Murthy, 2019). Centre for Monitoring Indian Economy estimated a jobloss of 11 million in 2018 (Nagraj, 2020; Vyas, 2019) and 27 million jobs were lost in age group of 20–30 years in April, 2020 (Sharma, 2020). Even with Government claim of economy picking up, after devastation caused by COVID-19 pandemic, the unemployment rate has risen to 9.2% for rural and 8.9% for urban areas (Chidambaram, 2021).

Unemployment in the educated workforce segments of graduates and technically qualified persons was high at around 8.7% and particularly for females in rural areas. Higher rates of unemployment of women between 5–7% in the long term and 8% on a daily basis and particularly in urban areas reflect the gender dimension. But even this level of unemployment of women is an underestimate as their work is "under reported, under counted and under-valued in National Statistics" (Ibid.: 67). Even where they are employed, it is largely in the informal sector with low income, insecure jobs and lack of social security. There was a steep fall in gender employment during 2005–2012 in rural areas, which has been attributed to other factors such as degree of distress in rural household income and access to education (Himanshu, 2011). These features continued and even aggravated in subsequent period. The latest labour force survey reports to sharp fall of 25 million female workers from the word force (Himanshu, 2019).

The other notable feature of the job market is the persistence of the unorganised sector which employs 83% of workers and when the informal workers in the formal sector are added, the workforce strength goes up to 92%. The employment in this sector is characterised by insecure jobs, low income long hours of work and absence of any social security. Regular wage workers form only 17.9% of total employment but only 6.8% of them are workers with regular jobs. Even though organised sector employment (UPSS) grew from 9.3% in 1999–2000 to 16.4% in 2011–2012, the workers with regular jobs only grew from 5.4 to 6.8% during this period, while the informal workers went up from 8.6% in 1999–2000 to 11% in 2011–2012. The increase in informal jobs persisted from 20.11.12 to 2017–2018 as most jobs are generated by micro and small units of unorganised sector. The number of and share of informal jobs within government/public sector also increased. Contract jobs without written contract increased massively in both government and private sector (Mehrotra & Padhi, 2019). This deterioration in quality of employment is due to sharp decline in public sector employment which reduced from 1.53% per annum in 1983 1994 to 0.057 per annum in 1994–2007. The increase in organised sector employment in private sector did not compensate it as it largely consisted of informal workers. Besides, the unorganised sector consists of a large segment of self-employed. Its widest prevalence is in agriculture where 62% are self-employed and 38% are casual workers. The non-agricultural unorganised sector consists of 72% workers of whom 63% are self- employed. Most of the self-employed rural or urban fare no better than wage workers in both sectors. Their earnings from their labour are also very low. This disconnect between work and income implies that higher worker productivity contributing to GDP growth is not translating into a corresponding increase in wages and incomes in the informal sector and workers there are self-exploiting (Bhaduri, 2008). The employment situation is also characterised by social segmentation (distinct from occupational skills segmentation). This is reflected in engagement of lower caste labour (Scheduled Caste (SC)/Scheduled Tribe (ST)/Muslims), poor households in unskilled manual and shop floor work, while supervisory and managerial jobs are held by people from higher castes (IHD, 2014). Mobility from the former to the latter is blocked not only by differential access to education and skills but also by widespread discrimination in hiring by employers even where the candidates from lower castes have comparable qualifications (Jodhka & Newman, 2007; Thorat & Newman, 2007). The gender dimension of this segmentation leads to lower labour participation rate, narrow sphere of work for women, lower earnings and limited upward mobility. Widely prevalent child labour, estimated at 10 million (Census 2001), reflects the level of poverty and vulnerability of rural households. Its decline to 4 million reported by NSSO (2011–2012) is difficult to reconcile with widely reported incidents of trafficking in children and brutalities practised on them by their employers. Bonded labour is the most distressed form of vulnerable employment with debt bondage as its most widely prevalent characteristic. The practice far from getting reduced with transformation of the economy has increased and mutated into new forms observed in brick kilns, stone quarries, and construction sector. Migrant labour is another segment of vulnerable labour (largely comprising marginalized communities) with most exploitative conditions of work, poor living conditions, low earnings, and even lack of access of basic services. Its percentage increased from 9.69 in 1982–1983 to 26.91 in 2009–2010 (Rodgers & Rodgers, 2011). The laws to abolish the bonded labour system, and regulate child and migrant labour virtually remain unenforced.

Have special employment programmes with public resources made any difference to the situation? One study carried out in the early 1990s brought out that hardly 1–4 weeks of employment in a year was provided and that too was unevenly distributed. The income earned by the beneficiaries was negligible. Payment was delayed by 2–3 weeks. (Tiwari, 1991). Inadequate allocation and huge implementation problems severely limited its potential. Besides, the programmes failed to raise elasticity of employment in agriculture through appropriate asset building (Rao, 2005). The position is not significantly better in the case of the Mahatma Gandhi National Rural Employment Guarantee Scheme (MNREGS). As against a guaranteed employment of a hundred days, on an average, 46 days of work has been provided. It has failed to stem distress migration and debt bondage. Timely payment has proved to be a much greater bottleneck due to channelling of payment through banks/post offices and insistence on Aadhar and Biometric authentication of worker's identity for participation in work besides inadequate allocations leading to huge unmet demand and rationing of employment. Recent changes in the Act and Policy guidelines have privileged infrastructural creation over provision of work to reduce corruption. The resulting delay in wage payment discourages workers from registering their demand or reporting for work and forces them to migrate in search of work.

This outline of the employment situation is hardly conducive to poverty reduction and improvement in the living standard of a large segment of population.

Wages

Not merely employment, the level of wage at which employment is available is crucial for reducing poverty and improving the living standard. The overall wage situation in India, however, is difficult to assess because of its specific characteristics. Only about half of the workforce constitutes wage workers about whom some data is available. The rest of the workforce is self-employed about whom there is no authentic data relating to income. Besides, wide variation in the structure of wages and income of wage workers across location, sector and size of the organisation on the demand side and skill level, social group, and gender on the supply side and differentiation in the self- employed by occupation and income also present difficulties in appraisal (IHD, 2014). Further, the task of evaluating the impact of economy on wage growth is extremely complex, given the diverse sources of data, concepts, definition, periodicity of availability, methodologies and survey design making comparability difficult (Himanshu, 2005). For example, the India Labour and Employment Report based on NSS data, concludes that there was overall average growth rate in wages of 3% per annum for regular and 3.2% for casual workers between 1983–2010. The growth rate was higher in respect of rural areas as compared to urban areas for both categories of workers. A similar trend was observed for agricultural wages, with a higher rise for casual workers (IHD, 2014). This is broadly confirmed by another study covering the period 1964–65 to 1999–2000 but only for male agricultural workers and less so in respect of female workers. The study, however, notes that there was a distinct slowdown in wage growth in the 1990s (Chavan & Bedamatta, 2006). But a study based on data from RLE (Rural Labour Enquiry) reports for 1983–2000 and from NSS for 2004–20 05 points to a sharply declining trend in growth rate of wages in agricultural operations from 60% during 1983 to 1987–1988, to 28% during 1987–1988 to 1993–1994 and further to 16% during 1993–1994 to 1999–2000 and a still lower 8% during 1998–1999 to 2004–2005 for male workers with a similar trend for female and child labour. This deceleration coincides with the agrarian crisis (Jha, 2006). This slowdown is also indicated in data presented in (Himanshu, 2005). NCEUS too has observed deceleration of already low rates of wages of agricultural (casual) labour during 1993–1994 to 2004–2005 from 2.9% per annum in 1993–1994 to 1.3% in 1999–2000 rising to 2.2% in 2004–2005 with average earning as low as 43 rupees per man day in 2004–2005 (NCEUS, 2007). The declining rates of growth in wages was also observed in rural non-agricultural work from 60% in 1980–1987 to 50% in 1993–1994 further to 22.9% in 1999–2000 and 14% in 2004–2005 (Jha, 2006). However, NCEUS confirms this decline in growth rates of wages outside agriculture during 1993–1994 to 2004–2005 in respect of regular workers only but not casual workers (NCEUS, 2007).

For the subsequent period, trends in real rural wages reported by labour bureau show a sharp slowdown since 2011–2012. Between December 2014 and December 2018, a growth of mere 0.5% of per year after adjusting inflation of 4.2% was witnessed in the real average wages of agriculture and rural workers compared to 6.7% a year in proceeding five years (Damodaran, 2019) indicating a near stagnation. Rising unemployment rate and decline in labour force participation accounts for this adverse wage growth in rural economy (Nagraj, 2020). Mehrotra and Parida study also concludes that real wages have not increased between 2011–2012 and 2017–2018 which in neither rural nor urban areas (Mehrotra & Parida, 2019). The 'virtual collapse' of wage growth resulting from slowing down of economy impacted by policy induced shocks during the period of 2011–2012 to 2017–2018 which even turned negative for many employment segments is attested by another study which also finds the collapse more dramatic among regular workers and in urban areas and in the higher decile of wage earners and not confined to informal sector or urban/rural poor (Srivastava & Padhi, 2020). This is corroborated by evidence on fall in per capita consumption, declining labour force participation, higher unemployment rate and a rise in absolute Poverty. After Covod-19 lockdown, the situation on wage growth would have only worsened.

Apart from declining growth in real wages in the reform period, the wage situation is also characterised by a high degree of disparities. Rural–urban disparity in wages has been a persistent feature. The wage of a casual worker in rural areas was 35% lower compared to urban areas and this disparity has only reduced to 20%. The gap in wages between the agriculture and non-agricultural segment has widened. The wage of a non-agricultural worker was more than twice the wage of an agricultural regular worker and 1.3 times that of a casual worker. The inequality in wages between casual and regular workers as well as across sectors increased during the reform period. The Gini co-efficient for aggregate wage inequality increased from 0.483 in 1983 to 0.510 in 2011–12 (IHD, 2014). Gender disparity is another dimension of the wage situation. This has featured in agriculture since the Green Revolution (Jose, 1988) and has increased over the years (Chavan & Bedamatta, 2006). This was both in respect of average wage as well as level of growth of real wages. The ratio of female wage to male wage has persisted at around 0.69. Overall, women workers get 20–50% lower wages than what men earn across most employment categories and locations (IHD, 2014). There are significant differences in wages for men too in different agricultural operations (Bhalla, 2007). The other dimension of wage disparity is regional inequality. There is considerable variation in wages across states. Daily wage of a casual worker in rural areas ranged from INR 87 in Chhattisgarh to INR 309 in Kerala in 2011–2012. In urban areas, it was INR 112 and INR 315 in the two states respectively. The most glaring disparity in wages relates to status of employment. There are huge wage differentials between workers in the organised and unorganised sectors, besides other aspects of the employment which characterise the disparity. Within the organised sector too, there is a huge difference in wages of a regular (permanent) worker and casual worker. The wage of a casual worker is only one-third of a regular worker (Bhalotra, 2002), while Das (2007) finds it even less than this. Wage inequality also exists among formal workers and is higher than in the casual workers. High income inequality is observed among women workers compared to male workers. Overall wage disparities increased in the post-liberalisation phase particularly between salaries of government employees and wages of regular and casual workers (Ibid.). A rural casual worker in 2011–2012 earned barely 7% of the wages a central public sector employee earned (IHD, 2014). The increase in wages in general over time is far less in the case of the poorest segment, rural casual workers when compared to public sector employees and managerial staff of the private sector. Casualisation of employment has contributed to this inequality. More disturbing is the wage differential across social groups for every type of work. It is particularly so for STs in rural areas who receive wages lower than even SCs and OBCs (Bhalla, 2007).

The most distressing aspect of the wage situation is that there are no minimum standards in fixation of daily wages in states and this has a negative impact on the earnings of casual workers. NCEUS has found the situation 'alarming'. The deplorable part is that even the low minimum wages fixed by states are not implemented. This situation prevails even where the central government has fixed minimum wages. Based on data from NSS (2004–2005), NCEUS found a significant proportion of workers to be not receiving minimum wages—85% of all casual workers in rural areas and 57% in urban areas (NCEUS 2007). As per NSS (2009–2010), 73% of rural farm workers and 37% of rural non-farm workers and 54% of urban non-farm workers received wages lower than the minimum fixed. In the case of women, it was 87%, 65% and 82% respectively (IHD, 2014). But 68% of workers in agriculture and 63% in the non- agriculture sector are self-employed. The income they earn from their enterprise is very low due to low capital, poor asset base, constraints of market and layers of exploitation by intermediaries. They fare no better than wage workers.

Considering that 92% of the workforce is in the unorganised sector and there is lack of adequate and decent employment, the level of income poverty and vulnerability even with high growth rates of the economy would require no further elucidation.

Conditions of Work

It is not merely the status of employment and level of wages but also conditions of work which contribute to poverty and low standard of living and vulnerability. The poor in the country (77% of populations as per NCEUS classification) share common characteristics—informal work status, low wages and oppressive working conditions and absence of social security. The latter position is briefly outlined here based on information sourced from NCEUS (2007) report.

Of the 256 million unorganised workers in the agricultural sector, 64% are farmers and 36% are wage workers. The latter constitute the largest segments of workers in the country. Their conditions are characterised by: (a) low income, (b) variation in availability of work, (c) long hours of back breaking schedule, (d) severe health risks with high fatality rates, (e) multifaceted exploitation, (f) high incidence of child and migrant labour, (g) low level of literacy and (h) lack of organisation. There is no social security or laws to protect them. The socio-economic position of non-agricultural workers who constitute around 38% of 167 million unorganised workers is characterized by (a) low level of schooling and lack of skills constraining mobility, (b) hazardous working conditions with serious risks to health in case of workers in diamond cutting, leather, metalwork, beedi rolling, underground mines, ship breaking, etc., (c) lack of even elementary facilities at work site, (d) sub-human living environment, (e) failure to implement labour laws (wherever existing) regarding wages, working conditions, etc. The vulnerability arising from low wage/remuneration and sexual exploitation of women workers is widespread in all categories of wage workers (NCEUS, 2007).

Self-employed workers dominate the Indian economy. Two-thirds of agricultural workers are farmers who are the largest segment of self-employed in the country. The crisis in the agrarian sector reflects their precarious survival (Jha, 2006). This crisis is characterised by (a) declining size of land per household, skewed distribution of land, increasing landlessness and marginalisation of land holdings, (b) low level or lack or education, and (c) average monthly income of a small and marginal farmer being lower than the average monthly expenditure leading to indebtedness. Their problems are compounded by virtual stagnation of output, non-viability of farming, high input cost and low returns and lack of access to bank credit. The condition of tenants is worse due to high rents, oral contracts and having to bear the entire risk of crop failure.

The self-employed workers in the non-agricultural sector consist of (a) own account workers (46%), (b) unpaid family workers 14.7%, (c) those hiring less than 10 workers, (9%). Most of them are own account workers who have low value assets, low scale operations and low remuneration. They suffer from lack of access to institutional credit and problems of marketing. Most of them are stagnating. Each category of self-employed worker suffers from problems unique to this section, which defines vulnerability. Handloom workers, the largest segment among them, suffer from very low income, decline in demand and constraints of raw material supply, deferred payments, indebtedness and outdated technology. Street vendors, another big segment in this category, face legal problems in their operation emerging from lack of a valid permit, eviction, confiscation of goods and lack of access to working capital. Rickshaw pullers, a large and significant group, face harassment from municipal staff and traffic police, have no shelter, pay high rent to owners and end up with disabling diseases. In the category of homemade workers, bidi rolling is the largest segment. The fragility of their survival is reflected in irregular work, low wages, rejection of products, wage deduction, irregular payment and non-implementation of minimum wages. They suffer from indebtedness and high health risks.

Poverty

Poverty is estimated on the basis of consumption expenditure required to obtain a calorie norm of 2400 cal per capita per day in rural and 2100 cal per capita per day in urban areas, with 1973–1974 as the base year. Poverty line is the money equivalent of this norm which is updated every five years using the latest data of consumption expenditure, adjusting it to consumer price index and price variation. Due to contestation about the methodology of estimation, it was modified in 1993 and used thereafter until recently. Based on the prevailing norm, poverty ratio was estimated at 54.93% in 1973 which declined to 51.32 in 1977–1978, further to 44.48 in 1983–1984, 38.86 in 1987–1988 and 35.97 in 1993–1994 and 27.5% in 2004–2005 (Government of India(GoI), 2012; Sankaran, 2008). In 2009, owing to widespread criticism about low estimates of poverty, the Expert Group to Review the Methodology for Estimation of Poverty—the Tendulkar Committee—looked into it and poverty ratios were revised on its recommendation to 45.3% in 1993–1994 and its reduction to 37.2% in 2004–2005 and 29.8% in 2009–2010 (GoI, 2009). Alternative estimates of poverty have been made by various agencies and individuals which are higher. Since 2010, UN sponsored Multi- dimensional Poverty Index has been developed according to which Poverty ratio is higher and India ranks 62 among 107 countries (PIB, 2020). Official estimates have been critiqued on various grounds. The most detailed one is by NCEUS using a different methodology and data source which conceptualises poverty as a graded phenomenon consisting of four categories 'Extremely Poor', 'Marginally Poor' and 'Poor' and 'Vulnerable'. The first three with consumption expenditure below US$1.25 per day per capita, the international norm for 'Extreme Poverty', constituted 41% of the population and along with 'Vulnerable' whose consumption expenditure is below US$ 2 constituted 77% of the population. A different approach was adopted for identifying the poor for effectively targeting Poverty alleviation programmes by carrying out a census of the poor in 2002, 2007, 2009 (Nayyar & Nayyar, 2016). This was replaced by a socio-economic and caste census in 2011. Currently, the results of this census are being used to reach the benefits of programmes to the deserving poor. But these estimates whether official or non-official are embedded in the conception of poverty as inadequacy of income. But poverty is also caused by other factors, the most significant of which is the historically entrenched inequalities based on social exclusion and discrimination. These inequalities affect the SCs, STs, Muslims and women and result in higher incidence of poverty and its slower reduction in them when compared to the rest of the population. This discrimination is driven by caste in the case of SCs, ethnicity in the case of STs, religion in the case of Muslims and patriarchy in the case of women and has not changed much over the years. Environmental degradation is another factor affecting poverty which imposes an additional disability on the poor and accentuates their vulnerability. This environmental stress is natural or manmade. In the former category are included drought- prone areas, desert and flood-prone areas while in the latter are areas degraded by water logging, industrial development, mining, etc. These factors affect productivity of land, cause loss of livelihood besides contributing to lower quality of life. The third factor of poverty lies in low Human Capital formation reflected in HDI—level of schooling and skills, access to health services, drinking water, sanitation and housing all of which contribute to poverty in addition to lack of employment and inadequate wages. State Interventions by way of programmes and schemes have been made to counteract these factors, but do not seem to have produced the desired results.

The officially claimed poverty reduction during the last two decades is highly contested. It has been argued that poverty reduction in the decade since 1993–1994 was lower than the 1980s despite higher rates of growth (Datt et al., 2003). The disjunction between growth, poverty and well-being has also been observed. Attention has been drawn to its urban tilt and un-equalising nature, which has held back poverty reduction, itself implying that the poor have been bypassed. The impact of growth during this period in terms of widening the nutritional gap resulting in shift in spending from food to non-food items (Sen & Himanshu, 2005), impoverishment of specific regions and social and economic groups, skewed access to health and education, decline in female-male ratio has also been brought out (Deaton & Dreze, 2002). In 2013 the Planning Commission (PC) announced further reduction of poverty ratio in 2011–2012 to 13.7% in urban areas and 25.7% in rural areas and a total reduction of 21.9%, with highest percentage of reduction in respect of SCs/STs and upper section of Muslims (GoI, 2013). This claim has been critiqued as grossly unrealistic in the context of current daily food and non-food costs which forces nearly 3/4th of the population to cut back on food, leading to reduced nutrition. Government is also accused of showing reduction in poverty by lowering the calorie norm by which it is measured and rationalising it as dietary diversification which is not valid in the case of the poor (Patnaik, 2007, 2013). The concentration of poverty has in fact increased in Jharkhand, Bihar, Odisha, Chhattisgarh, Madhya Pradesh (MP) and Uttar Pradesh (UP). where the share of the rural poor has risen from 50% in 1993–1994 to 65% in 2011–2012 while the annual rate of decline is the lowest, less than 1% in UP and Bihar (IDFC, 2013: 61). Even others, while conceding the higher rate of poverty reduction during 2004–2005 to 2009–2010, bring out its skewed distribution in terms of low rate of decline in respect of SCs, STs than others and wage labour households than self-employed (Thorat, 2014), unevenness across different social groups and states and urban tilt. Besides, this poverty reduction has been attributed to poverty alleviation programmes such as MNREGS and Public Distribution system in some states than to the growth process (Kannan, 2012). Social inequality continues to be entrenched in poverty and vulnerability and is also manifested in regional differentiation (Kannan & Raveendran, 2011).

As the controversy about the norm and estimate of Poverty did not subside, Government constituted another expert group headed by Prof. Rangarajan to review it which raised Poverty ratio in 2011 from Tendulkar based Poverty estimate of 21.9–29.5%. This was not officially accepted and vice-chairman, Niti Ayog was asked to look into it (Nayyar & Nayyar, 2016). There has been no estimate of poverty and inequality after 2011–2012. The report of the latest consumption survey 2017–2018 on the basis of which poverty is estimated was not officially released as it is reported to show a decline in per capita consumption expenditure in rural areas and a marginal increase in urban areas implying an overall increase in poverty. This correlates with other indicators such as unemployment and wages and income (Himanshu, 2020). This survey result accounts for rise in rural poverty by four percentage points between 2011–2012 and 2017–2018 and a decline in urban poverty by 5% points and on increase in overall poverty by nearly a percentage point to 23% in 2017–2018 (Bhattacharya & Devulapalli, 2019). COVID-19 could push nearly 400 million informal workers deeper into poverty (Singh, 2020).

Claims have also been made of improvement of 21% in the Human Development Index in the last decade, particularly in education and health, and convergence of SCs/STs/Muslims with an all India average on health, education and income indicators with the exception of nutrition and sanitation as also reduction in inter-state variation (Mehrotra & Gandhi, 2012). This claim is strongly contested (Chakraborty, 2011; Oommen, 2012). Education is characterised by increased inputs and school enrolment but poor learning outcomes, teacher absenteeism and severe lack of accountability. The health sector suffers from low spending, high child and maternal mortality rates in rural areas and alarming malnourishment, and low healthcare access. The disillusioned poor are turning to the private sector for these services which are unaffordable and land them in debt? As per the fifth National Family Health Survey, 2019–2020 between 2015 and 2019, many Indian States have suffered a reversal on several child malnutrition parameters. The impact of COVID-19 would have further worsened the position (Misra & Iqbal, 2020). As for social protection programmes, though National Food Security Act covers 75% of the households in rural areas and 50% in urban areas and nutritional programmes have been brought within its fold, PDS still suffers from exclusion, particularly caused by insistence on matching of Aadhar and bio-metric identification of ration card holders. Overall, the law has not registered the desired impact in eliminating hunger considering that India ranks 94 out of 107 countries in Global Hunger Index, 2020, behind Nepal, Pakistan, and Bangladesh (Global Hunger Report, 2020). The pension for elderly, widows and disabled has inadequate coverage, meagre assistance and disrupted payment. Mis-targetting, weak delivery and corruption are a common governance failure (Indian Development Finance Corporation (IDFC), 2013). Notwithstanding improvements registered by India in its HDI value, it ranks 129 out of 189 countries in UN Human Development Index. On the environmental dimension of poverty, the programmes to arrest degradation have failed to yield the desired results. The watershed development programme to address land degradation suffered from neglected livelihoods, lack of clear development goals, low community participation and poor post- maintenance. Organic farming to correct inappropriate input has negligible coverage (less than 1%). The wasteland development programme was iniquitous and unviable. Forest conservation programmes have ignored the interests of local communities, promoted commercial plantation and have failed to replace degraded forests. The enforcement of the Forest Rights Act has been subverted by rejection of many claims and ignoring community forest management. Water conservation efforts have not prevented the declining share of tanks and their state of disrepair and disuse. There is no effort to reverse discharge of mining and industrial waste into the rivers (IDFC, 2013). Environmental governance is weak as growth takes precedence over environment

(Srivastava & Kothari, 2012) and sustainability and employment generation fail to get integrated into it (Shah, 2012).

Thus, notwithstanding the official claims, neither in terms of employment and wages nor in terms of social, human capital and environment dimensions of poverty, do we get a social reality which lends credence to the scale of reduction in poverty. With continued higher inflation (particularly in food items) which matters the most to the poor (Himanshu, 2007) and slackening of growth, the situation got worse rather than better. It deteriorated further as a result of demonetization and ill prepared GST, COVID-19 and lockdown to prevent its spread has devastated the Poor with reverse migration, loss of employment increase in poverty, widening inequality and exposed them to greater vulnerability.

Inequality

The concern for reduction in inequality was reflected in distributive programmes and regulatory measures in the state policy during the four decades of the welfare political economy. The distributive dimension consisted of land reforms, public funded social services, reservation and enhanced financial allocation for SC/ST welfare, provision of subsidised credit and inputs to small and marginal farmers and small-scale enterprises, and a wide variety of poverty alleviation programmes. The regulatory measures included abolition of privy purses; restricted role of the private sector in economic activities; nationalisation of banks, insurance, some segments of trade and coal; and primacy given to the public sector in the economy. But, there was no attempt to reduce concentration of wealth and income of the rich (Vaidyanathan, 2005; Sengupta, 1998). These interventions failed to make a dent on the existing inequality. Land Reforms were poorly implemented. Subsidised benefits were cornered by more affluent sections among the poor. Low returns on public investment eroded the public sector's contribution to check private sector growth and expansion. Agrarian inequality could not be checked in the absence of tax on agricultural incomes. The 1980s witnessed an increase in overall income inequality, despite higher rate of growth and improvement in employment generation and real wages, due to declining capacity of agriculture to absorb labour force (Pal & Ghosh, 2007). With the onset of the market economy, the 1990s witnessed a significant increase in inequalities in consumption levels between the rich and the poor, urban and rural areas, social groups across states and regions within them (Deaton & Dreze, 2002; Pal & Ghosh, 2007). The features of this unequal growth include a lower level of employment generation with an adverse impact on incomes of agricultural labourers, increase in casualisation of workforce, higher labour productivity not leading to increase in salaries and remuneration, in respect of labour market. The agrarian features of the growth consist of declining viability of agriculture, concentration of operational holdings, increasing landlessness and worsening of outcomes in human development- health, education. The social development witnessed nutrition, declining per capita food consumption, and differentials in performance of states not related to poverty levels. The entrenched social inequalities seem to be consolidating rather than breaking. These features of inequalities are associated with levels of consumption, wage earning, distribution of wealth, pace of development across states and marginalised social groups, etc. (Pal & Ghosh, 2007).

The inequality in consumption is its most significant dimension the evidence of which has been brought out in the NCEUS report. In terms of its sixfold classification of populations, while 'Middle' and 'High' Income groups registered nearly 5% growth in monthly consumption expenditure between 1993–1994 and 2004–2005, the average growth rate of the 'Extremely Poor' 'Poor' and 'Vulnerable' was less than one percent. The former category of groups accounted for a disproportionately large share of total consumption expenditure. SCs and STs had the lowest Monthly Per Capita Expenditure (MPCE). The consumption deficit of the poorer sections among the lower expenditure groups was further aggravated by the larger number of dependents. The two higher income groups had an average MPCE of INR 1,388, while in the case of SCs/STs it was merely INR 303, and in the case of other poorer categories INR 321, less than one-fourth of the former (Sengupta et al., 2008). The gap in consumption share of top two and bottom two deciles is glaring. COVID-19 could enlarge this gap due to sudden shutdown of economy and rise in health expenditure (Nag & Geest, 2020).

This period of economic reforms has also witnessed a sharp increase in inequality in wage income; sharpest being between rural and urban settlements, casual and regular employment status and better off sections and vulnerable sections (Sarkar & Mehta, 2010). A study based on income tax returns has revealed that the income of the richest 0.01% segment of population was 150–200 times larger than the poorest bracket (Bannerjee & Piketty, 2005; NCEUS, 2007). Gini co- efficient of income inequalities increased from 0.44 to 0.47 in the post- reforms period (Hirway, 2012). The level of wealth also shows similar intensity of inequality with the top 10% of population having more than half of the total wealth (assets or net worth) of the country, while the bottom 10% have a mere 0.4% share (Jayadev et al., 2007). The wealth of Indian billionaires increased by 35% during lock down post COVID pandemic-2019 and by 90% since 2009 (Misra, 2021).

This skewed distribution of asset growth also characterises the higher income and lower income states pointing to the reinforcement of the structural inequalities of Indian society and disempowerment of the poor (Ghosh, 2005). Inter-state inequality has also shown a 70% increase during this period along with intra-state inequality both across social groups and between higher and lower income groups (Kannan, 2012) as well as rural and urban areas (Sen & Himanshu, 2005). Inequality between rich and poor are far higher when access to education and health, is taken into account (Dev, 2016). Social inequality far from narrowing is getting further aggravated by the growth process. SCs and STs continue to be at the bottom and Hindu upper castes are at the top of the hierarchical structure. This is manifested in under nutrition, underweight and stunting of the children of the former groups and widening disparities in educational and skill development levels of their youth (Kannan, 2012). Recent reort of Oxfam titled 'inequality virus'has observed that covid-19 pandemic has deely exacerbated existing inequalities in India and around the world. (Misra, 2021) But regulatory measures to reduce these inequalities are not on the agenda of policy and governance. The palliatives in terms of Poverty Alleviation Programmes cannot neutralise them and even as palliatives these programmes suffered from design flaws and poor implementation, which affected their outcomes (Rao, 2005).

Vulnerability

Vulnerability in this context is a condition where a household is ill- protected and is in danger of sliding down the ladder of economic and social status. Landlessness or land poor status, low income, irregular work, hazardous and oppressive working conditions, subhuman living environment, low level of educational attainments, limited access to social goods and social discrimination based on caste, ethnicity, gender and religion, all tend to produce this vulnerability. There is a high degree of congruence between poverty, informal work status, low educational attainments and vulnerability. The vulnerability increases with a sudden shock like serious illness requiring costly treatment, death or disability of the main earner of household, asset loss etc. compelling the household to borrow and fall into a debt trap. These conditions characterise farm and non-farm wage and self-employed workers in varying degree.

As for wage workers in this segment of population, there has been a perpetual deficit of employment and the inability of the economy to absorb the labour force. Even for those who are fortunate enough to get some work, the duration of work does not show consistency and continuity in many cases, indicating intermittent unemployment. Neither slow economic growth of the welfare economy nor the high economic growth of the market economy has eliminated the uncertainty of work which renders the job seekers highly vulnerable to exploitation in terms of level of wages and conditions of work, and exposes them to perpetual poverty, spells of hunger, under nutrition, debt bondage and poor quality of life. Low level of schooling/illiteracy forecloses all options for higher mobility in status of work and enhancement of level of wages. Lack of access to social goods, nutrition and health in particular, lowers their productivity which impinges adversely on their efforts to improve their income. The termination of work in the absence of social security is nothing short of a disaster in these conditions. The targeted interventions fail to reach them and regulatory provisions to counteract these conditions do not get enforced. Lack of organisation increases their manipulation and consequent vulnerability in these circumstances. Their vulnerability which had aggravated due to the slowing down of economy, rising unemployment has worsened with pandemic and ensuring lockdown affecting 364 million or more workers and could continue for a long time (ILO, 2020) The self-employed among them are not much better off. Most of them share the characteristics of wage workers—low income and consumption, low level of schooling, indebtedness, health risks, exploitation by intermediaries and lack of social security an economic status below the poverty line. They face additional constraints—low value of productive assets, uncertainty of demand for goods they produce, supply of raw material, lack of access to credit and marketing, deferred payment, wage deduction, etc. The increasing stagnation in their enterprises reflects their plight. These vulnerabilities seem to have increased in the period of high growth, more particularly resulting from exposure to the global market and flooding of the local market with cheap goods from other countries which have driven some of them to suicide.

Development Policies

Development policies are embedded in the prevailing political economy. Under the state-controlled political economy, development policies were oriented towards welfare of the poor, elimination of poverty, provision of employment and reduction in inequalities in income, wealth and consumption. This was sought to be achieved through regulatory measures and higher public expenditure in favour of the poor through a host of programmes. In the period of market economy since 1990, the economy was liberalised from constraints of state regulation and the welfare of the poor was sought to be achieved primarily though faster economic growth. Major reforms were introduced in the structure of the economy—fiscal policy, financial sector, foreign and domestic Investment. Reforms in Fiscal Policy were effected through reduction of fiscal deficit, and cut in direct and indirect taxes. The former resulted in lowering of central government expenditure as a share of GDP from 7.02% in the late 1980s to 2.74%, leading to reduced public investment in infrastructural development and social services, which negatively impacted on poverty alleviation and employment generation. The tax reforms resulted in reduced transfers to the state government thereby contributing to scaling down of social and rural development programmes. Reduced food subsidy resulted in curtailment of eligibility under PDS and higher cost of food grains under PDS for Above Poverty Line (APL) families, leading to lower off take of food grains from PDS and decline in per capita food availability from 501 g in 1991 to 458 in 2000. Downsizing of government establishment translated into less employment generation in the public sector (Rao, 2005). Closure of loss making public sector undertakings (PSUs) and exposing other PSUs to market competition had the effect of reducing access to certain essential services. Introduction of user charges in certain social utilities affected access of the poor to them. The lower tax revenues from tax reforms reduced government's capacity to undertake public expenditure on infrastructure and social services. The reforms in banking led to drying up of credit to small and marginal farmers and small industries and increasing reliance on non-institutional credit, resulting in increased cost of cultivation, reduced viability of farming and indebtedness. Liberalisation of foreign and domestic investment manifested in skewed investment distribution across states and consequent increase in regional inequalities. It also led to sectoral bias of investment in favour of consumer goods for the rich with lower potential for employment (Pal & Ghosh, 2007), and urban bias in project selection at the cost of rural areas thereby increasing rural–urban disparity. The deregulation of investment and licensing privileged developed regions which have solid infrastructure and disadvantaged backward and poorer states which lacked it, thus reinforcing existing regional inequality. Trade liberalisation exposed farmers to volatility of input and output prices, inflow of cheaper commodities from other countries and thus forcing many of them to commit suicide. A similar effect occurred in respect of small and medium industries whose products are driven out by cheaper imports. The reduced role of the state also implied withdrawal of programmes for skill development, market support and transitional security for retrenched workers (Pal & Ghosh, 2007).

The post-reform period has contributed to poverty, unemployment and inequalities through other policies as well. One of them relates to acquisition of land for development projects leading to massive displacement of farmers from their land, livelihood, habitat, environment and social networks. The pace and ambit of acquisition has increased manifold due to the opening up of areas to foreign direct investment and enactment of the Special Economic Zone (SEZ) Act. As per unofficial estimates, from 1947 to 2000, state-displaced 60 million people, of whom more than 40% were STs and 20% SCs (Fernandes, 2006). This does not take into account acquisition by corporates directly from people through market transactions. The projects implemented on their land do not give them employment nor are they designed and required to do so. The scale and pace of acquisition has continued after 2000. In the absence of rehabilitation, most of these displaced peoples filled the ranks of unemployed and were exposed to the destitute labour market for precarious survival. The situation has not significantly changed after enactment of the new law on land acquisition. The social and ethnic nature of this displacement reinforces and accentuates the structural and social dimension of poverty which is not even partly neutralised by any affirmative programme.

Another facet of this development policy is the huge and increasing environmental degradation which affects the poor and the disadvantaged the most. This environmental degradation has increased manifold in the globalised economy. From 1999 to 2007, there was an annual diversion of 53,000 hectares of forest and the process continues (Srivastava & Kothari, 2012). Infrastructure creation and extraction of minerals have diverted a huge quantum of agricultural land, common land and forest. The latter two are resources on which the poor, particularly the tribals, depend for their survival. Mining has not only destroyed productive potential of agricultural land and forest in the vicinity, deprived people of their livelihoods and lowered quality of their life due to polluted water resources and air, it also uses up millions of tonnes of water for its operations otherwise used for irrigating crops and meeting drinking water needs. The affected poor persons are not compensated by either provision of employment or welfare measures. Between 1991 and 2004, the value of mineral production increased fourfold while employment in the area declined by 30% (Srivastava & Kothari, 2012). The regulatory mechanism, in any case, is weak and ineffective and regulatory agencies ignore glaring violations of legal and ethical norms so as not to hurt growth.

Export orientation of the economy has led to over exploitation of resources of the ecosystem and rapid resource exhaustion. This has disrupted livelihoods of fisherfolk, damaged farmlands and salt pans in coastal areas resulting from salinity ingress. Shrimp farming has led to virtual extinction of local fish, a regular food item of the local people. The import of hazardous and toxic waste—metal scrap, electronic hardware, depleted uranium and thorium and ship breaking—poses a serious threat to the lives and health of people engaged in handling it. Globalisation of the economy has also promoted production and consumption of energy intensive material products and consequent increase in carbon omission and unequal energy consumption between classes and regions and thereby accentuating climate change. The state's stand in climate change negotiations has privileged growth over preservation of ecological balance. Its victims are largely the poor as they have no means to protect themselves from its adverse impact (Ibid.).

The state's labour policy in the post-reform period has greatly contributed to the poverty and exploitation of 92% of its labour force which is in the unorganised sector. This is on account of the government's tilt towards employers, which has undermined labour rights and delegitimised collective bargaining. This tilt is reflected in giving a free hand to the employers in respect of retrenchment, lockouts, closure and anti-union measures and non-interference in lay off of workers or voluntary retiring them to reduce the workforce. The recent regressive labour reforms carried out to attract investors would turn many secure workers in the formal sector into informal workers (Srivastava, 2020). The state has also used its coercive power to curb protest/resistance by workers against these measures. This repression is against peasants and other occupants of land resisting its acquisition and workers against management in industrial establishments. A similar tilt is also evident in judicial decisions. The corporates have succeeded in subverting labour laws and achieving a flexible labour market even without government changing them (Gill, 2012).This policy environment has deactivated and de-motivated trade unions as there is limited space to operate. With 92% of its workforce in the unorganised sector, the prospects of extricating it from poverty, exploitation and social degradation are bleak.

Conclusion

The state at the time of independence had articulated a well crafted agenda of development to dissolve the toxic combination of poor development policies and programmes, unfair economic arrangements and bad politics. From the foregoing, it is evident that this commitment to the people—a kind of social contract as it were, in terms of improvement in living standards, provision of employment at an adequate wage, and reduction in inequalities in income and wealth remains unrealised irrespective of whether the economy was state- controlled or market-driven. This failure to achieve development goals was attributed to the slow rate of growth in the former while in the latter it is due to the nature of growth. The latter period has unmistakably increased the toxicity of the combination of exclusionary economy, adverse development policy and unresponsive politics. In the welfare economy there was at least one mitigating factor, i.e. the state had relative autonomy to design development policies to address the needs of its vast sections of poor and vulnerable population, had the power to regulate the economy for this purpose and was far more responsive to the people (electorate) than to the capital or the business class. This liberty is not permitted to a state in a globally integrated market economy. To reverse the current distorted, exclusionary, un- equalising and environmentally degrading growth and development policies promoting it, a radical shift is needed in both the economy and development paradigm. The changes to be effected in development policies would require that the state does not take away the existing livelihood resources of the poor, provides productive and secure employment at an adequate wage to all, prioritises elimination of hunger and malnutrition, makes available without discrimination public funded social goods like quality education, drinking water, healthcare, sanitation and social security, makes determined efforts towards removal of discrimination and exclusion of SCs, STs, minorities and women and bridges multi-dimensional inequalities. The changes in economy would need to integrate redistribution and environmental protection and regeneration in the growth process and ensure that its macro-economic policies significantly contribute to the pursuit of these development goals. Such a shift can only emerge when the 77% of the population, described as poor and vulnerable (NCEUS, 2007) become central to the politics of the country and dominate its concerns in governance.

References

Ahluwalia, I. J. (1998). State of the economy. In V. A. Pai Panandiker (Ed.), *Fifty years of swaraj: Highlights and shadows*. Konark Publishers.

Banerjee, A., & Piketty, T. (2005). Top Indian incomes: 1956–2000. In A. Deaton, V. Kozel (Eds.), *The Great Indian poverty debate*. MacMillan.

Bhaduri, A. (2008). Predatory growth. *Economics and Political Weekly, 43*(16), 10–14.

Bhalla, G. S. (2007). *Indian agriculture since independence*. National Book Trust.

Bhalotra, S. (2002). The impact of economic liberalisation on employment and wages in India. Paper submitted to the International Policy Group, International Labour Office, Geneva, January 31.

Bhattacharya, P., & Devulapalli, S., (2019). India's rural poverty has shot up. Live Mint 3 December 2019.

Chakraborty, A. (2011, December 17). Human development: How not to interpret change. *Economic and Political Weekly, 46*(51), 16–19.

Chandra, N. K. (1982, April 17). Long-term stagnation in the Indian economy, 1900–1975. *Economic and Political Weekly, 17*(14–16).

Chavan, P., & Bedamatta, R. (2006, September 23). Trends in agricultural wages in India 1964–1965 to 1999–2000. *Economic and Political Weekly, 41*(38), 4041–4051.

Chidambaram, P. (2021, January 31) Across the aisle: No expectation, no disappointments. *The Indian Express*.

Damodran, H. (2019, March 1). Rural distress deepens: Wage growth dips, non-farm jobs hit. *Indian Express*.

Das, P. (2007, December 15). Wage inequality in India: decomposition by sector, gender and activity status. *Economic and Political Weekly, 47*(50), 58–64.

Datt, G., Kozel, V., Ravallion, M. (2003, January 25). A model-based assessment of India's progress in reducing poverty in the 1990s. *Economic and Political Weekly, 38*(4), 355–361.

Deaton, A., & Dreze, J. (2002, September 7–13). Poverty and inequality in India: A re-examination. *Economic and Political Weekly, 37*(36), 3729–3748.

Dev, S. M. (2016). *Economic reforms, poverty and inequality*. Indira Gandhi Institute of Development.

Dev, S. M., & Mooij, J. E. (2004). *Patterns in social sector expenditures: pre and post reform (Working Paper No. 43)*. Centre for Social and Economic Studies.

Dev, S. M., & Ravi, C. (2007, February 10–16). Poverty and inequality: All India and States, 1983–2005. *Economic and Political Weekly, 42*(6), 509–521.

Dubey, A., & Thorat, S. (2012, March 10). Has growth been socially inclusive during 1993–1994 to 2009–2010? *Economic and Political Weekly, 47*(10), 43–53.

Fernandes, W. (2006). Liberalisation and development induced displacement. *Social Change, 36*(1), 109–123.

Ghosh, J. (2005). The Indian economy (1970–2003). In D. Kumar (Ed.), *The Cambridge economic history of India* (Vol. 2, pp. 1757–2003). Orient Longman.

Gill, S. S. (2012). Distribution of income and share of wages in India: Labour under a globalisation economy. *The Indian Journal of Labour Economics, 55*(1).

Global Hunger Report (2020) Global Hunger Index 2020 October 16, 2019. Express Website October 19, 2020

Government of India. (2009). *Report of the expert group to review the methodology for estimation of poverty*. Planning Commission.

Government of India. (2012). *Economic Survey (2012–13)*. Ministry of Finance.

Government of India. (2013). *Press note on poverty estimates 2011–12* (July 22). Planning Commission.

Government of India, Ministry of Labour and Empowerment (2016) *Report on fifth annual employment—unemployment survey 2015–2016* (Vol. 1). Labour Bureau

Himanshu. (2005). Wages in rural India: Sources, trends and comparability. *The Indian Journal of Labour Economics, 48*(2), 375–406.

Himanshu. (2007, February 10). Recent trends in poverty and inequality: Some preliminary results. *Economic and Political Weekly, 42*(6), 497–508.

Himanshu. (2011, September 10). Employment trends in India: A re-examination. *Economic and Political Weekly, 46*(37), 43–59.

Himanshu. (2019, August 1). The seriousness of the problem of unemployment in India. *Live Mint*.

Himanshu. (2020, April 15). Freedom struggle was about combating poverty: There has been a setback. *Indian Express*.

Hirway, I. (2012, May 19). Inclusive growth under a neoliberal policy framework: some critical questions. *Economic and Political Weekly,* 47(20), 64–72.

IDFC Rural Development Network. (2013). *India rural development report 2012–2013*. Orient BlackSwan.

Institute of Human Development (IHD). (2014). *India labour and employment report*. Academic Foundation.

International Labour Organisation. (2016). *Indian labour market update*. ILO Country Office for India.

International Labour Organisation. (2020). *Rapid assessment of the impact of COVID-19 crisis on employment*. ILO Brief India.

Jayadev, A., Motiram, S., & Vakulabharanam, V. (2007, September 22). Patterns of wealth disparities in india during the liberalisation era. *Economic and Political Weekly, 42*(38), 3853–3863.

Jha, P. (2006). Some aspects of the well-being of India's agricultural labour in the context of contemporary agrarian crises. *Indian Journal of Labour Economics, 49*(4), 741–764.

Jitendra. (2019, June 4). It is official: Unemployment rate in rural, urban India is highest in 47 years. *Down to Earth*.

Jodhka, S., & Newman, K. S. (2007, October 13–19). In the name of globalisation; meritocracy, productivity and hidden language of caste." *Economic and Political Weekly, 42*(41), 4125–4132.

Jose, A. V. (1988, June 25). Agricultural wages in India. *Economic and Political Weekly, 23*(26), A46-A51+A53-A58.

Joshi, S. (2006, January 28–February 3). Impact of economic reforms on social sector expenditure in India. *Economic and Political Weekly, 41*(4), 358–365.

Kannan, K.P. (2012). How inclusive is inclusive growth in India? *The Indian Journal of Labour Economics, 55*(1).

Kannan, K. P., & Raveendran, G. (2009, March 7–13). Growth sans employment: A quarter century of jobless growth in India's organised manufacturing. *Economic and Political Weekly, 44*(10), 80–91.

Kannan, K. P., & Raveendran, G. (2011, September 17). India's common people: The regional profile." *Economic and Political Weekly,* 46(38), 60–70.

Kannan, K. P., & Raveendran, G. (2019, November 9). From jobless to job loss growth: Gainers and losers during 2012–2018. *Economic and Political Weekly, LIV*(44), 38–44.

Kumar, A. (2013). *Indian economy since independence: Persisting colonial disruption.* Vision Books.

Mehrotra, S., & Gandhi, A. (2012, April 7). India's human development in the 2000s: Towards social inclusion. *Economic and Political Weekly, 47*(14), 59–64.

Mehrotra, S., & Parida, J.K. (2019). India's employment crisis: Rising education levels and falling non-agricultural job growth. In *CSE working paper 2019–04 October*. Centre for Sustainable Employment—Azim Premji University.

Misra, U., & Iqbal, N. (2020, December 21). Reading of NFHS data: Why findings of the latest round are of concern. *Indian Express.*

Misra, U. (2021, January 25). COVID deepened inequalities: Wealth, education, gender. *The Indian Express.*

Murthy, V. S., (2019, September 12). Demonetisation, Faulty GST implementation behind slow down, Says Manmohan Singh. *Business Line.*

Nag, B., & Geest, W. (2020). *Economic impact analysis of COVID-19 implications on India's GDP, employment and inequality, working paper*. Indian Institute of Foreign Trade.

Nagraj, N. (2020). TIF-Understanding India's economic slowdown, February 7, 2020

National Commission for Enterprises in the Unorganised Sector (NCEUS). (2007). *Report on condition of work and promotion of livelihoods in the unorganised sector*. NCEUS.

Nayyar, D. (2006, April 15–21). Economic growth in independent India: Lumbering Elephant or running Tiger. *Economic and Political Weekly, 41*(15), 1451–1458.

Nayyar, G., & Nayyar, R. (2016, August 29). India's 'poverty numbers', revisiting measurement of poverty. *Economic & Political Weekly, LI.*

Oommen, M. A. (2012, February 18). Understanding human development. *Economic and Political Weekly, 47*(7), 4–5.

Pal, P., & Ghosh, J. (2007, July). Inequality in India: A survey of recent trends. *DESA Working Paper* 45.

Pappola, T. S. (2014). The question of unemployment. In B. Jalan, *The Indian economy: Problems and prospects.* Penguin.

Patnaik, U. (2007). *The Republic of hunger and other essays.* Three Essays Collective.

Patnaik, U. (2013). The dishonesty in counting the poor. *The Hindu,* July 30, 2017.

Press Information Bureau. (2020). Global Multidimensional Poverty Index, UNDP, 2020, September 07, 2020, Delhi

Pre-and Post-reform periods. *Economic and Political Weekly,* 45(37), 45–55.

Rao, C. H. H. (2005). *Agriculture, food security, poverty, and environment: Essays on post-reform India.* Oxford University Press.

Raychaudhury, T. (2005). The Mid-eighteenth century background. In D. Kumar (Ed.), *The Cambridge economic history of India* (Vol. 2, pp. 1757–2003). Orient Longman.

Rodgers, G., & Rodgers, J. (2011, June 4). Inclusive development? Migration, governance and social change in rural Bihar. *Economic and Political Weekly, 46*(23), 43–50.

Sankaran, S. R. (2008). Planning for the poor: Indian experience. In K. S. Bhat (Ed.), *Towards social development*. Rawat Publications.

Sarkar, S., & Mehta, B. S. (2010, September 11). Income inequality in India: Pre-and post-reform periods. *Economic and Political Weekly, 45*(37), 45–55.

Sharma, Y. S. (2020). 27 million youth in age group of 20–30 years lost jobs in April. *The Economic Times E paper*, 13 May 2020.

Sen, A., & Himanshu. (2005). Poverty and inequality in India. In A. Deaton & V. Kozel (Eds.), *The Great Indian poverty debate*. MacMillan.

Sengupta, A. (1998). Fifty years of development policy in India. In H. Karlekar (Ed.), *Independent India: The first fifty years*. Oxford University Press.

Sengupta, A., Kannan, K.P., & Raveendran, G. (2008, March 15–21). India's common people: Who are they, how many are they and how do they live? *Economic and Political Weekly 43*(11), 49–63.

Shah, A. (2012). Environment, employment and labour: Pathways to sustainable development. *Indian Journal of Labour Economics, 55*(1).

Singh, B. P. (2020) Impact of COVID-19 on rural economy in India. MPRA Paper No. 100530 20 May 2020: 39 UTC

Srivastava, R., & Padhi, B. (2020). Collapse in wage salary income growth in India, 2011–2012 to 2017–2018. Institute for Human Development, Working Paper–01/2020.

Srivastava, A., & Kothari, A. (2012). *Churning the earth: The making of Global India*. Penguin.

Srivastava, R. (2020, October 5). There is much in the labour codes that needs to be discussed and debated. *The Indian Express*.

Thorat, S., & Newman, K. S. (2007, October 13–19). Caste and economic discrimination: Causes, consequences and remedies. *Economic and Political Weekly, 42*(41), 4121–4124.

Thorat, S. (2014). Tackling social exclusion and marginality for poverty reduction: Indian experiences. In J. von Braun & F. W. Gatzweiler (Eds.), *Marginality: Addressing the nexus of poverty, exclusion and ecology*. Springer (Open Access at SpringerLink.com).

Tiwari, R.K. (1991). Growth and its pro-poor character in India during 1993–94—2009/10: Lessons for making growth more inclusive July 18, 1991, Durgabai Deshmukh Memorial Lecture. Council for Social Development.

Vaidyanathan, A. (2005). The Indian economy since independence (1947–1970). In D. Kumar (Ed.), *The Cambridge economic history of India* (Vol. 2, pp. 1757–2003). Orient Longman.

Vyas, M. (2019). 11 million jobs lost in 2018. Centre for Monitoring Indian Economy, January 9, 2019. Business Today online, January 4, 2019.

World Health Organisation. (2008). *Closing the gap in a generation: Health equity through action in the social determinants of health* (Commission on Social Determinants of Health, Final Report). WHO.

Chapter 18
Water Governance and Supply in Urban Areas

Dunu Roy, Vasudha Akshintala, and Ruchika Sharma

Water is a basic human resource and one that requires efficient management; and its distribution should be based on principles of equality, conservation, and sustainability. One of the most pressing issues in the contemporary search for better standards of living, social justice, and environmental conservation is the allocation and use of water. However there is an increasingly uneven distribution of safe and adequate water, especially for marginalised social groups.

The Hazards Centre has been providing technical and professional assistance to many community groups and organisations working with the poorer sections of society, mainly in the urban areas. Through this endeavour it has become clear that one of the major problems faced by the deprived sections is the lack of water and sanitation. This is, in turn, related to the pattern of water governance emerging in urban areas, and its major determinant is the policy package that drives urban renewal. The attention of the Centre was drawn to this determinant in December 2005, when the Jawaharlal Nehru National Urban Renewal Mission (JNNURM), the biggest initiative in urban renewal, was launched in 63 cities of million-plus population, with a funding support of $ 6.4 billion from the Asian Development Bank (ADB) (Ministry of Urban Development, 2011). The objectives of the JNNURM were linked to making urban infrastructure and services more 'efficient' and 'accountable'. Apart from solid waste management, drainage, transport, parking, and heritage sectors, the largest allocations under JNNURM were earmarked for 'water supply and sanitation' (Hazards Centre, 2009).

While the central government was committed to provide 35–90% of the funds required for these projects, depending upon the size of the city, it was expected that the remaining capital would come from private and market sources. Hence, JNNURM was inextricably linked to 'investor-friendly' changes in urban governance and these were termed as 'reforms' that had to be undertaken by the local governments who constitutionally control land and urban development. In order to provide legal teeth to

D. Roy (✉) · V. Akshintala · R. Sharma
Hazards Centre, New Delhi, India

I. Qadeer et al. (eds.), *Universalising Healthcare in India*,
https://doi.org/10.1007/978-981-16-5872-3_18

Governance Reforms

Property	Governance	People
Repeal ULCRA	City planning by ULB	74th Amendment
Reform Rent Control	Double entry accounts	Participation Law
Reform Property tax	E-Governance	Public Disclosure Law
Certify Property Title	*User charges for O & M*	*Service to poor*
Computerise Registration	Budget for BSUP	*(water, sewerage, sanitation,*
Simplify conversion	Rain water harvesting	*heath, education, social security)*
Streamline construction	Recycle water	20-25% EWS/LIG in housing projects
	Encourage PPP	

Mandatory – have to be done in the firat couple of years
Optional – have to be done within the Mission period of sevey years

Fig. 18.1 Reforms under JNNURM

these changes, state governments and Urban Local Bodies (ULBs) were also required to sign Memoranda of Agreements before they could access central funds.

Since JNNURM has now been officially declared as a 'success', it is now being extended in its second phase to all the 5000-odd urban settlements in India (Planning Commission of India, 2012).[1] It is in this context that it becomes important to understand the score of mandatory and optional 'reforms' that the ULBs are forced to accept if they want financial support for building the necessary infrastructure (Fig. 18.1).

One-third of these reforms have to do with easing the purchase and sale of land as a commercial commodity, including repeal of the Urban Land Ceiling and Regulation Act, reform of the Rent Control Act, and reform of property taxes, so that the ULBs can raise revenues from the only asset that they possess, and enable them to repay the loans from the Centre as well as the market. Another one-third relate to city planning, double entry accounting systems, special budgetary provisions for the poor, and e-governance, with stricter norms for raising user charges to pay for operation and maintenance. Along with making rules for water harvesting and recycling, these reforms are also directly linked to directions for encouraging Private Public Partnerships (PPPs). The remaining one-third helps in formulating the laws for ensuring participation and disclosure and access to services and housing, especially for the poor. But since all these are linked to property rights, the eventual access mechanism is controlled by the possession of papers that prove ownership—something that most urban poor do not possess.

A quick look at the distribution of investments across the 63 JNNURM cities reveals that half the projects sanctioned are for water supply and sewerage, and the cost of these projects is roughly 70% of the total budget (Fig. 18.2).

In other words, the basic infrastructural requirements for better health are determined by the manner in which investments will be made. But if one selects a random set of cities from Agra to Vadodara, for which data is available on the website of the Ministry, their City Development Plans indicate that all of them have large slum

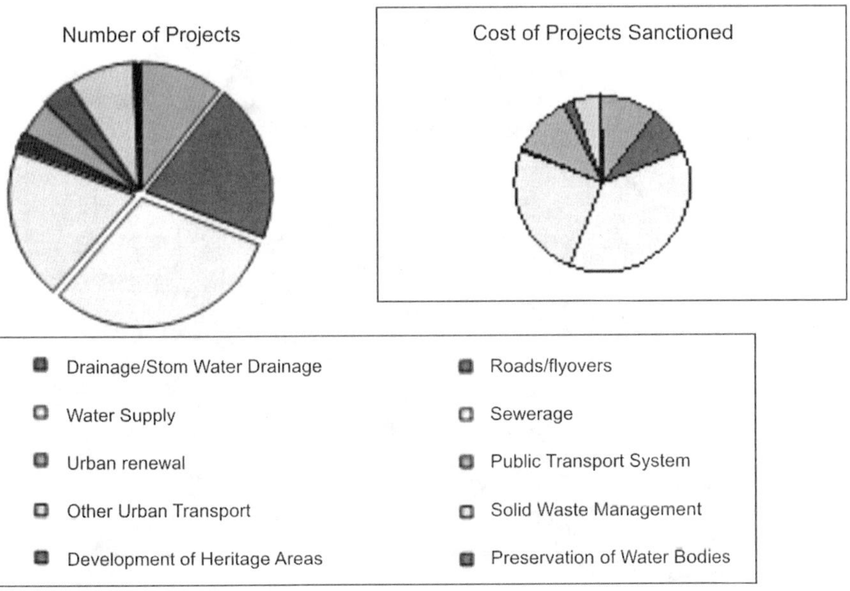

Fig. 18.2 Allocation of JNNURM funds for infrastructure demand and supply

populations of 1–20 lakhs, and the majority are currently unable to provide access to water supply to more than half the slum population (Ministry of Urban Development, n.d.a).

Simultaneously, every city or town is planning to expand in ever larger circles to accommodate projected urban 'growth' in the tertiary sector. Thus, Bangalore has moved away from garment manufacture to information technology and electronics with major inputs of foreign direct investment while declaring its 540 slum settlements as 'shadow areas' because they cannot be properly serviced. Hyderabad, with 1630 slums, has followed a similar trajectory into 'Cyberabad'. Modern Ahmedabad has unsuccessfully tried to attract its textile magnates to invest in slum networking in its 710 slums, while property taxes have boomed threefold. Almost all other cities have aspirations of attaining the 'world class' status.

The case of Delhi is symptomatic of this global disease. Since 1990 the administration, emboldened by a series of viciously anti-poor judgements by the courts and a pervasive vision of a 'slum-free city', has been demolishing hutments and moving the poor out to the periphery of the city into 'resettlement' colonies on land which had been considered unfit for human habitation (Map 18.1).

Service availability and provisioning is far worse in these colonies than in the original settlements. Thus, if one considers the supply of water to the entire city, officially 42% is sourced from ground water and—given the location of the resettlement colonies in low-lying areas—much of it is heavily polluted (Hazards Centre, 2007).

In addition, with a hopelessly unrealistic supply norm of 360 L per capita per day (lpcd), the city has never been able to meet more than 60% of its requirement and the

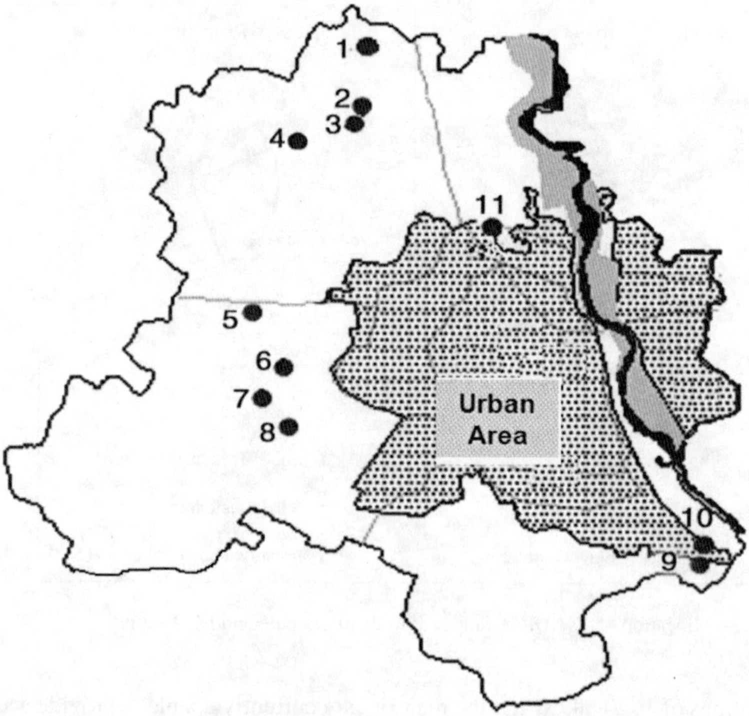

Map 18.1 Delhi-resettling the poor at the periphery. 1. Narela; 2. Holambi Kala; 3. Holambi Khurd; 4. Bawana; 5. Bakkarvala; 6. Hastsaal; Kakraula; 8. Pappankala; 9. Molarband; 10. Madanpur Khadar; 11. Bhalaswa. *Source* Compiled by Hazards Centre from newspaper reports

norm has been arbitrarily reduced to 225 lpcd for slums and resettlement colonies—though the Delhi Jal Board further slashes it to 42.5 lpcd. Surveys conducted by us in 1998 revealed that actual supply is as low as 33 lpcd in the poorer settlements, and as high as 400 lpcd in the affluent areas. Another 2002 survey in 3000 flats built by the Delhi Development Authority for high, middle, and low income groups also yielded a norm of 100 lpcd with which all families appeared to be content—and this is well within the actual availability of 120 lpcd (TRIPP, 2000).

This also means that there is corresponding pollution of the effluent, with the difference that the sewers and drains carry about 90% of it away in the regular colonies while in the slums one-third is disposed of on land and thereby leaches into the shallower aquifers. A study of 77 samples taken from 5 slum clusters and 6 resettlement colonies in 2005 bore out this hypothesis, since only 8% of the samples in the pre-monsoon season and 22% during the monsoon were found to be potable and, while both types of colonies had terrible water supply, the officially planned resettlement colonies were 'more' polluted than in the 'illegal' slums (Fig. 18.3) (Hazards Centre, 2005–2006).

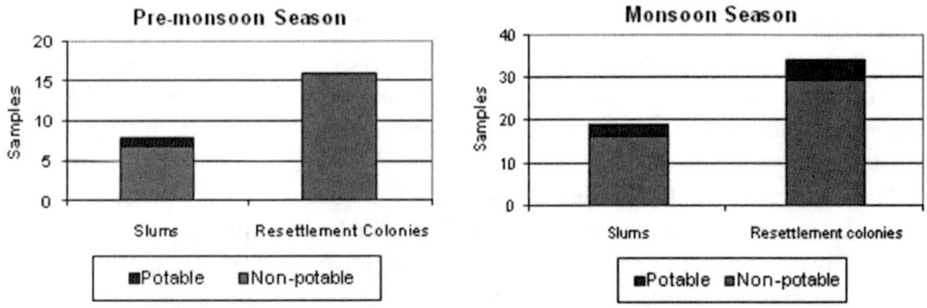

Fig. 18.3 Quality of drinking water in slums and resettlement colonies in the pre-monsoon season. *Source* Hazards Centre (2005–2006)

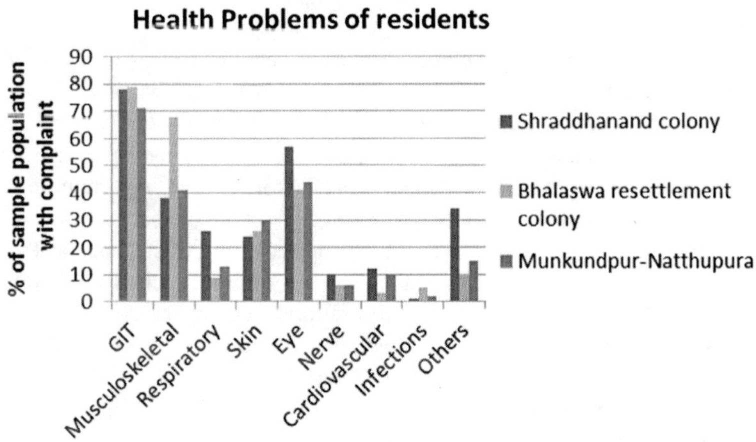

Fig. 18.4 Health problems of residents around the Bhalaswa Landfill. *Source* Bhalaswa Lok Shakti Manch and Hazards Centre (2012)

Yet another study was performed in 2008 of 15 ground water samples in one of the 'model' resettlement colonies settled in 2000, with 20,000 evicted families from 11 different slums, located right next to one of the three landfills that are still operational in Delhi. This study clearly indicated that toxic leachates (dissolved solids, faecal coliform, and heavy metals like zinc, cadmium and lead) had infiltrated into the ground and severely polluted the water supply, with the wells closer to the landfill being far more polluted than those further away. During the health survey, the people complained of various problems such as gastro-intestinal diseases, musculo-skeletal pain, skin and eye irritation, and respiratory problems (Fig. 18.4) (Bhalswa Lok Shakti Manch and Hazards Centre, 2012).

Regular contact with the polluted groundwater for use in domestic chores such as bathing, washing utensils and clothes, had obviously led to many people suffering from skin and eye irritations and itching. There was considerable reporting of these conditions in the media and community groups also sent delegations to the Chief

Minister and the water utility. The response of the Jal Board to the hue and cry was to paint all the hand pumps red. Yet the irony is that the resettled families are located on tiny plots on a 10-year 'license' and already, there are indications that the people may be moved again since the land is surrounded by a golf course, a lake, a park, and a housing complex.

This leads us to ask two questions: why is water quality so bad in these colonies? And why is it worse in resettlement colonies which are supposed to be properly planned by the authorities prior to relocation of people from slums? It may be because both slums and resettlement colonies are inhabited by the same poorer classes who do not have the political claim to resources unlike the wealthy citizens. Additionally, 'resettlement' may not be to make life better for the poor, but merely evict them from where they have already contributed in improving the land and made it 'valuable', and thus locate them in the undeveloped periphery where they can repeat the same process all over again.

This explains why the 'world class' city has to become "slum-free" and why the poor are considered an environmental menace, so that they can be easily dumped outside the city. Then, as the city expands and develops, and the land at the periphery becomes valuable because of their efforts, they can be picked up and flung out. Additionally, there is a propensity to make a profit from everything, including waste. Thus, in Delhi, privatisation of waste has been carried out, and earlier ways of waste management that actually helped in reducing and recycling waste, such as the waste pickers, have been made illegal. National policy and schemes such as JNNURM drive centralisation, and encourage private corporations, thereby discouraging existing decentralised and efficient mechanisms, which also offered routes for livelihoods for the urban poor.

Following the above study, we carried out a study in 2009, to focus on the quality of water in surface water sources, hand pumps, bore wells, and tankers, as well as Ranney wells and piped water supply at the nearest point to the water treatment plants (Figs. 18.5, 18.6, 18.7 and 18.8) all over Delhi.

During this study, 53 water samples were taken at points throughout the city, and analysed for various parameters. It was observed that, of the 53 samples, only 2 water samples had potable water. Seventy-two percent of the samples had faecal contamination, another 72% had fluoride levels above permissible limits, some had high levels of iron, lead, and cadmium, and in others, organo- chloro and organo-phosphorous pesticides were present. Even 87.5% ground water samples had faecal contamination (Hazards Centre, 2012). This again raises questions about the sustainability of the current system in managing sewerage and the efficiency of completely centralised water management. The current debate on sanitation restricts itself to talking about toilets. However, construction of toilets at every site can only ensure greater use of water, all of which—in the absence of adequate treatment and disposal—eventually reaches the surface as well as ground water sources. This is evident from the fact that piped water had faecal contamination in 46% of the samples taken in Delhi and this water is supplied to people who are socially and economically less capable to cope with the health hazards. Thus, there is a need to look at alternative models for water supply and waste disposal.

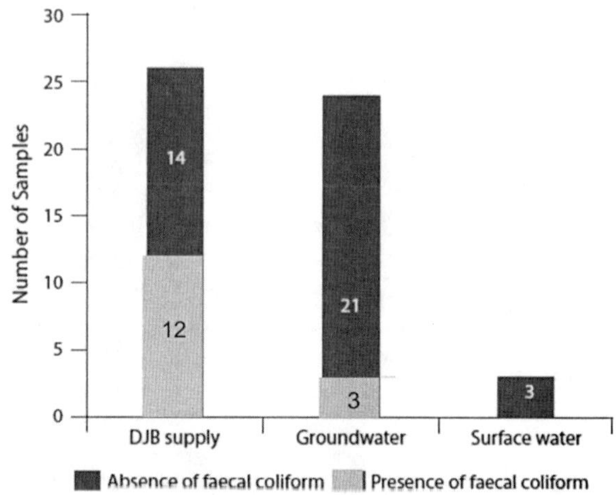

Fig. 18.5 Faecal coliform in supply

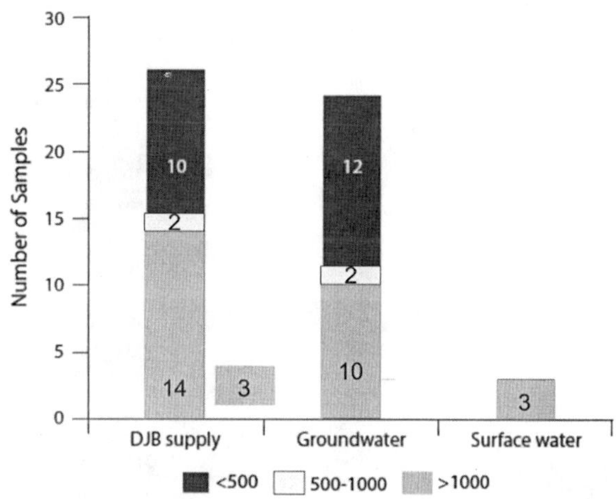

Fig. 18.6 Bacterial colony count

Water and sanitation are only part of the social determinants of health. Not surprisingly, health services also seem to follow the same trajectory as the supply of these services. Thus, in Delhi, all hospitals, maternity homes, and other health centres are concentrated in the core of the city (Map 18.2).[2]

The periphery, to which the poor are being forced to move, does not have adequate health services, where they can only avail of medical services from the dispensaries run by the Government of Delhi, and even these are poorly maintained and understaffed. This leads to the question as to who has rights over health, water, sanitation, and all other infrastructures in a region. Is access to health eventually conditioned by wealth and the political clout it commands?

The social determinants of health in urban areas are clearly rooted in the investment policies that are driving the processes of 'urban renewal' and 'economic

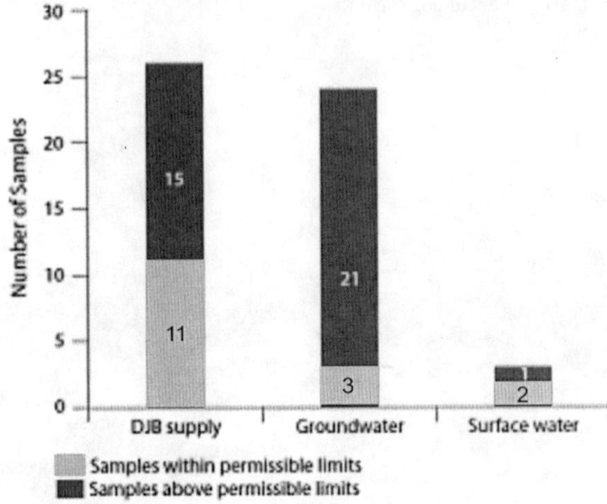

Fig. 18.7 Fluoride contamination

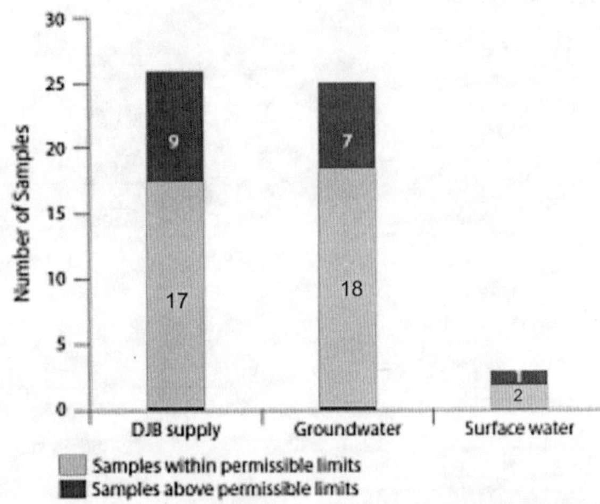

Fig. 18.8 Arsenic contamination. *Source* Figures 18.5, 18.6, 18.7 and 18.8 Hazards Centre (2012)

growth'. In the vision of the policy-makers, urban development is solely defined by the growth in Gross Domestic Product (GDP). Hence, all urban policies are accompanied by a set of 'reforms' that heighten user charges and favour the privatisation of services. The returns on investment, however, mainly accrue from land and property and, consequently, cities expand to shift from manufacturing to services and informal labour is driven to the periphery. However, the immiserated working population, already underserved in the slums, gets a harsher deal in the new resettlement colonies. Eviction from the core of the city ensures even less access to water, sanitation, transport, livelihoods, and all other services. Pollution mitigation technologies (such as water and waste treatment)—that may enhance GDP growth—are inaccessible to the majority of the urban poor. The policy-driven attempt to invest and

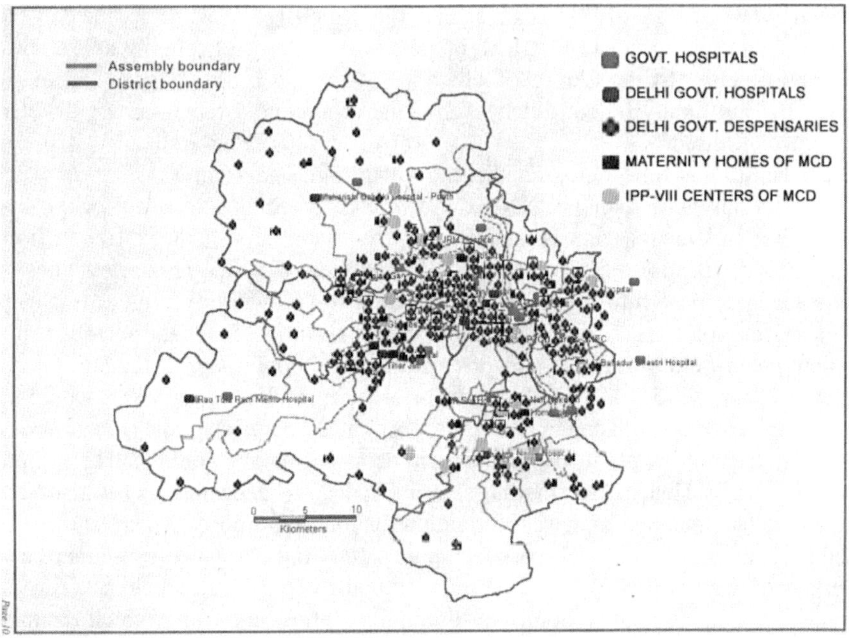

Map 18.2 Distribution of health services in Delhi. Compiled from: List of hospitals on website of Government of Delhi, http://www.delhi.gov.in/wps/wcm/connect/doit_health/Health/Home/Directorate+of+Health+Services/, accessed on April 26, 2010

make profits requires that externalities are passed on to the underprivileged sections of the population whose 'exclusion' is central to this mode of 'development' that neglects all other aspects of sustainability.

Hence, if healthcare is to be assured to all sections of the people then this mode of development has to be challenged. Mere targeting of the poor, or providing them with cash coupons, or talking of 'inclusive' development is not sufficient enough to address the processes of exclusion. Livelihoods, homes, food, water, and sanitation are all contributors to the state of health of a family. Health for all will remain a distant and elusive dream as long as supply and governance mechanisms ensure that these are not accessible.

Postscript

The JNNURM model of urban renewal meandered to a close in 2013, after which the new government at the Centre offered a triple-rainbow palette of Smart Cities (Ministry of Urban Development, 2015a), Atal Mission for Rejuvenation and Urban Transformation (AMRUT), and Sardar Patel Urban Housing Mission. The announcement of INR 48,000 crore for the development of 100 'smart' cities, in particular, created a wave of curiosity in an expectant public which had been disappointed by the "world-class" cities under JNNURM, in spite of the release of roughly INR 47,000 crore for 65 cities by the Centre, of which the States and Union Territories actually used 73%, but finally failed to deliver the kind of smoothly functioning cities that had been promised.

The question now becomes whether the 'smart' cities have more to offer for water supply and sanitation than the JNNURM 'world class' cities did. In this regard, one has to first understand what is 'smart' about them and how is that different from the earlier conception of 'world class'. On the face of it, the 'smartness' lies in using Geographical Information Systems (GIS) for providing optimum transport and services, solid and liquid waste management facilities. Since these cities could be new green field ones, or a part of existing urban conurbations, the key infrastructure of these cities like roads, traffic, electricity, water, sewage, etc. would be completely covered with cameras and sensors, that are connected to a control centre through a technology platform, so that rapid decision-making could lead to optimal use of resources. Hence, the 'smartness' is embedded in the technology being used to collect, collate, manage, and use information for control purposes. Smart software is used to represent the physical space occupied by city infrastructure, using maps and overlays. Smart sensors capture real-time data on roads, water and electricity, gas, crimes, revenue, air quality, home consumption, lighting, and so on, which can then be used to regulate each of those systems. Smart applications can analyse the use of such systems of public transportation, healthcare, education, safety, registration, welfare delivery, housing, maintenance, and the status of vulnerable groups. Smart cell phones can be used to both track down micro-activity as well as disseminate macro-information.

Different control centres in the city can manage its energy, water, transport, airport, and infrastructure in such a manner that there can be a 20–30% reduction in energy use, water loss, transport cost, health expenditure, educational investment, and street crime. A 'smart' city thus begins to replace the priority given to roads and flyovers, bridges, buildings, railways, water and sewer lines with critical investments in broadband networks, mobile towers, cameras, wireless and satellite communication, mass transport, net-based delivery services, and compact data access centres; thereby saving on the use of public resources such as land and making city administration more accountable and transparent.

Here, in one swipe of the magnetic card, therefore, is the ideal dream of a city that is 'efficient', 'liveable' and 'sustainable'. Its carbon footprint surges down because computers regulate and balance energy use with supply matching demand all the time, and renewable energy becomes widespread. All homes, offices, and shops are connected electronically to a 'smart' grid that controls the utilities. Traffic jams are a distant memory. So are pollution, waste, unsavoury sounds and smells and sights. There are no jostling crowds either competing for scarce commodities. And, most dramatically, so much value has been created that investments bring in handsome returns while jobs are aplenty.

These returns are, therefore, central to the sustainability of the 'smart' city because the 'smart' decisions to invest or not, by the institutions that control capital, will be made on the basis of an assessment of what profits can be made out of the commodities in a competitive market. The vision of revenues that will flow in the future will determine investment decisions that are made in the present. It is such an attractive vision that the present government has relaxed the requirement of built-up area and capital conditions for Foreign Direct Investment (FDI). Corporations from all over the world are expected to come flocking in with large purses and high competencies in building infrastructure, as is reported to be happening in Dholera, the proposed iconic 'smart' city in Gujarat located on the Delhi-Mumbai Industrial Corridor, where the state government declared a Special Investment Region in 2009 to arm itself with more powers to acquire land.

But what is it that drives the idea of the 'smart' city and makes it seem possible at this stage of urban evolution? Firstly, the current existence of supremely fast technological capacity to gather and process massive gigabytes of data has an important role to play. The other is the demonstrated capacity of this technology to provide a very healthy return on investment. The third is the opening up of opportunities to market the technology that centralises decision-making at the scale of the interlinked urban conurbation. The fourth is the anticipated shift of 40% of the population from rural to urban areas to contribute 75% to growth in GDP. And the fifth is the assessment that private finance capital is willing to invest in these 'engines of growth'.

As suggested by a report from McKinsey and Company (originally a firm providing finance and budgeting services), India will need 20 to 30 new cities every year in the next ten years to house this migrating population (McKinsey Global Institute, 2010). In the same vein, International Business Machines (IBM), formed out of a merger of three companies involved in tabulating, recording, and computing data, estimates that India will need 500 new cities in the next twenty years (D'Monte, 2015). It is curious how firms such as McKinsey, IBM, Cisco, Oracle, Microsoft, TCS, L&T (all of whom have entered the electronic software or hardware business) have become experts in urban development, as they jostle with each other to bid for projects, and team up with the builder lobby to build 'smart' cities. But will they bid for supplying minimum water to the public or to gain maximum profit for selling it?

Some of the same central ideas seem to permeate the Atal Mission for 500 other than 'smart' cities (Ministry of Urban Development, 2015b). AMRUT proclaims that providing basic services to households and building amenities in all cities will improve the quality of life for all, especially the poor and the disadvantaged, and this is a national priority. According to the AMRUT concept, a High Powered Expert Committee estimated as early as in 2011 that INR 39,20,000 crore was required for creation of such an urban infrastructure, including INR 17,30,000 crore for urban roads and INR 8,00,000 crore for services (including water), with an additional estimate of INR 19,90,000 crore for operation and maintenance of created infrastructure and services 'every year'. The purpose of AMRUT is to (i) ensure that every household has access to a tap with assured supply of water and a sewerage connection; (ii) increase the amenity value of cities by developing greenery and well maintained open spaces; and (iii) reduce pollution by switching to public transport or constructing facilities for non-motorised transport. The pursuit of better outcomes will not stop with the provision of taps and sewerage connections to all. After achieving the benchmark of universal coverage, a process of 'incrementalism' will be set in motion to achieve other benchmarks gradually according to national priorities. For instance, the construction and maintenance of storm water drains is expected to reduce, and ultimately eliminate, flooding in cities, thereby making cities resilient. AMRUT also plans to make 'States equal partners in planning and implementation of projects, thus actualising the spirit of cooperative federalism'. Therefore, capacity building and a set of reforms have also been included in this Mission. The Mission statement optimistically declares that 'Reforms will lead to improvement in service delivery, mobilisation of resources and making municipal functioning more transparent and functionaries more accountable, while Capacity Building will empower municipal functionaries and lead to timely completion of projects (Ibid.). The Mission will focus on the 'Thrust Areas' of water supply, sewerage, septage management, and storm water drains; non-motorised and public transport facilities; and enhancing amenity value of cities by creating and upgrading green spaces. Water supply under AMRUT includes the augmentation of existing water supplies, water treatment plants, and universal metering—the last being of particular importance if greater revenues are to be recovered from users and the maintenance costs met. Rehabilitation of old water supply systems and rejuvenation of water bodies is also on the agenda; as is special water supply arrangements for difficult areas, hill and coastal cities, including those having water quality problems (such as arsenic, fluoride). Recycling of water for beneficial purposes and reuse of wastewater has been itemised. Faecal sludge management is supposed to be done in a 'cost-effective manner.' But questions of how the costs are to be met have not been answered in any detail (Ibid.).

The total outlay for AMRUT is INR 50,000 crore for five years from 2015 to 2020 and the Mission will be operated as a Centrally Sponsored Scheme. The annual budgetary allocation for the Mission will consist of four parts: 80% for project fund; 10% as incentive for reforms; 8% for state administrative expenses; and 2% for Ministry administrative expenses. The 'incentive' for reforms is of more than academic interest since, very much as in the case of JNNURM, the 11 reforms are for e-governance, accounting, planning, devolution, changes in bye-laws, audits, and the iconic 'Swachh Bharat' (for sanitation), but all tied together to improvements in the levy and collection of user charges and better credit ratings. As the base document states, the reforms (are) to improve service delivery, 'mobilise resources', and make municipal functioning more transparent and functionaries more accountable (Ibid. 5–6, authors' emphasis).

Which of the above objectives is of priority has already been suggested for the Smart Cities Mission, and is further clarified for the (Sardar Patel) Housing for All by 2022 scheme covering all 4,041 statutory towns in stages (Special Correspondent, 2014). This scheme has the following components: (a) Rehabilitation of Slum Dwellers with 'participation of private developers using land as a resource'; (b) Promotion of affordable housing for weaker sections through 'credit linked subsidy'; (c) Affordable housing 'in partnership' with public and private sectors and (d) 'Subsidy' for beneficiary-led individual house construction or enhancement. As the portions in single inverted commas show the emphasis on sale of land as a commodity, the involvement of private parties with their profit motivations, housing loans with their interest payments over 15 years and linked to the Jan Dhan Yojana (the Bank savings accounts of the beneficiaries), will ensure that only those who have adequate financial capacities will be able to access the 'affordable' housing.

Private firms are, of course, greatly welcoming of such an approach. A 2014 report by the National Real Estate Development Council (an association of real estate and infrastructure developers) and KPMG (the Indian arm of the Dutch accounting firm, Klynveld Peat Marwick Goerdeler) titled 'Decoding Housing for All by 2022', considers the US $ 2 trillion anticipated investment as an 'innovation' that 'has infused new life into' the real estate sector (KPMG & NAREDCO, 2014). Provided, of course, a set of reforms, necessary for the sector to 'mobilise such huge resources', are put in place. These 'reforms' are centred around streamlining the approval process, relooking at building development norms, promoting the PPP framework, revising the 2013 Land Acquisition Act, 'channelising higher (public) funding in housing', and 'empowering' EWS/LIG households (by providing them with credit) (Ibid.).

In other words, the private sector wants to make it easier for it to access public funding in housing for its own profits. Since water supply is, or should be, an integral part of all this housing, it would be interesting to understand how water is also enmeshed in this participation by the private sector in what is essentially a public service. A study on 'Trends in Private Sector Participation in the Indian Water Sector' by the Water and Sanitation Program (WSP) administered by the World Bank in 2011 is quite revealing in this respect since the purpose of the WSP is ostensibly 'to support poor people in obtaining affordable, safe, and sustainable access to water and sanitation services' (Water & Sanitation Program, 2011). The study covers 26 successful as well as failed PPP attempts in the public domain in both industrial and domestic water supply in urban areas since 1990 (Ibid.). Half the projects were awarded in the five years after 2005, and half in the 15 years before. The early PPPs during the 1990s were largely in the southern states of the country but the trend changed after 2004. The study found that the availability of 'public' funding under schemes such as JNNURM enabled a wider cross-section of states/cities to initiate projects on their own. But most pertinent are the changes that took place in the nature of the contracts during this period. The bulk water supply system PPPs during the 1990s gave way to mere operation and maintenance (O&M) PPPs in the early 2000s, on the curious grounds that this would 'emulate the operational efficiencies of the private sector' (Ibid. 7). Further, the Build Operate Transfer (BOT) models with 100% private financing, yielded ground to management contracts with long-term concessions (Ibid.). While 'there was strong advocacy by multilateral funding agencies to develop water projects on a PPP basis' during the 1990s and several projects of the 2000s decade depended heavily on financial aid from these multilateral funding agencies, since 2005, however, most water PPP projects were 'initiated by the project sponsoring authority', i.e. the public bodies. The study found that 'Projects which were being developed during the 1990s and early 2000s were based on PPP structures which envisaged private financing', but later the PPP projects relied heavily on publicly financed JNNURM and Urban Infrastructure Development Schemes for Small and Medium Towns (UIDSSMT) schemes (Ibid.:8). Municipalities were required to contribute a share of the project cost, and the appraisal process deliberately encouraged PPP-based projects. Thus, clearly, the private firms learnt to leverage public finance to reduce their financial exposure and protect their returns.

The key question, therefore, is whether these plans will succeed and, at the very least, provide necessary water, sanitation, and health for the citizens? A review of the performance of the earlier JNNURM, that also had several 'smart' reforms at its core, such as e-governance, enhancement of collection of property taxes and user charges, computerisation of registration of land and property, and administrative reforms showed that project completion was dismal, with Gujarat heading the list of project completion rates at 56% and Uttar Pradesh at the tail with a mere 12%. Even Delhi and Maharashtra, touted to be the most modern, 'smart' states, had a completion rate of only 17% and 26% respectively. But most cities claimed enhanced tax revenues (Government of India, 2013). These higher returns were thus not based on better performance, but on higher taxes and tariffs for civic services (Ministry of Urban Development n.d.b).

So what is the basis for claiming that the 'smart' city will be any better than the 'world class' one? Is it that the quantum of money will be much higher? That does not seem to be the case, as JNNURM had allocated an annual average of INR 330 crore per city as compared to the annual average of INR 100 crore being set aside now per city. Is it that the capacities of the urban local bodies and state governments to use the money will be much higher now? This too does not appear to be a realistic scenario since none of the capacity-building measures to be taken up under the second phase of the now-abandoned JNNURM have been put in place. Or will the political zeal and administrative acumen of this government be far superior to that of the previous one, as will the much-touted 'participation' of the people?

These are difficult questions to answer but this much is certain— that there has been no basic change in policy formulations between the two periods. The same mode of 'development' is still being pursued, but now perhaps with an added measure of aggression. The targeting of the poor, providing them with cash transfers, and talking of 'inclusion' has acquired a bombastic edge. Supply and governance mechanisms will, therefore, continue to ensure that basic facilities, including water sanitation and shelter, are not accessible, and health for all will meet the same fate as housing for all. And grassroots movements, such as the Jameen Adhikar Andolan in Dholera (Our Representative, 2015), Gujarat's first iconic 'smart' city, may once again come to the fore to assert their fundamental rights to land, livelihoods, and water. The future awaits.

Notes

1. National Urban Renewal Mission (JNNURM); Vols. I & II, Grant Thornton India, New Delhi, March 2011.
2. Lists of hospitals on website of Government of Delhi; http://www.delhi.gov.in/wps/wcm/connect/doit_health/Health/Home/Directorate+of+Health+Services/, accessed on April 2010.

References

Bhalaswa Lok Shakti Manch and Hazards Centre. (2012). Ground Water Quality and Health Impact in Bhalaswa. New Delhi: Hazards Centre. Anonymous. 2014. 10 Cities that are Helping India Prosper; Delhi Tops. Report, Rediff.com, Business. 25 November. Accessed May 4, 2018. http://www.rediff.com/money/report/special-10-cities-that-are-helping-india-prosper-delhi-tops/20141125.htm

D'Monte, L. (2015, June 19). Turning India City-Smart. *Live Mint.*

Government of India. (2013). *Report of the comptroller and Auditor General of India on performance of the Jawaharlal Nehru National Urban Renewal Mission. Report No.15 of 2012–2013 (Performance Audit).* Ministry of Urban Development.

Hazards Centre. (2005–2006). *A study on potability of available water source of five JJ clusters and six resettlement colonies in Delhi.* Hazards Centre.

Hazards Centre. (2007). *A fact-finding report on the eviction and resettlement process in Delhi.* Hazards Centre.

Hazards Centre. (2009). *Half time or time out: Citizens' Review; Jawaharlal Nehru National Urban Mission–A collective view from below.* Hazards Centre.

Hazards Centre. (2012). *Ground water quality and health impacts in Bhalaswa.* Bhalaswa Lok Shakti Manch and Hazards Centre.

KPMG and NAREDCO. (2014). *Decoding housing for all by 2022.* KPMG. Accessed May 4, 2018. https://assets.kpmg.com/content/dam/kpmg/pdf/2014/09/Decoding-Housing-for-all-2022.pdf

McKinsey Global Institute. (2010). *India's urban awakening: building inclusive cities, sustaining economic growth.* McKinsey & Company India. Accessed April 4, 2018. https://www.mckinsey.com/~/media/McKinsey/Global%20Themes/Urbanisation/Urban%20awakening%20in%20India/MGI_Indias_urban_awakening_full_report.ashx

Ministry of Urban Development, Government of India. (2011). *Revised guidelines, Jawaharlal Nehru National Urban Renewal Mission.* Ministry of Urban Development.

Ministry of Urban Development, Government of India. (2015a). *Smart city, mission statement and guidelines.* Ministry of Urban Development.

Ministry of Urban Development, Government of India. (2015b). *Atal mission for rejuvenation and urban transformation, mission statement and guidelines.* Ministry of Urban Development. Accessed February 21, 2017. http://amrut.gov.in/writereaddata/AMRUT%20Guidelines%20.pdf

Ministry of Urban Development, Government of India. (n.d.a). Jawaharlal Nehru National Urban Renewal Mission, City wise CDP. Ministry of Urban Development. Accessed May 10, 2012. http://jnnurm.nic.in/citywise-cdp.html

Ministry of Urban Development, Government of India. (n.d.b). Reforms, Jawaharlal Nehru National Urban Renewal Mission. Accessed August 16, 2015. http://jnnurm.nic.in/reforms.html

Our Representative. (2015, October 13). Farmers to protest Gujarat government move to 'hand over' 28,000 ha for proposed Dholera smart city. *Counterview.* Accessed October 30, 2015. http://www.counterview.net/2015/10/farmers-to-protest-gujarat-government.html

Planning Commission of India, Government of India. (2012). Report of the committee on JNNURM-II, Clean Bastis, safe communities and people's cities. Yojana Bhavan.

Special Correspondent. (2014, October 9). Sardar Patel urban housing mission: Housing for all by 2022. *The Hindu.*

Transport Research and Injury Prevention Program-TRIPP. (2000). *Water consumption, use and problems in DDA flats of Delhi.* Indian Institute of Technology.

Water and Sanitation Program. (2011) *Trends in the private sector participation in the Indian water sector: A critical review.* Water and Sanitation Program. Accessed May 4, 2018. http://www.wsp.org/sites/wsp.org/files/publications/WSP-Trends-Private-Sector-Participation-India-Water.pdf

Chapter 19
Challenges of Reclaiming the Public Health System: Experiences of Community-Based Monitoring and Planning in Maharashtra

Abhay Shukla and P. M. Arathi

In the second half of the twentieth century as a part of post-independence promises of a 'welfare state' countries of the South Asian region did significantly expand a wide variety of public services. These large public delivery systems were expected to fulfil the wishes of the majority of the people. The state governments with the new optimism and energy derived from the struggle for independence were supposed to be dedicated to provisioning of certain basic services to its people. However, the actual records of the state run public services of these countries—instead of being genuinely accountable and responsive to the needs of the majority—have often been mixed.

These systems in areas such as healthcare have largely tended to be controlled by unaccountable bureaucracies, which have been subject to dominance by national elites, who are themselves subjugated to an inequitable global order and unequal power relations in the international order. These public systems have often become increasingly distanced from the people they are supposed to serve, and are in varying degrees influenced by vested interests, which frequently have used these systems as opportunities for expanding corruption and misusing public resources. This is the background against which, during the last few decades, powerful international forces and their national allies have managed to push the neoliberal agenda of further weakening public systems in the name of 'austerity' and 'fiscal responsibility', along with promoting privatisation and commercialisation. Public services have been starved

A. Shukla
SATHI, Pune, India

National Convener of People's Health Movement, New Delhi, India

National Rural Health Mission, New Delhi, India

P. M. Arathi (✉)
School of Indian Legal Thought, Mahatma Gandhi University, Kottayam, Kerala, India

I. Qadeer et al. (eds.), *Universalising Healthcare in India*,
https://doi.org/10.1007/978-981-16-5872-3_19

of funds, have often been partly privatised, or have been 'hollowed out' and significantly replaced by private provisioning on the ground. This situation has led to a veritable crisis in systems like the public health services in India.

With this background, and increasingly large sections of people being deprived of basic social services, the direction forward now, cannot be privatisation. This has proved to be only promoting a system 'of the elites, for the elites, by the elites'. Neither can a return to largely unaccountable and unresponsive bureaucratic public systems be the answer. The way forward in the early twenty-first century must be based on a process of citizens collectively 'reclaiming public systems', forging a new relationship between society and state, where people occupy the central place as active protagonists, and the state is held accountable for all its actions, where the people from grassroots level play a significant role in public decision-making. This inevitably implies development of a new kind of work ethic and public spirit among public officials and providers, accompanied by a qualitatively different level of consciousness and action regarding public entitlements by organised people.

Deepening Democracy to Strengthen Public System

The discussion on people's participation in governance or 'deepening democracy' arguments basically poses questions like who is a citizen? and what should be the appropriate level of involvement of citizens in democratic practices?

In the neoliberal and globalised world, the idea of citizenship has been radically reshaped in the last two decades (Gaventa, 2010). The definition of citizenship is influenced and rearticulated by the relationship of citizens with market, state, democracy and civil society. Gaventa (2010) describes two contradicting and conflicting ways in which citizenship is being understood: one, to see citizens as active actors in the development process and the other, to see citizens as products shaped by other forces (economic and political) that make them consumers, users, voters or beneficiaries. He argues that the relationship between citizen and state or market is multi-dimensional and created by spaces of multiple identities. He critiques the role/capacity of Non-Governmental Organisations (NGOs) to represent citizens and suggests that they should see citizens as actively engaging with markets, states or with civil society and as rights-bearing actors. He differentiates between 'speaking for the citizens' and 'working with citizens', the latter being a model for deepening democracy or the state-society relationship. He situates the 'citizen-centred approach' as a contrast to four major approaches influenced by neoliberal ideology: namely the 'neoliberal market based approach', 'narrow state reform approach', 'a thin democracy approach' and 'a thin civil society approach'. Kabeer's (2003) work on Bangladesh demonstrates how neoliberalism has led the NGOs to focus on market participation as the route to empowerment.

Neoliberalism and globalisation have thus drastically altered the terrain of citizenship. The neoliberal market approach rearticulates the citizen's relationship with the state as consumers in the global market (Dagnino, 2005; Munck, 2005). The option of 'Exercising power through the market' is available only to the affluent class and not applicable to the poor sections of society. Neoliberal approaches reform the state and weaken the focus of the state as a provider, arbiter, deliverer and protector of rights. Agreeing with the argument of Cornwall and Coelho (2007), Gaventa challenges the idea that mere civil society participation can be an effective instrument to make the state accountable. He suspects that the simple creation of new spaces for institutionalised participation with the state does not alter the power relationships, whereas in fact it may reinforce the status quo (Gaventa, 2010).

Another change in the focus of democracy brought by neo-liberalism is from the voices of resistance and the struggles of citizens to the 'uniform institutionally designed approaches to elections, representation and the rule of law'. Kabeer (2005) critiques the nature of the neoliberal state, in the context of Bangladesh. For her, 'the state does not merely fail to protect the rights of the citizens; it actively contributes to their violation'.

The discussion on how neoliberal discourses have depoliticised the understanding on engagement of civil society and the participation of the citizens is described through the concepts of 'diminished democracy' (Skocpol, 2003) and 'downsizing of democracy' (Crenson & Ginsberg, 2002).

An alternative to the dominant approaches is 'seeing like a citizen approach'. Gaventa explains this approach as "rather than focusing on institutional designs as a starting point, it starts with the perceptions of citizens themselves and asks how they interact and view the institutions from which they are expected to benefit" (Gaventa, 2010: 63). This approach of people's participation in democracy thematically relies on the framework of the right-based approach to development, focuses on the issue of inclusion, participation through organised collective action, and development of democratic institutions. The 'seeing like a citizen approach' visualises citizenship as civil, political and social rights gained through participatory processes and struggles. In other words, citizen participation itself becomes a social right, an instrument to claim and realise all other rights. Gaventa (2010) claims such an approach to citizens' participation, which is an 'actor- based approach', re-politicises our understanding of participation and transforms citizens from being mere beneficiaries to 'right bearing citizens' where citizenship moves beyond assigned passive roles of voters, beneficiaries and consumers to 'makers and shapers of policies' (Cornwall & Gaventa, 2001).

In this political process, Gaventa (2010) emphasises the importance of stretching the idea of citizenship beyond engagement with the nation state. The singular vertical relationship between the state and citizen is being challenged in his work. His imagination of citizenship adds to the traditional vertical relationship with the state and is based on both vertical and horizontal social relationships. He argues in every day practice citizenship is an 'assemble of identities, affiliations and forms of action'.

Cornwall and Coelho's (2007) work in Brazil is empirically grounded in public health practice. A study on health councils, tests the significance of synchronised action of three components namely, committed public managers, civil society activism and an appropriate institutional design in building more inclusive healthcare services. This could be an example of seeing like a citizen approach Gaventa (2010) that leads to deepening democracy.

By citing different experiences (related to privatisation of water, waste management, transport and telecom) from different parts of Latin America (Uruguay and Brazil) and Europe (Italy, Norway, Germany, France and England), Wainwright (2013) argues that the struggle to defend 'principles of commons' like water, beaches, forests and 'social commons' like health education and knowledge is essentially a struggle to transform the state. The different experiences of trade unions and other movements with people's participation around the globe to oppose privatisation and for 'remunicipalisation' demonstrate how such an initiative can become a force to make public services genuinely serve public interests and ensure transparency. Valuing people's experience and knowledge paves the way for sharing power with the public. Wainwright (2013) identifies this process as similar to the feminist concept of 'prefiguring' an alternative (creating experience of the future that we would like to see in the present).

Public Health Experience from India

The National Rural Health Mission (NRHM) was launched in India in April 2005 with a view to bring about architectural corrections and strengthening of the rural public health system, towards improving health services for the rural population. The NRHM aimed at strengthening public health services by ensuring increased funds and a wide range of reforms at the healthcare delivery levels. While strengthening the healthcare system has been essential, it has been recognised that this was not sufficient to attract people back to public health facilities, who had in many areas largely given up on government health services. Healthcare delivery level improvements must be accompanied by enhanced articulation of needs and demands from the beneficiaries of these services and processes. Hence, in order to increase the accountability of the health system, to increase people's participation in public health services, and to convince people that they should avail of these services as a right, a novel process was introduced in the NRHM called Community Based Monitoring and Planning (CBMP) of Health Services. NRHM envisaged CBMP as an intensive accountability to ensure services to people (Garg & Lasker, 2010). With facilitation by civil society organisations and support from the state NRHM, community members and grassroots activists have been involved in organising a range of processes for accountability of public health services. CBMP was an outcome of consistent efforts taken by the People's Health Movement, Jan Swasthya Abhiyan.

By acknowledging the relevance of community-based monitoring as 'an extremely positive development', NRHM allots the central role and allocates the task of active and regular monitoring to the community members.[1] This is perhaps the first effort of its kind by the official health system in the country to institutionalise community monitoring of health services. The NRHM framework document declares that community-based monitoring relies on 'right to healthcare approach' and rightly qualifies participation as: 'Besides ensuring accountability, it would also promote decentralised inputs for better planning of health activities, based on the locally relevant priorities and issues identified by various community representatives' (Government of India (GoI), 2013). The document emphasises the relevance of people's participation in strengthening the public health system. To this effect, the NRHM framework document asserts that, "…Bringing the public back into public health by allowing community members and their representatives to directly give feedback about the functioning of public health services, including giving inputs for improved planning of the same" (Ibid.: unpaged).The document stresses capacity building of actors outside the health department and thereby strengthening the community monitoring system. NRHM document defines a 'joint facilitation role' of the health department with civil society groups and panchayats.

However, even though the NRHM theoretically agrees to the framework of 'right to healthcare' in implementing the community-based monitoring system, it still envisages a blend of 'neoliberal market based approach', 'narrow state reform approach', 'a thin democracy approach' and 'a thin civil society approach' in practice. This contradiction is reflected on the ground in people being assigned passive roles as beneficiaries and consumers although the NRHM theoretically agrees with the framework that envisages a more proactive role for people as citizens. The NRHM document acknowledges this reality by conceding that a genuine community-based monitoring and planning actually involves 'a change in the balance of power in the health sector, in favour of people.' The NRHM policy document places CBMP as:

> It need not be reiterated that this entire exercise carries meaning only if ordinary people and their spokespersons in the form of both Panchayat representatives and community based organisations, gain a degree of authority to identify gaps and propose priorities and influence decision making regarding health system. It is difficult to imagine that this significant shift in balance of power which involves making health officials and functionaries directly accountable and answerable to people can be carried out exclusively by the agency of the health department without any additional facilitation, although their central involvement at every stage would of course be essential (Ibid.: Unpaged).

Here, we discuss how this change in balance of power is taking place at grassroot level practices and whether our existing power structures are receptive to the change in power relationships. Is this shift really possible in a society where inequality is manifested in every single public action of the state, which also reiterates and silently promotes all the existing hierarchical relationships? The discussion also addresses how the "deepening democracy approach" functions in a highly class-driven, caste-divided and gender-discriminated society like India.

Overview of the CBMP Framework and Processes in Maharashtra

CBMP of health services is being implemented in selected areas of Maharashtra, among certain other states in India, as a component of NRHM since mid–2007.

CBMP processes are organised at the village, Primary Health Centre (PHC), block, district and state levels. A state nodal NGO (SATHI in the case of Maharashtra) coordinates the CBMP activities across districts, in collaboration with the district and block nodal NGOs, working with the state health departments. A multi- stakeholder monitoring and planning committee at each level collates the findings from the level below, monitors the health system at its own level, and passes these results up to the next level once or twice a year. Such CBMP committees have been formed in implementation areas at PHC, block, district and state levels.

Scale of CBMP in Maharashtra

CBMP has been implemented in five pilot districts, (Amaravati, Nandurbar, Osmanabad, Pune and Thane), initially covering 15 blocks and 225 villages. Encouraged by the emerging model of CBMP, in 2009 the state NRHM extended the process to additional blocks and villages, so that currently around 370 villages in 18 blocks are covered by the CBMP process in these districts. Since March 2011, the process has been further extended to eight new districts (Solapur, Gadchiroli, Kolhapur, Chandrapur, Nashik, Beed, Raigad and Aurangabad) so currently; the CBMP process covers over 600 villages across 13 districts. Within these 13 districts, a total of 30 civil society organisations are involved in collaboratively implementing the CBMP process.

Key Processes in Community-Based Monitoring and Planning

Formation/Expansion and Capacity Building of Community-Based Committees

A key activity in the CBMP process is building awareness among communities regarding basic health entitlements related to NRHM. Following this, Village Health, Nutrition, Water Supply and Sanitation Committees (VHNWSCs) have been significantly expanded with inclusion of active community members selected in village meetings. These village committees have been activated and members have been oriented to carry out CBMP activities. Similarly, multi-stakeholder CBMP committees have been formed from the PHC level to the state level in the CBMP areas. Such CBMP committees include panchayat members, health officials, civil society representatives and certain delegates from lower level committees. Members of these committees have been given training related to health services in the context of NRHM, health rights and entitlements, CBMP processes and promoting people's participation.

Community Data Collection and Filling Health Report Cards

At the core of CBM is the process of recording and reporting the state of public health services in villages and facilities as experienced by the people. Based on orientation, the village committee members have been involved in the process of filling up village health report cards, with active guidance from facilitators and coordinators of the nodal NGO/ community based organisation. Information is collected on indicators like village level disease surveillance services; maternal and child health services including immunisation, antenatal care and postnatal care; curative services at the village level; use of village untied funds, etc. Once they are filled, the village report cards are displayed in a prominent place in the village, and a copy is sent to the PHC level monitoring committee for further dialogue and action. Similarly data is collected and report cards are prepared at the level of sub-centres, PHCs and CHCs.

People's Tribunals: Jan Sunwai or Jan Samvad

These are mass events attended by large numbers of local community members, people's organisations, NGOs, government officials and prominent persons from the region. At Jan Sunwais or Jan Samvads, people are invited to report their experiences of health services and denial of care, as well as findings included in the health report cards. The authorities present then respond to these testimonies and findings, stating how the problems will be addressed. As part of CBMP in Maharashtra, public hearings have been organised at the PHC level, block level and district level; hence nearly two hundred public hearings have been organised so far as part of the CBMP process.

Periodic State Level Dialogues

Prior to the development of CBMP there were no regular forums for community level groups to raise issues at the state level in ways that could elicit action. Currently, officially mandated dialogues between the state health officials, district and block health officials, and civil society representatives are organised on an annual basis. These dialogues help to address issues that have not been resolved at lower levels and reinforce the commitment of the entire health department. The participation of health officials from various levels helps to assign responsibility to take corrective actions, which is often declared during the meeting itself.

Community-Based Planning

In continuation of community-based monitoring, to help tackle various local and facility level issues, promotion of decentralised community-based planning of health services has been initiated in five districts since 2011. It was observed that Patient Welfare Committees—Rogi Kalyan Samitis (RKS)—were not aware of their expected role in deciding about the utilisation of flexible funds related to NRHM. In this context, workshops on community-based planning for Monitoring and Planning Committee members including panchayat representatives and RKS members were organised at various levels regarding how flexible funds should be used for genuine patient welfare. This has led several RKSs to address the key issues emerging from community monitoring in their facility-based plans.

Indicators of Positive Impact: People are Returning to the Public Health System

Significant Rise in Positive Ratings of Public Health Services in CBMP Areas

Village level health committees have used report cards to assess the state of health services. Four rounds of assessment were undertaken by the respective committees till 2010 by collecting information in 195 villages and 32 PHCs from four pilot districts. The committee members rated health services as either 'Good', 'Partly Satisfactory' or 'Bad'.

Analysis of information compiled through the village report cards shows an increase in 'Good' rating in successive rounds of community monitoring. In the first round (mid–2008), 50% of the services were given 'Good' rating, which increased to 63% by Phase 4 (end–2010). Thus, there has been a consistent overall improvement in village health services related to the CBMP process. There has been major improvement in 'Good' ratings to certain services from first to fourth rounds, like Antenatal care (58% increased to 72%) and immunisation (65% increased to 89%).

Similarly, the data collected from PHCs can be divided into four categories: infrastructure, services, personnel and medicines. Analysis of information compiled from 32 PHCs in five districts reveals that in the first round, only 44% of PHC services received 'Good' rating. By the fourth round there was a significant improvement, with 75% of services being rated as 'Good'.

Significant Increase in Utilisation of PHC Services: Evidence from Thane District

Generally there has been an increase in utilisation of health facilities after implementation of NRHM. Moreover, there is a higher level of increase in CBMP areas. We studied three key utilisation indicators: outpatient attendance, inpatient admissions and institutional deliveries for three years—2007–2008, 2008–2009 and 2009–2010 in Thane district. These trends, related to the utilisation of PHCs covered by CBMP, were analysed and compared with the average trends for PHC utilisation in the entire district, and it clearly shows greater increase in the utilisation in PHCs in CBMP areas.

Community Monitoring Process Has Promoted and Increase in OPD Attendance: Between 2007–2008 and 2009–2010, the average increase in OPD attendance for PHCs in the entire Thane district was 17%, whereas increase in OPD utilisation in CBMP covered PHCs was significantly higher at 34%.

Higher Increase in Utilisation of Inpatient Admissions: Similarly, between 2007–2008 and 2009–2010, the average increase in inpatient admissions for PHCs in the entire district was 50%, whereas the increase in CBM covered PHCs was significantly higher at 73%.

Greater Increase in Institutional Deliveries: Between 2007–2008 and 2009–2010, the average increase in deliveries in PHCs in the entire district of Thane was 48%, whereas the increase in deliveries in CBMP covered PHCs in the district was significantly higher at 101%.

It can be concluded that NRHM related improvements have led to some overall increase in utilisation of PHCs in recent years. Further, in PHCs covered under the CBMP process, increased community awareness along with additional improvements in services promoted by public dialogue and other accountability processes seem to have induced more people to access PHCs for various types of care, indicating a movement from private providers to the public health system.

Selected Stories of Change Related to Community-Based Monitoring in Maharashtra[2]

Community Monitoring Helps to Complete the Half-Built Sub-Centre

It is a story known to everyone, even though the details might change from place to place. People in Jamshet village in Dahanu block of Thane district required a health sub-centre. The sub-centre was sanctioned; but the 'politically connected' contractor, who was supposed to build the sub-centre, delayed the construction which stretched on for over two years, resulting in a half-built useless structure. The villagers went to the block level authorities and complained, but there was no response. In this scenario, the CBMP process made a difference. The village level members of the CBMP discussed the issue in a series of Gram Sabhas, and then raised this at the Block level monitoring committee meetings on repeated occasions. Further, given the inaction of the contractor, one day scores of mobilised community members took their implements and arrived at the sub-centre to 'complete' the construction on their own through 'Shramdaan'! This moved the local authorities and contractor into action. The sub-centre building got completed and it has become fully functional. Even an additional ANM was posted at this sub-centre and at present it is a full-fledged sub-centre which is actively used by the community. The ANM, Ms. Vasawale, reports that 'in the last six months, there have been 83 deliveries in this sub- centre'.

Community-Based Planning Leads to Major Improvements in Nasarapur PHC

Based on issues identified during community monitoring, capacity building of RKS members including Panchayat Raj Institutions (PRI) representatives and on suggestions given by CBMP civil society organisations, several issues were addressed in Nasarapur PHC in Bhor block of Pune District. These improvements took place within a few months following initiation of community-based planning:

- Lack of drinking water was identified as a major problem. Now to provide drinking water to patients, a water storage tank with inbuilt water filter has been installed.
- In order to make the laboratory properly functional, a tank for water storage has been purchased and a new pipe line for the laboratory has been installed.
- People complained that there was no board with the name of the PHC, and it used to be difficult for new patients to find it. Now an appropriate board has been put up through RKS funds.
- The post of sanitation worker was vacant in Nasarapur PHC, which resulted in a lack of cleanliness. So to maintain clean premises, the RKS committee has now decided to locally appoint a sanitation worker.
- Workshops on 'Right to Health' and 'role of adolescents in village development' are now being conducted for groups of adolescents in nearby villages, with support from the RKS fund.

Kavita Chooses the PHC for Her Delivery and 'Trupti' is Born

CBMP is gradually winning people back to the public health system, helping them to escape impoverishment from healthcare expenditure. The failure of the public health system in many areas to convince even poor people about its quality of services is an ongoing tragedy. No wonder Gopal Sonar, a poor landless labourer in Ajarataluka of

Kolhapur District sold his only buffalo for fifteen thousand rupees, anticipating the expenses that would be required for his daughter's first delivery in a private hospital. His daughter Kavita, during her pregnancy, attended some meetings conducted in the village under CBMP. The local activist Shivaji briefed her about the improved functioning of the PHC due to CBMP and about her entitlement to free delivery care. Kavita was convinced that her delivery should take place at the PHC and not in a private hospital, even though her father was reluctant. Repeatedly assured by Shivaji, the family took Kavita to the PHC when the labour pains began, and she delivered normally at the PHC. Gopal was jubilant as he had to pay just five rupees at the PHC for that delivery, as against the anticipated sizeable amount expected in a private hospital. The newborn girl was named Trupti (meaning 'satisfaction')!

Some Further Steps and Decisions Required to Carry Forward Community Action Processes

CBMP is a nascent and emerging process, which involves 'cooperation with assertive dialogue' to promote health system strengthening and reorientation. Despite positive impacts, since this process generates social momentum for positive change, some degree of resistance is encountered from certain health officials who are unable to respond to the need for change and accountability. Hence a key challenge in this process is to ensure continued improvements in health services and enhanced responsiveness of the health system over time. This depends to a significant extent on health officials at various levels taking ownership and getting actively involved in the process, as well as adequate space being given to civil society organisations and community-based activists to effectively promote pro-people change.

Building on and in order to carry forward the positive process of community-based monitoring and planning in Maharashtra, further action on several fronts is required:

Constraints Being Placed on Representation of Civil Society Organisations in the CBMP Process Need to be Removed: It has been observed during the last two years that the mandate/proportion of civil society organisations in key CBMP bodies (such as state and district mentoring committees) has been reduced. Civil society role in key communitisation bodies must be broad based and participatory instead of being 'official centred'. The reduction of this role tends to constrain important multi-stakeholder processes. Instead, adequate and effective civil society representation must be ensured.

Need to Widen Spaces for Decentralised Health Planning Activities: While CBMP committee members have taken initiative to give inputs to local health planning processes, medical officers often continue to dominate these, allowing only minimal inputs from PRI members and inadequate space for involvement of community representatives and civil society activists. Further, in states like Maharashtra, although several community-based planning suggestions for inclusion in the annual PIP have been endorsed by officials at lower levels, these seem to have been eliminated from the final state PIP, apparently due to decisions taken at higher levels. This is a situation that needs to change if community-based planning is to become a reality concerning the PIP development process. Much more receptivity, transparency and openness on part of most of the health officials is required to make health planning under NRHM genuinely decentralised and communitised.

Need to Plan Phased Modification of Civil Society Inputs Instead of Eliminating these Inputs: The CBMP process in Maharashtra is based on people's participation, and community-based organisations with the help of grassroots NGOs. The later are playing a crucial role in capacity building, facilitating various types of collection of information and analysis, as well as ensuring dialogue with and response from healthcare providers at various levels. It also needs to be recognised that community action is primarily a collective process, where local organisations play a key role in mobilising people and articulating their issues. Given this situation, while the civil society organisations need to modify their role to make it less intensive in the first phase areas (where community level processes have been underway for over four years), if the officials plan an 'exit' of these facilitating civil society organisations, this is likely to seriously damage the CBMP process.

At the same time, provisions which can enable community members to directly demand accountability, such as wide display of guaranteed health services, publicising health entitlements through mass media, toll free help lines for persons seeking care in public health facilities, institutionalising participatory forums like Jan Samvads and much more effective and responsive grievance redressal systems, need to be operationalised. Such measures would encourage ordinary people to ask for their health rights, requiring progressively less intensive inputs from civil society organisations.

Addressing Systemic and Structural Health System Issues: Community- based monitoring activities have so far been maximally effective regarding local health service*s* (e.g. village, sub-centre, PHC levels), whereas actions and decisions at higher levels (district, state) have so far been less amenable to community accountability. Similarly, community-based planning has also been allowed some space at local levels, such as incorporating suggestions related to spending of RKS funds. However, despite action on local implementation issues, key health system issues raised through the CBMP process need to be addressed much more effectively. The recent formation of the state monitoring and planning committee is a positive step to address such issues. NRHM needs to develop a specific set of strategies to ensure that genuine systemic issues being raised though the CBMP process, such as medicine procurement or vacant posts, are effectively addressed in a timely manner.

Experiences of Experiments on Deepening Democracy in Public Health

Based on the process of CBMP, now people are getting involved in revitalising health services. All role players involved in this process now need to ensure that this process of restoring people's confidence in the public health system, along with improving and reorienting public health services, is given maximum support and priority at all levels. Such commitment backed by action can ensure that the 'public' comes to the centre of the public health system.

The NRHM document on suggested broad process of initial facilitation of capacity development addresses the tensions that are created by community-based monitoring in rural India. The document reflects an anxiety about the 'potentially disruptive situations' and 'demotivation of health functionaries' and highlights the importance of having 'appropriate checks and balances in the methodology'. The health officials do not have the capacity to take in assertive actions from community representatives on deficiencies, gaps and denial of healthcare, which leads to 'virtual breakdown of dialogue' and 'complete polarisation'.

'Democracy' is the concept/language used by a wide spectrum of ideologies and institutions; from military powers to social movements. The idea of deepening democracy is a derivation from the debates between the Athenian democracy[3] of classic democratic theory and expansive democracy[4] of standard liberal democracy. The definitional issues of community participation in primary healthcare are analysed through 200 case studies by Rifkin (1986). Gaventa (2006) describes processes of deepening democracy with instances of 'focus on the politically empowered monitoring groups, through village assemblies, by making existing structures more inclusive of excluded groups' (Ibid.). Meaningful people's participation can be ensured through a combination of all these examples. For such participation, it is important to understand the social practices of engagement and concepts like deliberation, participation and decision-making process in the local cultures. This understanding further evokes fundamental questions related to analysis of power relations in a stratified society such as 'where does real power reside, how power is being exercised on an everyday basis and so on' (Gaventa, 2010).

Numerous works[5] articulate the actualisation of deepening democracy demanding a 'deliberative democracy' in which 'citizens address public problems by reasoning together how best to solve them'; and where the conceptualisation relates 'equal citizens as the dominant force in democratic life'. The CBMP ideologically and practically demands deliberative democratic interventions and the political will to achieve its spirit and goals. Citizens' juries like the Jan Sunwai are a representative sampling of the citizens, who deliberatively argue and propose more reasoned solutions to the public issues.

The notion of community participation in health is strongly emphasised in the Alma Ata Declaration, 1978 by envisaging the role of people in planning and implementing healthcare programmes both as a duty and as a right (Madan, 1987). In Madan's analysis, community participation is hampered by a wide range of factors including geographical specialties, non-egalitarian social structures and non- cooperation of the bureaucrats and medical professionals. The Kerala experiment of the people's plan programme is one of the success stories from India which tried to transcend the existing limitations for the purpose of ensuring people's active participation in the level of planning.

T. M. Thomas Isaac and Richard W. Franke (2002) call it 'a remarkable radical experiment in democracy'. Isaac and Franke counter the neoliberal argument that decentralisation implies 'downsizing the state' and argue that decentralisation is, in fact, a means of making the state more effective and is a strategic response to an 'affirmative democratic state'. In their study they argue how Kerala's campaign for democratic decentralisation leads to "possible structures of resistance to international neoliberal policies" (Isaac & Franke, 2002: 9). Planning as an instrument of social mobilisation, mass participation[6] and transparency is the distinctive feature of Kerala's experiment on decentralisation.

In India, the context of deregulation, privatisation, reduction of social services, curtailment of state spending on services and the overall shift of the state from being the watchdogs of democracy to stewardship of market requires attention to the importance and relevance of the concept of deepening democracy. This context demands people to shift their roles from being mere participants in the democratic process to more responsive, creative and effective forms of engagement with the state (Fung, 2003). Fung and Wright demonstrate that the panchayat reforms in West Bengal and Kerala have created both direct and representative channels that develop substantial administrative and fiscal development power to individual villages. This democratic decentralisation process is seen as 'basic reform of devolution—for accountability'. The limitation of the process of deepening democracy is cited in a study on democratic deepening in India and South Africa. Heller (2009) argues that subordinate groups have limited opportunities for meaningful engagement with the state. Another study by Heller et al. (2007) suggest people's participation as the good model for development. An analysis of local governance system in Karnataka identifies failure of a centralised system of governance and planning to resolve local problems as the thriving force for the introduction of the idea of decentralisation. In India, the limited experiences with the concept of deepening democracy in Kerala, West Bengal, Karnataka and Maharashtra show that the major form of experiment is decentralisation of planning through the Panchayat Raj system. These experiments had a narrow focus on public health planning and the CBMP is a different experiment in comparison.

It is in this context that CBMP of health services supported by the NRHM has emerged in certain states of India as a type of regular participatory audit of public health services, which facilitates active involvement of people in the public health system. Community monitoring is conceptualised as a strategy for ensuring that health services reach the people who need them, and for ensuring public accountability to check service delivery failures. In other words, while efforts are being made to strengthen the supply side of health services by other components of NRHM, the demand of health services from the community is sought to be ensured through the community-based monitoring and planning process. The present status of NRHM turned National Health Mission (NHM) and its future is still uncertain in matters related to CBMP. Focusing only on healthcare delivery through CBMP is a limited action in itself, unless there is an effort to initiate and strengthen people's participation as part of the developmental agenda in all aspects of policy making. However, the concept and practice of CBMP, and experiences from Maharashtra indicate the potential for transforming the power relationships in democratic processes. Conceptually, this CBMP is based on the theme of deepening democracy. CBMP is closely related with proactive expansion of democratic processes, with a growing role for citizens in the monitoring of bureaucracy and state functionaries and restoring to collectives of citizens a central role in the governance of public services with the exercise of people's power. Experiences are emerging in various countries, especially in Latin America, demonstrating how citizens may take collective initiative to reclaim public systems, reshaping their functioning while challenging and reversing neoliberal trends towards privatisation.

Deepening of democracy also envisages levelling of power relations between people and the bureaucracy; the conventional hierarchical relationship between public systems and ordinary people, particularly rural and marginalised communities, is challenged and is sought to be transformed into a more equitable relationship. Hence CBMP is a step in the right direction towards democratisation, seeking to challenge the hierarchy between hitherto powerless common people and unaccountable officials, by mediating an accountability process that gives citizens and communities both voice and agency. Moving beyond the traditional liberal discourse which is focused on individual citizens, CBMP places communities and collectives of citizens at the centre of accountability processes. As a process of expanding democracy, it has a vision of changing the relations of power in the health system and beyond; it is focused on challenging the unaccountable power of the health bureaucracy, and promotion of people's collective power to shape health related decision-making.

Notes

1. Community members includes beneficiaries, community-based organisations and NGOs working with communities and panchayat representatives.
2. Thirty-five such stories of change in the context of CBMP processes have been documented in Marathi in detail and the collection has been published in the form of a book.
3. The major proponents are Lukham, Schumpeter, John Stuart Mill, G.D.H. Cole and Carole Patman.
4. The idea of expansive democracy is a reinvigoration of many earlier participatory theories as suggesting "increased participation in and control over collective decision-making, whether by means of direct democracy in small-scale settings or through stronger linkages between citizens and institutions that operate on broader scales" (Gaventa 2006: 12).
5. See the works of Cohen and Sabel (1997) and Dryzek (2000).
6. 'Mass participation is not limited to elected representatives or voluntary agencies, but includes ordinary people assembling in gram sabhas with non-official

experts and volunteers. Officials have to work alongside non-officials' (Isaac & Franke, 2002: 19).

References

Cohen, J., & Sabel, C. (1997). Directly-deliberative polyarchy. *European Law Journal, 3*(4), 313–342.

Cornwall, A., & Coelho, V. S. (2007). *Spaces for change? Participation.* Zed Books.

Cornwall, A., & Gaventa, J. (2001). Bridging the gap: Citizenship, participation and accountability. *PLA Notes, 40*(2001), 32–35.

Crenson, M. A., & Ginsberg, B. A. (2002). *Downsizing democracy: How American sidelined its citizens and privatized its public.* The John Hopkins University Press.

Dagnino, E. (2005). We all have rights, But ... Contesting concepts of citizenship in Brazil. In *Inclusive citizenship: Meanings and expressions.* Zed Books.

Dryzek, J. S. (2002). *Deliberative democracy and beyond: Liberals, critics, contestations.* Oxford University Press on Demand.

Fung, A. (2003). Thinking about empowered participatory governance. In A. Fung, & E. O. Wright (Eds.), *Deepening democracy: Institutional innovations in empowered participatory governance* (Vol. 4, p. 3).

Garg, S., & Laskar, A. R. (2010). Community-Based monitoring: Key to success of national health programs. *Indian Journal of Community Medicine: Official Publication of Indian Association of Preventive & Social Medicine, 35*(2), 214–216. https://doi.org/10.4103/0970-0218.66857

Gaventa, J. (2006). Triumph, deficit or contestation? Deepening the 'deepening democracy' *Debate.* Working Paper 264 in conjunction with LogoLink and the Citizenship DRC. Institute of Development Studies, University of Sussex.

Gaventa, J. (2010). Seeing like a citizen? Re-Claiming citizenship in the Neoliberal World. In A. Fowler, & C. Malunga (Eds.), *NGO management: The Earthscan companion.*

Government of India. (2013). *National Health Mission: Communitisation: Suggested broad process of initial facilitation and capacity development.* Available at http://nrhm.gov.in/communitisation/community-action/suggested-broad-process-of-initial-facilitation- and-capacity-development.html. Accessed on March 19, 2015.

Heller, P. (2009). Democratic deepening in India and South Africa. *Journal of Asian and African Studies, 44*(1), 123–149.

Heller, P., Harilal, K. N., & Chaudhuri, S. (2007). Building local democracy: Evaluating the impact of decentralisation in Kerala, India. *World Development, 35*(4), 626–648.

Isaac, T. M. T., & Frankie, R. W. (2002). *Local democracy and development: The Kerala People's campaign for decentralised planning.* Rowman and Littlefield Publishers.

Kabeer, N. (2003). Growing Citisenship from the grassroots: Nijera Kori and social mobilisation in Bangladesh. *The Bangladesh Development Studies, 29*(3/4), 1–20.

Kabeer, N. (2005). Editorial introduction. In N. Kabeer (Ed.) *Inclusive citizenship: Meanings and expressions* (Vol. 1). Zed Books.

Madan, T. N. (1987). Community involvement in health policy; socio-structural and dynamic aspects of health beliefs. *Social Science and Medicine, 25*(6), 615–620.

Munck, R. (2005). Neoliberalism and politics, and the politics of Neoliberalism. In *Neoliberalism: A critical reader* (pp. 60–69).

Rifkin, S. B. (1986). Lessons from community participation in health programmes. *Health Policy and Planning, 1*(3), 240–249.

Skocpol, T. (2003). Doubly engaged social science. In J. Mahoney, & D. Rueschemeyer (Eds.), *Comparative historical analysis in the social sciences* (pp. 407–428).

Wainwright, H. (2013, February). Participatory alternatives to privatisation. *Speech given to social movements in Greece.*

Chapter 20
Constrained by Purchasing Power: The Story of Calorie Intake in India Post-liberalisation

Sourindra Mohan Ghosh

Introduction

Low consumption and availability of food have been perennial features of the Indian economy. It was a saddle of the colonial era that India carried when it embarked on its journey as a free country. In the early 1950s, the national monthly per capita total availability of food grain remained below 12 kgs. As early as the Second Five Year Plan (1956–1961), the policy makers recognised low food availability as a challenge to the country's development and introduced the Public Distribution System (PDS) in the late 1950s to enhance access to basic food. In the later years, PDS was further strengthened with the initiation of procurement of agricultural produce through the Food Corporation of India (FCI) at a guaranteed price fixed by the Agricultural Prices Commission. It also induced more food grain production. The food stocks with the FCI provided a buffer during lean or drought years. As a result of these interventions, the later part of the 1970s and the 1980s witnessed some success in overcoming food shortages, as by 1991 monthly per capita total availability of food grains increased to more than 15 kgs. However, a lot was yet to be achieved in terms of securing food consumption sufficiency for the majority of the population. Even in the early 1990s more than 70% of the rural population and 58% of the urban population was still consuming fewer calories than the government's own standards of daily per capita Recommended Dietary Allowances (RDAs) of 2400 kcal/day and 2100 kcal/day for rural and urban areas respectively.

On entering the liberalisation era in 1990, the policy focus on improving food availability fizzled out. The emerging policy framework—reduction of government expenditure—truncated the PDS from its universal nature to a targeted one in 1997. As the trend of neglect of the agricultural sector and food security system set in, not only food grain availability but caloric intake as well began to fall. As we shall see later in this chapter, the secular decline of calorie intake continued unabated throughout

S. M. Ghosh (✉)
Centre for Economic Studies and Planning, Jawaharlal Nehru University, New Delhi, India

I. Qadeer et al. (eds.), *Universalising Healthcare in India*,
https://doi.org/10.1007/978-981-16-5872-3_20

the 1990s and during the first decade of the 2000 as well, till a turnaround in 2011–2012. Instead of critical reflection and course correction, several explanations were offered to prove that there is nothing to worry about such declines of per capita calorie intakes; on the contrary it was claimed to reflect India's social and economic development. Arguments were put forward claiming that increased mechanisation had reduced physical activity and hence biological demand for energy, leading to voluntary reduction in calorie intakes (Deaton & Dreze, 2009; Rao, 2000). International experiences, ranging from the then newly industrialised Britain of the eighteenth and nineteenth century to a more recent one of China during the 1980s–1990s were also mobilised to show similarity with the Indian experience, where advent of improved technologies in the production sphere coincided with declining calorie intake (Deaton 2010). However, there are evidences of increased calorie intake with increasing income in Britain as it moved up from rural poverty of the 1780s and 1790s to 1830s and 1860s. In a cross-sectional sample of different families of workers in Britain in 1889–90, the lower income heavy industry workers' families were found to have considerably lower levels of calorie intake (2071 kcal daily per capita), than higher income textile workers' families (2415 kcal daily per capita), who presumably had 'lighter' work than the former (Clark et al., 1995). Regarding China, we can end up with misleading interpretations if we ignore the fact that firstly, China's daily per capita calorie intake was considerably higher (by almost 200 kcal) than that of India's during the same period i.e. in the early 1990s (Du et al., 2002); secondly, the reduction in China's calorie intake in the 1990s was attributable to the retreat of state welfare, retrenchment of labour and rapidly increasing food prices (Meng et al., 2004). Those who have tried to explain declines in calorie intake in terms of increasing mechanisation of the economy have missed the point that while 'biological calorie demand' depends on requirement, and hence on the level of physical activity, actual 'intake' levels depend, among other things, on purchasing power of the consumer. It is the interaction of these factors that determines the amount of food a person consumes. As a matter of fact, any conceptual framework that does not take into account the interaction of different social and economic forces will lead to incorrect inferences drawn from circumstantial associations. For example, only going by the 'work-requirement' channel, would have us believe that low calorie intake of an unemployed person is because of her inactivity; however, nothing can be further from the truth.

A great deal of literature has drawn attention towards sluggish employment growth in the post-liberalisation period of the 1990s, followed by an employment growth of low quality and un-remunerative jobs in the first half of the 2000s, followed by the period of the last half of the decade of 2000 till 2009–2010 when employment virtually stagnated (Chandrasekhar & Ghosh, 2007; Papola & Sahu, 2012). It is precisely this entire period of the post-liberalisation era which experienced secular declines of calorie intake. Conversely, as the employment growth rate improved in 2011–2012, so did calorie intake. This chapter attempts to find out whether there is any link between deteriorating livelihoods—and hence purchasing power—and decline of calorie intake in India during the post-liberalisation period. The 2011–2012 departure from the declining trend will provide us a counter check on the validity of our inferences. Section two of this chapter documents trends in calorie intakes and the extent of under-nourishment in terms of calories. Sections three and four explore determinants of calorie intakes in India; the fifth is the concluding section.

Trends in Calorie Intake

The unit level data of five large sample Consumption Expenditure Surveys (CES) rounds of the National Sample Survey (NSS) between 1993–1994 and 2011–2012 were analysed. The NSS records household monthly consumption of all food items (its schedule covers approximately 150 individual food items). From the quantity of individual food items consumed,[1] we have calculated the calories those food items provide and added up at the household level to get the total household calorie intake in a month. For comparisons, we have calculated per consumer unit[2] equivalent of average calorie intakes of individuals which makes our analysis invariant of age-sex composition change in population over time. The methodological shift in the NSS 55th Round of CES rendered it incomparable with the other NSS rounds. To make it comparable, we have incorporated adjustments as suggested by Sen and Himanshu (2004a, b).

Average Calorie Intake

The decades of 1990 and 2000 experienced a gradual decline in calorie intake. As shown in Fig. 20.1, in rural India calorie intake fell from 2694 kcal in 1993–1994 to

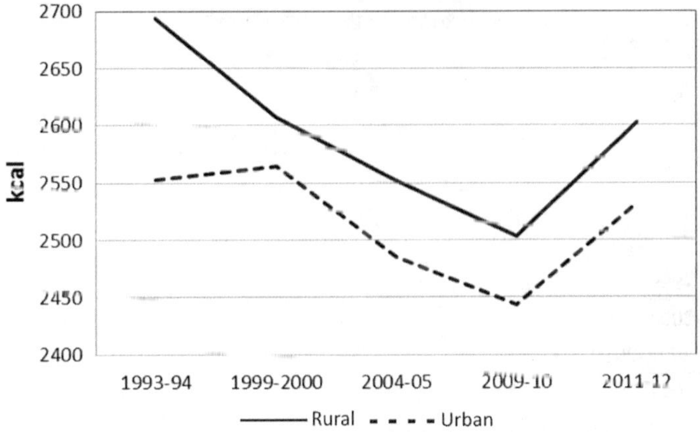

Fig. 20.1 Average per consumer unit calorie intake of individuals: all India. *Source* NSS unit data, various rounds. Author's calculation

2503 kcal per consumer unit per day in 2009–2010, a decline by 7.1% from 1993 to 1994. In urban areas, calorie intake declined from 2553 kcal to 2443 kcal per consumer unit per day during the same period, a decline by 4.3%. The years 2011–2012 saw a reversal of the declining trend as calorie intake increased to 2603 kcal and 2532 kcal per consumer unit per day in rural and urban areas respectively, thus registering an increase by 4% and 3.7% from 2009 to 2010. Even with a lowered base of 2009–10, such an increase in calorie intake is still quite substantial and, though it could not quite reach the early 1990s level, it did manage to get considerably close to the levels of 1999–2000. Thus, the average calorie intake level of 2011–2012 is the highest in the last decade.

Percentage of Persons Above Calorie Cut-Off

As Table 20.1 depicts, during the period of declining calorie intakes, percentage of individuals with intake of 2700 kcal (or more) per consumer unit per day—which the NSS defines as the minimum calorie requirement for a consumer unit—also gradually reduced from 43 and 35% in 1993–1994 to 31% and 28% in 2009–2010, in rural and urban areas respectively. In 2011–2012, percentage of individuals with such calorie sufficiency increased to 37% in rural and 33% in urban areas, which is the highest since 1993–94. It is also noteworthy that percentage of persons with calorie intake of less than 80% of the 2700 kcal norm is the lowest for 2011–12 in the last two decades, indicating that 2011–2012 improvements have taken place particularly among those who are at the lower end of calorie intake.

Table 20.1 Percentage of individuals with sufficient per consumer unit calorie intake: time trends (rural and urban India)

		Calorie < 80%[a]	Calorie 80–100%[a]	Calorie 100% or more[a]
Rural	1993–1994	26.4	31.1	42.6
	1999–2000	32.5	32.2	35.3
	2004–2005	31.5	35.5	33.0
	2009–2010	30.9	38.3	30.9
	2011–2012	24.3	38.6	37.1
Urban	1993–1994	31.9	33.0	35.2
	1999–2000	36.4	33.6	30.0
	2004–2005	34.4	36.4	29.2
	2009–2010	35.3	36.9	27.8
	2011–2012	29.5	38.0	32.5

[a]As percentage of 2700 kcal, per consumer unit per day
Source NSS unit data, various rounds. Author's calculation

Intake of such low levels of calories in the increasing percentage of poorly fed people during 1993–1994 to 2009–2010 is a matter of concern. Undernourishment has many negative physiological effects on the body such as susceptibility to disease and infection, reduced ability of the body to work, grow, or to heal/recover from illness. For infants, children or pregnant women—i.e. those with special requirements of nutrients—effect of undernourishment can be particularly damaging. Also, prolonged undernourishment can lead to reduction of body sizes due to homeostatic adaptation. The issue of increasing undernourishment in India in the post-liberalisation period is something that cannot be ignored.

Factors Influencing Calorie Intake

It is important not only to understand the factors that have led to declining calorie intakes, but also the conditions that reversed it in 2011–2012. This section is dedicated to that discussion.

Increasing Mechanisation?

There are certain scholars who do not see such declines of calorie intake as an indication of increasing undernourishment; instead they see it as a natural outcome of the development process, particularly, increasing mechanisation of work leading to less requirement for energy and hence less demand for calories. However, on the face of it, the 'increasing mechanisation' (Deaton & Dreze, 2009) argument to explain the declining trend of calorie intake in the 1990s and the 2000s is inadequate at least on one ground. First of all, technological improvement in the production sphere over time is not unique to the 1990s or the 2000s; one would generally agree that such relative improvements did take place in the 1970s or in the 1980s as well. Secondly, there had been a gradual shifting-out of the share of workforce from agriculture, which is generally considered to be the heaviest form of work, to services and industry right throughout the 1970s and 1980s as well, as was the case with the later decades (Papola & Sahu, 2012). Hence, even if we accept that, over time, activity level of the population as a whole has gone down, it is not something unique to the 1990s or the 2000s; it has happened in the 1970s and 1980s as well. Yet, in 1970s, calorie intake increased (Radhakrishna et al., 2004) (daily per capita 2268 kcal and 2107 kcal in 1972–1973 to 2364 kcal and 2379 kcal in 1977–1978, in rural and urban areas respectively); and so it did in our most recent year of 2011–2012, when the level of calorie intake was even lower than those in 1972–1973 (2020 kcal and 1982 kcal in 2009–2010 to 2099 kcal and 2058 kcal daily per day per capita in rural and urban areas). So, increasing mechanisation cannot sufficiently explain decline in calorie intake in the post-liberalisation period.

Expenditures and Calorie Intake

While the work-requirement channel, as examined above, cannot consistently explain the trends of calorie intake, it may be useful to turn our attention towards other explanations. Is it possible that over time, increasing preference for 'better food' shifted people away from cheaper sources of calories to costlier ones, resulting in decline in calorie intake? Exploring the relation between the level of spending and calorie intake might give some insight into this proposition. Deflated by Consumer Price Indices[3] (CPI), expenditure (at constant prices) has increased for the entire period from 1993–1994 to 2011–2012 (Table 20.2). From 1993–1994 to 2009–2010, calorie intake declined, apparently showing a negative relation between expenditure and calorie intake over time; on the other hand, from 2009–2010 to 2011–2012 cal intake increased, which apparently shows a positive relation between the two. It appears that there is no stable relation between expenditure and calorie intake over time. The question that arises is: what can reconcile this apparent confused relation between expenditure and calorie intakes?

Engel Curves

We can examine the calorie-expenditure relation in another way. When we plot calorie intake per consumer unit of a large population against their MPCE (at constant prices), both in logarithmic terms[4] (Fig. 20.2a and b), we find a positive relationship between the level of expenditure and calorie intake. This relationship is depicted by positively sloped calorie Engels curves for each year in Fig. 20.2a and b. During the period of 1993–1994 to 2009–2010, there has been a gradual downward shift of the calorie Engel curves, so for a given level of expenditure, calorie intake has fallen during this period. What is really shocking is the fact that even the individuals of poorer households reduced their calorie intake even though they had quite low levels of calorie intake to start with. The 2011–2012 cal Engel curve stops the downward drift; as we can see, calorie Engel curves of 2009–2010 and 2011–2012 almost overlap with each other, indicating unchanged levels of calorie intake for same levels of expenditure during this period. The increase in average intake of calories in 2011–2012 from 2009 to 2010 is depicted by the rightward shift of the calorie Engel

Table 20.2 Average yearly monthly per capita expenditure (MPCE) growth rate (percent), using CPI as deflator: rural and urban India

	1993–1994 to 1999–2000	1999–2000 to 200420–05	2004–2005 to 2009–2010	2009–2010 to 2011–2012
Rural	3.1	1.9	1.8	6.7
Urban	2.3	1.8	2.7	6.1

Source NSS unit data, various rounds. Author's calculation

curve, because of a positive shift of the entire expenditure distribution (with both minimum and maximum levels of 2011–12 expenditure higher than their 2009–2010 counterparts).

The expenditure Engel curves—plotting log food expenditure against log MPCE (both at constant prices)—show that the decline of calorie intake occurred because, at a given level of total expenditures, expenditure on food declined during 1993–94 to 2009–10, causing reduction in food consumption and intake of calories, which does not support the possibility of 'increasing preference for costlier food'[5]; on the other hand during 2009–10 to 2011–12 expenditure on food remained the same for a given total expenditure (Fig. 20.3a and b). The rightward shift of the expenditure Engel curve depicts increase of calorie intake in 2011–12, as observed before as well. Evidently, an increase in expenditures is what has caused increase in calorie intakes in 2011–12; and a reduction of it had caused declines of calorie intake in the previous period. The question is: what prevented the fall of food expenditures for a given level of total expenditure during the period of 2009–10 to 2011–12, unlike what we observed during 1993–94 to 2009–10? To answer this, we examine the role of purchasing power.

Role of Purchasing Power

One of the plausible reasons for the decline of food expenditures for a given level of total expenditures during the larger part of post- liberalisation India could be reduction of purchasing power of the people. This can explain the pattern of calorie intakes. As mentioned earlier, a similar experience of declining calorie intake was observed in China in the early 1990s in the post economic reforms era. The same phenomenon could have happened in India, as increasing impoverishment of the general population (due to lack of remunerative jobs, particularly in the rural sector) and withdrawal of state welfare in the post-reform era eroded people's purchasing power (Patnaik, 2013). Over the years, there has been a gradual change in the consumption expenditure pattern in India as the share of spending on non-food items in total expenditure has increased, from the 1970s till date (Table 20.3), compared to spending on food (Government of India (GoI), 2001, 2014b). This entire period which has seen an increasing share of non- food spending in total expenditure has seen both downswing and upswing phases of calorie intakes. Since increasing share of non-food spending in total expenditure did not always necessarily mean falling calorie intakes, the downswing phases of calorie intake must have been those when inadequate rise in incomes in the face of increasing pressure of essential non-food items have failed to maintain food expenditures, resulting in reduced purchase/consumption of food items and hence an increasing proportion of the population falling below minimum cut-off levels of calorie intakes. We are hypothesising that non-food expenditure as a proportion to income bears a direct relationship with proportion of persons who are falling behind the required calorie norm. We present some evidence for this hypothesis.

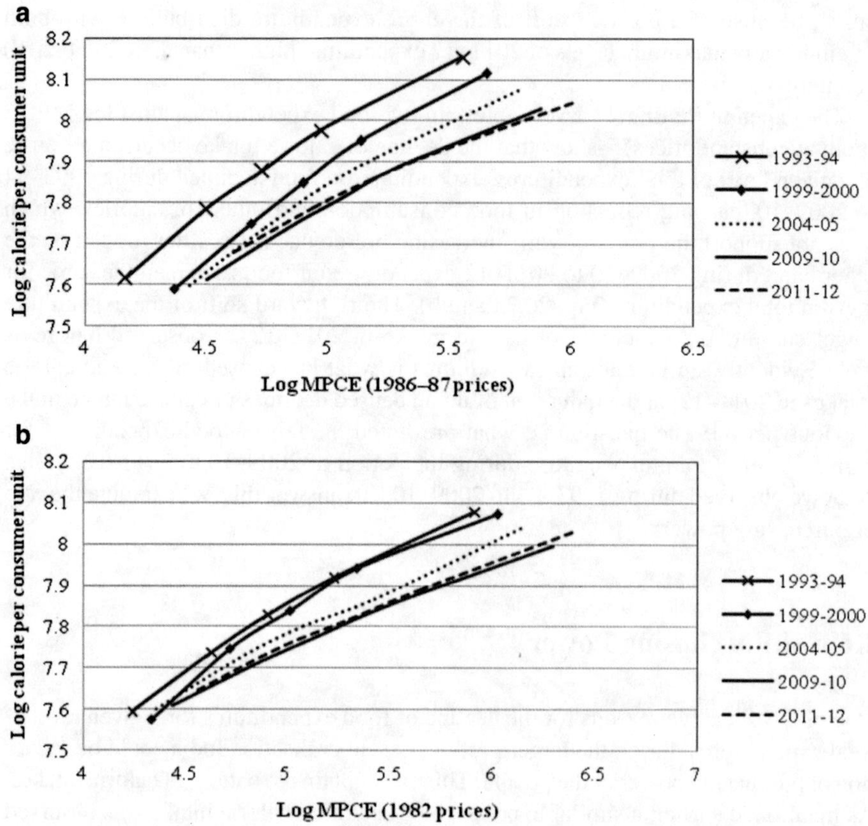

Fig. 20.2 **a** Calorie Engel Curves: All India Rural **b** Calorie Engel Curves: All India Urban. *Source* NSS unit data, various rounds. Author's calculation

Relation Between Income and Calorie Intake

There is no income data available at household level against data on actual expenditure. So there is no direct or straightforward way to calculate actual expenditure shares in income. However, the NSS Employment and Unemployment Surveys (EUS) of the same CES rounds give us daily wages of casual labourers and regular wage/salaried workers. The casual labourers in rural areas constitute over 35% of the overall workforce (GoI, 2014a); and even in larger proportion in the lower MPCE deciles. In the urban areas though they constitute just over 14% of the workforce, and have quite a significant presence in lower deciles (nearly 35% in lowest 0–10% deciles to over 20% in 20–30% deciles). Apart from that, the behaviour of casual labourer's wages will probably be a good proxy for that of the income/wages of other poorer sections of the population. Non-food expenditure as a proportion of the casual labourer's income thus has explanatory importance in our hypothesis in both rural and urban

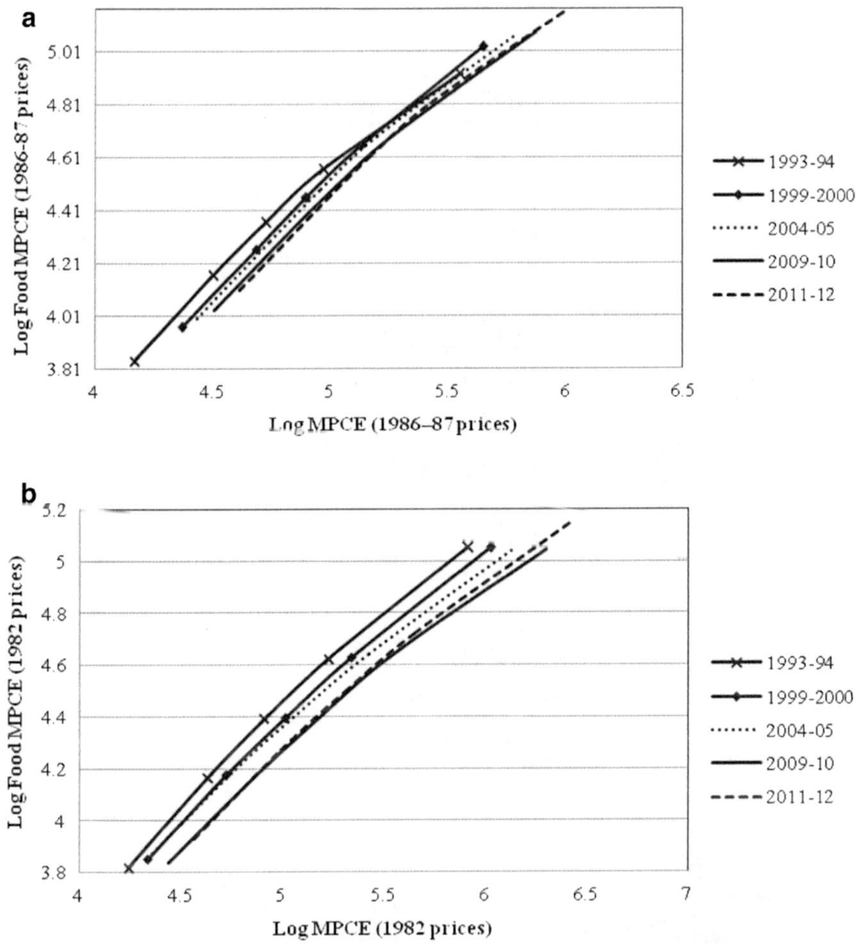

Fig. 20.3 **a** Expenditure Engel Curves: All India Rural **b** Expenditure Engel Curves: All India Urban. *Source* NSS unit data, various rounds. Author's calculation

sectors, given that they are perhaps the most vulnerable among the working class. The regular wage/salaried workers on the other hand constitute only around 7% of work force in rural areas and very few of them appear in the lower or middle deciles Hence they are not important for our hypothesis for rural area. In the urban area, however, regular wage/salaried workers constitute around 43% of the workforce, and the lower-middle and middle deciles have a good proportion of them (around 40–50%) in the total work force. So their income has explanatory importance in our hypothesis for urban areas. We must bear in mind the fact that wage of regular wage/ salaried worker might have a relatively high dispersion, with its average value being upwardly biased by the earnings of the high wage/salary categories. So the average wage of this category might not strictly correspond to those who are at the calorie

Table 20.3 Percentage share of different non-food Items in MPCE

		1972–1973	1977–1978	1983	1987–1988	1993–1994	1999–2000	2004–2005	2009–2010	2011–2012
Rural	Fuel and light	5.6	6.0	7.1	7.4	7.4	7.7	10.2	9.5	9.2
	Clothing and bedding	7.0	8.7	8.6	6.7	5.4	7.0	4.5	4.9	6.3
	Footwear	0.5	0.7	1.0	1.0	0.9	1.1	0.8	1.0	1.3
	Miscellaneous goods and services	8.8	10.3	12.5	14.4	17.3	20.0	23.4	24.0	26.1
	Durable goods	2.2	7.0	2.3	3.6	2.7	2.7	3.4	4.8	6.1
	Non-food total	24.1	32.8	31.5	33.1	33.7	38.5	42.3	44.2	49.0
Urban	Fuel and light	5.6	6.4	6.9	6.7	6.6	8.0	9.9	8.0	7.6
	Clothing and bedding	5.3	7.1	7.7	6.0	4.7	6.2	4.0	4.7	5.3
	Footwear	0.4	0.6	1.1	1.1	0.9	1.2	0.7	0.9	1.2
	Miscellaneous goods and services	19.2	14.6	20.4	23.5	27.5	32.0	37.2	37.8	39.7
	Durable goods	2.2	8.9	2.7	4.2	3.3	3.7	4.1	6.7	6.3
	Non-food total	32.7	37.6	38.9	41.5	43.0	51.1	55.9	58.1	60.1

Source: NSS unit data, various rounds. Author's calculation

cut-off margins. Interpretations in this regard will be somewhat affected by this limitation. We have made several improvisations and assumptions in constructing the per person incomes:

(a) We have assumed that a rural worker works roughly 22 days per month and an urban worker works 23 days per month (GoI, 2014a).
(b) In an average family of five members, the number of earning members is calculated from respective year's Worker Population Ratio.
(c) Wage multiplied by number of earning members gives the total income of a family of five members. Income per person is accordingly derived.

These assumptions were used to draw the separate rural and urban per person income lines from respective daily average wage rates (GoI, 2014a). Per person expenditure on non-food items within 10% neighbourhood of 2700 kcal per consumer unit per day is calculated as a percentage of the two income lines. We chose this group as they are at the cut off margins of calorie levels and observing their non-food expenditure against the income lines that we have constructed would show the stress that their trend of non-food requirement would create on the food budget, if they are faced with such incomes. The real object of observation is not the actual percentage of non-food expenditure in casual labour income/regular salaried income, but the trend of proportional relation between the two.

Stress of Non-Food Requirements

We observe that the period of rising non-food expenditure as percentage of income (1993–1994 to 2004–2005) is marked by steadily increasing proportion of calorie deficient people (Fig. 20.4). With increasing pressure of non-food requirements, stress on the food budget increased leading to declining intakes of calories. Hence the mismatch between changes in non-food requirements and incomes is a strong reason for declines in calorie intake.

Pressure of Burgeoning Food Prices

However, increase in the proportion of calorie-deficient people (or decline in calorie intakes) is not limited to the period of increasing non- food requirements, relative to income. It continued during 2004–2005 to 2009–2010, despite stagnating/declining non-food expenditure's proportion to income. An important reason appears to be accelerating food price inflation during this period (Fig. 20.5), which eroded additional nominal disposable income for spending on food that became available due to slackening of non-food expenditure (relative to income).

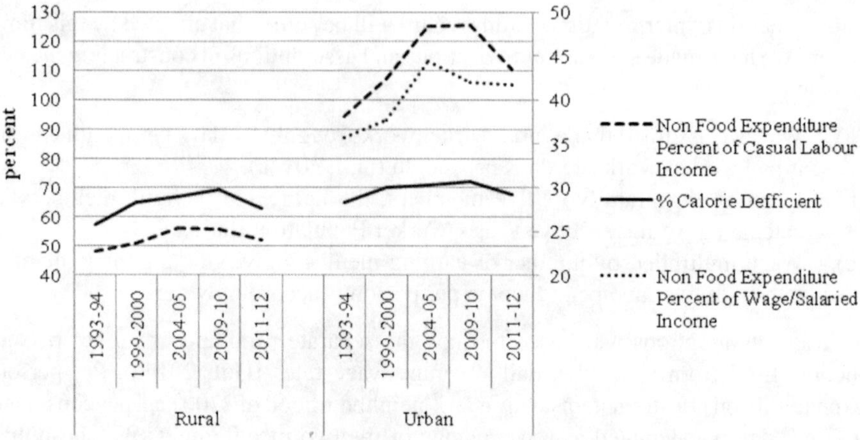

Fig. 20.4 Non-food expenditure as percentage of income and percentage of calorie deficient persons. *Source* NSS unit data, various rounds. Author's calculation

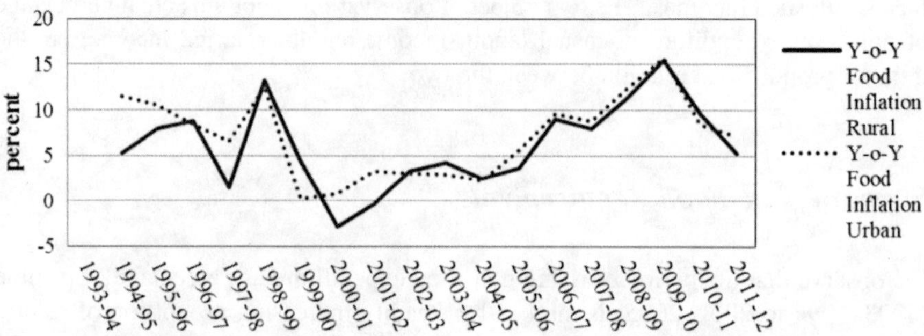

Fig. 20.5 Year on year food inflation. *Source* NSS unit data, various rounds. Author's calculation

Effect on Food Budget

The combined effect of these two factors, non-food requirements and food prices, appear to determine the food budget that an individual can afford. Any income increase will not translate in increase in food budget if income increase gets absorbed by the increase of non-food requirements and food prices. If we assume that the average of increase in non-food requirements and food prices represents the stress on food budget, only an income increase that can overcome this stress can increase food consumption and calorie intakes. It is only in 2011–2012 that income increase outstripped the combined increase of non-food requirements and food prices (Fig. 20.6). The year 2011–2012 saw a considerable increase in expenditure on food compared to 2009–2010 (Fig. 20.7), resulting in an increase in calorie intakes and decline in proportion of calorie-deficient people.

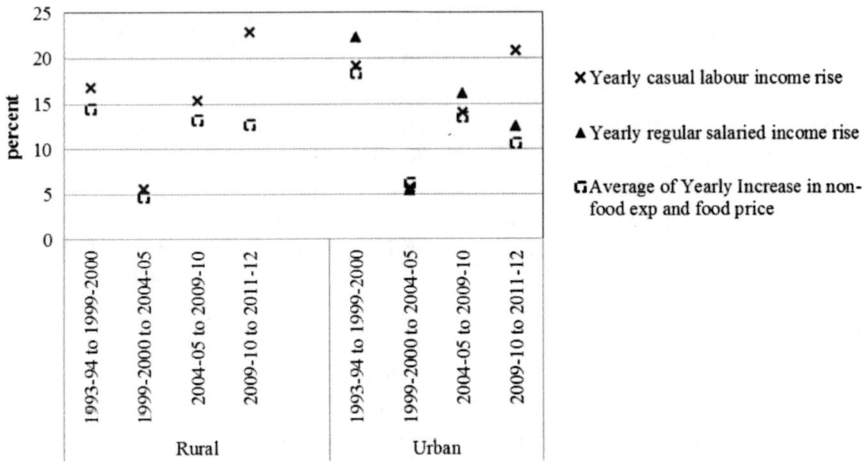

Fig. 20.6 Increase in income vs. non-food expenditure and food inflation. *Source* NSS unit data, various rounds. Author's calculation

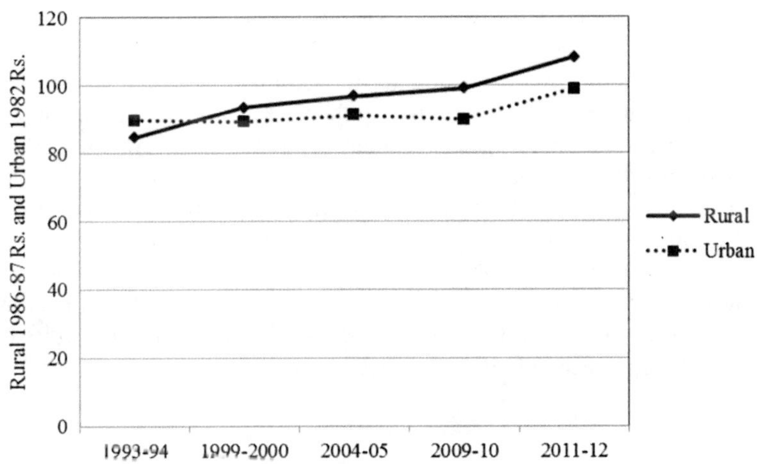

Fig. 20.7 Real average expenditure on food. *Source* NSS unit data, various rounds. Author's calculation

Conclusion

Thus evidences show that the increasing pressure on food budget in the 1990s and the 2000s caused decline in calorie intakes resulting in increasing proportions of people falling below cut off level of calorie intake. A substantial rise in wages particularly of the poorer sections of workers like casual labourers, in both the rural and urban areas, in 2011–2012 compared to 2009–2010 seems to be a major contributing factor to improvement in calorie intake in 2011–2012, which is consistent with our earlier observation that such improvement has taken place even at the lower end. Two things become clear with these evidences. First of all, declines in calorie intakes in the 1990s and 2000s can in no way be termed as voluntary—in the sense that people are choosing to spend more on non-food items by sacrificing calories 'under no constraint'— because in 2011–2012, calorie intakes increased even with increasing share of non-food expenditure as wage rise (coupled with decelerating food inflation) could accommodate both. Secondly, it is amply clear that people would prefer to increase their food intake if they can afford, indicating a state of insatiable hunger that exists in our country. The only factor that is contributing to it is the lack of purchasing power among the country's vast majority of population.

The importance of crucial welfare programmes in protecting people's purchasing power needs to be emphasised here. Because there are ample evidences that improvement of purchasing power and calorie intakes in the latest year of 2011–2012 was due to relative strengthening of some of the social welfare programmes in the recent years. Two welfare programmes, the National Rural Guarantee Scheme (NREGS) and the PDS, particularly stand out as important factors enhancing people's purchasing power through providing livelihood security and protecting against increasing food prices. The initiation of the rural employment guarantee scheme, though far from playing its role to the desired extent, has had a positive impact, particularly on infant and maternal nutrition (Dev 2011; Nair et al., 2013). With such high rural-to-urban migration rates, with the migrant urban labour having familial ties in rural areas, such rural welfare schemes have positive impacts on urban areas as well. On the other hand, PDS, even in its truncated, 'targeted' form as compared to the previous 'universal' form has improved in efficiency since mid-2000 (Basu & Das, 2015). Both these programmes are now under threat of dilution, or worse, of being dismantled. While NREGS is showing signs of getting weakened with expenditure cuts, the new Expert Committee is advocating dismantling of the PDS. Such a notion of 'development' that subverts important components of social and economic welfare of the majority of the population can by no means be called pro-people or inclusive in its nature. This policy direction can only impede universal healthcare, not strengthen it.

Notes

1. For a few food items, nutrient conversion is based on its value (INR) consumption.
2. Taking the calorie requirement of an average male in the age group 20–39 doing sedentary work as the norm, the average calorie requirements of males and females of other age groups are expressed as a ratio to this norm. For more details, see GoI (2014c: 8).
3. Monthly Per Capita Expenditure (MPCE) is deflated by Consumer Price Indices. Consumer Price Index for agricultural labourers and for industrial workers were used for rural and urban areas respectively.
4. The use of logarithm makes it possible to condense large individual data sets from different NSS rounds for each year.

5. Increasing preference for costlier food items—that give fewer calories per rupee spent (at constant prices)—can be visualised as a situation where at a given level of total expenditure, calories decline even with food expenditures remaining the same; however, it makes no sense that there is an increasing preference for costlier food yet food expenditure itself is falling.

References

Basu, D., & Das, D. (2015, 17 February). A flawed approach to food security. *The Hindu.*

Chandrasekhar, C.P., & Ghosh, J. (2007,March 20). Self-employment as opportunity or challenge. *The Hindu Business Line.*

Clark, G., Huberman, M., & Lindert, P. (1995). A British food puzzle, 1770–1850. *The Economic History Review, 48*(2), 215–237.

Deaton, A. (2010). Understanding the mechanisms of economic development. *Journal of Economic Perspectives, 24*(3), 3–16.

Deaton, A., & Dreze, J. (2009). Food and nutrition in india: Facts and interpretations. *Economic and Political Weekly, 44*(7), 42–65.

Dev, S. M. (2011). *NREGS and child well-being* (Working Paper 4). Mumbai, Indira Gandhi Institute of Development Research.

Du, S., Lu, B., Zhai, F., & Popkin, B. M. (2002). A new stage of the nutrition transition in China. *Public Health Nutrition., 5*(1A), 169–174.

Government of India. (2001, May). *Level and pattern of consumer expenditure in India 1999–2000.* Report No. 457 (55/1.0/3). National Sample Survey Organisation, Ministry of Statistics and Programme Implementation.

Government of India. (2014a, January). *Employment and unemployment situation in India 2011–12.* Report No. 554(68/10/1). National Sample Survey Organisation, Ministry of Statistics and Programme Implementation.

Government of India. (2014b, February). *Level and pattern of consumer expenditure in India 2011–2012.* Report No. 555 (68/1.0/1). National Sample Survey Organisation, Ministry of Statistics and Programme Implementation.

Government of India. (2014c, October). *Nutritional intake in India 2011–12.* Report No. 560 (68/1.0/1). National Sample Survey Organisation, Ministry of Statistics and Programme Implementation.

Meng, X, Gong, X., & Wang, Y. (2004). Impact of income growth and economic reform on nutrition availability in urban China: 1986–2000. *Economic Development and Cultural Change, 57*(2), 261–295.

Nair, M., Ariana, P., Ohuma, E. O., Gray, R., De Stavola, R. B., & Webster, P. (2013). Effect of the Mahatma Gandhi National Rural Employment Guarantee Act (MGNREGA) on malnutrition of Infants in Rajasthan, India: A mixed methods study. *PLoS ONE, 8*(9), e75089. https://doi.org/10.1371/journal.pone.0075089

Papola, T.S., & Sahu, P. P. (2012, March). *Growth and structure of employment in India: Long-term and post-reform performance and the emerging challenge.* Institute for Studies in Industrial Development, Indian Council of Social Science Research.

Patnaik, U. (2013, October 5). Poverty trends in India 2004–05 to 2009–10: Updating poverty estimates and comparing official figures, 48(40), 43–58.

Radhakrishna, R., Hanumantha Rao, K., Ravi, C., & Reddy, S. B. (2004, July 10). Chronic poverty and malnutrition in 1990s. *Economic and Political Weekly, 39*(28), 3121–3130.

Rao, C. H. H. (2000, January 22). Declining demand for food grains in rural India: Causes and implications. *Economic and Political Weekly, 35*(4), 201–206.

Sen, A., & Himanshu. (2004a, September 25). Poverty and inequality in India (II) widening disparities during the 1990s. *Economic and Political Weekly, 39*(39), 4361–4375.

Sen, A., & Himanshu. (2004b, September 18). Poverty and inequality in India (I),' *Economic and Political Weekly, 39*(38), 4247–4263.

Chapter 21
Is There an Escape Route from the Smog of COVID-19 Pandemic?

Imrana Qadeer and Sourindra Mohan Ghosh

Responses to COVID-19 differ across countries depending upon their socio-cultural, economic and political contexts and the strength of their health systems. The pandemic unfolded in India over the months of February and March 2020 amidst a great social and political turmoil. Except for Kerala the response of the initially affected States was slow. Around mid-March, a high powered policy making and monitoring committee was set up and the 123 year old Epidemic Diseases Act (EDA) 1897—giving unlimited powers to the state—was promulgated. The Disaster Management Act-2005 was invoked to provide the administrative framework for a 21 day nationwide lockdown from 25th March. Together they made the pandemic control a highly centralised, harsh, bureaucratic exercise; led by the Home Ministry and its police, while the professional inputs remained docile and compliant with official assurances of health coverage. The WHO welcomed the Indian strategy as pioneering. The vocabulary of aggression, fighting a war, control and elimination dominated the political as well as the scientific language with a focus on international travellers and the Indians abroad. A fact ignored was that the new viruses are a part of our destructive relationship with the environment where biological control through technology may help ignore significant relational distortions in society because of business interests.

The Indian health system that normally deals with emergency situations was itself in a crisis with long standing conflicts of interest of a society riddled with caste and class contradictions that had distorted the post- independent dream of an integrated health service sector providing basic care irrespective of people's capacity to pay.

This chapter is based on a published paper titled, "Covid-19 Beyond biological Dynamics", Social Change July 24, 2020.

I. Qadeer (✉)
Council for Social Development, New Delhi, India

S. M. Ghosh
Centre for Economic Studies and Planning, Jawaharlal Nehru University, New Delhi, India

I. Qadeer et al. (eds.), *Universalising Healthcare in India*,
https://doi.org/10.1007/978-981-16-5872-3_21

The shift from welfare state policies to a neo-liberal order in 1990s under Structural Adjustment and Health Sector Reforms (HSR) meant transforming health service into a commodity, thereby increased inequality of access, shrinking public sector with corporatisation and commercialisation, public private partnerships, and health insurances. The result was higher costs of medical care, neglect of primary care, receding access forthe poor and declining quality of services. The economy too was already shaky with decelerating real wage growth since 2014 (Kundu, 2018) and rising unemployment in the more recent period. It was in such a context that COVID-19 pandemic (declared a public health emergency of international concern by the WHO on 30 January) reached India. Its first case was reported on 30 January jumping to a hundred by 14 March. Three days later WHO declared it a Pandemic.

The challenge as understood by the experience elsewhere was an early containment of prevalence to restrict further spread of a very fast spreading pathogen which, even though harmless for 80% affected, can lead to serious morbidity in 15–20% of the affected population calling for hospitalisation; of these 4% may need critical care. High prevalence could lead to stress on health services and higher fatalities among older age groups. These proportions depend upon the rate at which the virus reproduces (R0), efficiency of case detection and care provided. Given the inadequate attention the Pandemic received over February and March and facing the possibility of exponential growth, a stringent national lockdown was implemented without taking people into confidence or organising for the subsistence of the working population in the cities.

This paper deals with both the delay and the handling of the pandemic under the lockdown when science and rationality were overshadowed by political expediency in India. It then explores the post lockdown period to look at what institutional shifts took roots and the contemporary thrust of policy. Based on these some conclusions are drawn.

The Delay

Surveillance was initially restricted to airport disembarkations at metropolitan cities (leaving all other modes of transport) and limited to temperature screening. The airports were not strict. Household tracking and contact tracing mostly left out service staff of the households of international travellers. Indian Council Medical Research (ICMR) guidelines for testing were narrow, testing only those with breathlessness and flue like symptoms. The number of tests done and the available laboratories were inadequate. The efforts at making personal prevention possible through washing hands, maintaining physical distance, and avoiding crowds were relevant only for those who had the means to do so as the majority of the urban working class living in slums and congested colonies did not have the luxury of adequate housing, water supply and sanitation, nor the ability to procure sanitizers. The administration was busy with confronting citizens' secular protests regarding government's new policies on citizenship, preparing for the US president's first visit to India, and 'handling' the unique virus of communalism that was provoked in Delhi by the end of February.

Hit by the quick doubling of COVID-19 by mid-March and prompted by the desire to be in control and appear to act decisively, the political leadership's knee jerk reaction was a national lockdown that hit the 92 million urban informal workers out of the total 401 million informal non-agricultural workers (ILO, 2018). The inability of public health experts to assert alternative plans for investing to improve surveillance and community participation, strengthen services, or to insist on a limited lockdown that protected smaller vulnerable productive units and ensured subsistence for the vulnerable, was conspicuous by its absence.

The Lock Down: A One Dimensional Golden Arrow

While people were exhorted to fight a war against an evil enemy (the virus) and not politicise the crisis, the shaming and pointing of fingers, as in the case of the TablighiJamaat in Delhi (an Islamic missionary movement that promotes the practice of Islamic principles by its members) that was blamed for spreading COVID 19, was used to encourage exclusionary practices against Muslims (Ellis-Petersen & Azizur Rahman, 2020). Even camps set up for the victims of violence in Delhi were arbitrarily wound up, at the same time as the young protesters of the movement against NPR, NRC and CAA (Karnad, 2020) were rounded up. Lockdown thus became a multipurpose instrument of ill-liberal governance—an antithesis of trust building and promoting participation. The war was in fact turned against a section of the citizens and the unsuspecting working class who had no prior information of what was to come. The 64,000 international travellers and their privileged class thus appropriated all existing basic services in the urban space while a large section of the urban informal workers were left high and dry. Their choice of returning home reflected that they no more trusted the promises of shelter and food that came as an afterthought. Social distancing—a brutal fact of Indian life—was thus reasserted. Of the men women and children who walked miles towards the security of their homes, some died in accident, some of hunger and disease, and many were sprayed with inappropriate antiseptic, herded and humiliated by the new public health guardians—the police. Those who reached home discovered that the livelihood issue followed them home. The government then declared that there is no data on these workers and therefore it cannot even give compensation to the next of kin of those who died (PTI, 2020a).

Throughout these months the middle class fully supported the lockdown and blamed the mind set of this untrusting lot. It was only after the exodus of urban workers began that an allocation for relief came—too little, too late. A meagre sum of 15,000 Crores was allocated for the strengthening of health services (PTI, 2020b). No details were provided regarding its actual distribution. The use of police and the draconian EDA 1897 to discipline the public by beating, humiliating and forcing decisions in the name of greater public good highlighted the loss of the very essence of public health—public participation and trust in the state machinery.

When the pandemic did not relent by early April, the Prime Minister himself started asking the States to suggest plans for staggering the lock down. In the process the centre absolved itself of the responsibility for withdrawal, extending it to May 3rd. For the containment of the pandemic under the lockdown the participation of private laboratories was encouraged. These labs legally fought for a hike in remuneration with the support of ICMR officials-against the recommendations of their own experts, who wanted free testing for all with government subsidies. Yet the bulk of testing was done by 156 government labs while 69 private labs contributed marginally. Production of ventilators, PPEs, sanitizers became incentives for private industry participation (Laxmanan & Nayyar, 2020; Sathish, 2020). The Minister of Petroleum and Natural Gas proposed using surplus grain for ethanol production for hand sanitisers (SNS, 2020) while families rendered jobless went without food. Instead of strengthening the public sector infrastructure, even for clinical management of serious COVID-19 cases and its comorbidities, the private sector was encouraged. As of March 17, there was one isolation bed per 84,000 Indians in government hospitals, and one quarantine bed per 36,000 Indians (Ghosh, 2015). Their total bed strength was 727,341. Although they handled only 10% of the critical COVID load according to the reports (Raghavan et al., 2020), yet, for the government, promoting the private sector came first even though their cost was very high. Reports also came in that in some private hospitals, cost for ten days in the wards was Rs. 110,000 and for a day in the ICU it was Rs. 50,000 (Ganguly, 2020). The Ministry's advisory for the rural areas made it clear that no additional resources were available, that they had to depend on what they had though the workload of front level workers was increased and no additional remuneration or protection was to be given (GoI, 2020). Due to the paucity of services, non-COVID-19 emergencies were neglected along with critical routine maternal care and preventive services (Ghosh & Qadeer, 2020). Hunger added to this crisis by increasing human vulnerability as has been established by studies of its role in tuberculosis and Malaria (Bhargava et al., 2014; Zurbrigg, 2019).

The States were not consulted despite health being a State subject and each State being the best judge of local conditions and resources; planning thus was highly centralised. Despite the low level of testing rates, the Health Ministry projected the apparent linear rise in prevalence charts as evidence of the doubling rate slowing under lockdown. An extension of the lockdown was justified to break the chain of infection (Perappadan, 2020). This was the real goal according to the chair of the expert committee, and would be lost "if the lockdown ends abruptly" (PTI, 2020c). The Health Ministry and the ICMR officials also refused to accept that community transmission was occurring even when their own researchers published evidence (Koshy, 2020).

Not only there was no transparency of data, there was evidence of lack of cooperation and often conflict between the scientific and the administrative wings of the government (Krishnan, 2020). Open access as well as reporting by investigators that ensures that information is shared was not encouraged. The government went to the Supreme Court pleading that journalists should publish data on COVID-19 only after official clearance, to avoid false alarm. Though the court rejected this, it did advise-news channels to refer to and publish government data (EDT, 2020), thus absolving the government for not keeping the public informed on its own.

The prolonged lockdown perhaps caused greater harm than the pandemic itself. It destroyed the economy and not only harmed the workers and their families but also the health of all the elderly, chronically ill, pregnant women and children. COVID-19 actually started peaking once the lockdown was gradually withdrawn. The economy of the cities could not revive given the exodus of workers and the losses incurred by the small entrepreneurs. Joblessness due to economic breakdown increased further, and people's ability to cope with this morbidity load as well as food shortages grew weaker. Yet, it was proposed to use the harvested rice for production of sanitisers Unemployment rose to 27.1 in early May, 127.1 million lost work of which 91.3 million were daily wage labourers, hawkers and small traders, the rest being salaried workers (Vyas, 2020). Harvesting and procurements of the Rabi wheat crop were affected due to distances, market protocols and labour shortage that made selling difficult and farmers incurred losses (Vohra, 2020).

The criticism of the lockdown mounted and inevitably its unlocking began from June 1 by which time already 3,76,305 cases were reported, that climbed to 5,66,840 by lockdown two announcing further concessions on first of July. Maharashtra, Tamil Nadu, Delhi and Gujarat remained the leading states (Babu Nikhil, 2020). On the 29th of August 2020, the lockdown was further restricted to the Containment Zones by the Ministry of Home Affairs with its guidelines for activities permitted. The issues of shortage of medical personnel, infections and deaths among doctors and health workers, their ostracisation by the public, non-payment of salaries by institutions, and work overload with consistently rising daily cases were making the situation difficult to cope with[1] despite all attempts of the state to engage the private sector. A major question therefore that needs to be answered was, how did India use the time that it gained by imposing the lockdown?

Building and Strengthening Infrastructure

The 2019 scores on the Global Health Security Index reflect pandemic preparedness and capacity and ranked India 57th out of 195 countries; much lower than Asian middle-income, Indonesia, and Thailand.[2] This was also the period when the Niti-Aayoghad come out with a "Scheme to link new and/or existing private medical colleges with functional district hospitals through PPP". Fifty percent beds were to be privatised charging market rates, with the justification that this will subsidise the remaining 'regulated beds' (Jha, 2020). Apart from running the district hospitals, the PPP model was also to create more hospitals in tier 2 and tier 3 cities to be empanelled under the Ayushman Bharat scheme in 112 aspirational districts. The model was to apply to medical colleges as well.[3] This step got a thumbs up from the industry.

An analysis of the pre-COVID-19 year in terms of proportion of vacant beds to handle additional load of patients, patient perception of in-patient care, non-availability of well-equipped ICUs in adequate numbers in some states and, state spending on public sector health leaves much to be desired (Ghosh & Qadeer, 2020). This undermining reflected lack of preparedness of public sector health services. By May 2020, 60,948 ventilators were purchased but only 23,699 were installed in public hospitals across India (Sharma, 2020) reflecting laxity to take advantage of the lockdown period to prepare the country's dilapidated public sector health infrastructure. We are told now that for each case of diagnosed case there may be 100 infections and that deaths recorded are underestimates (Chatterjee, 2020). The poverty of our infrastructure despite its well refurbished private sector therefore is evident.

The government has borrowed from the AIIB and the World Bank US $ 0.5 billion and 1.0 billion respectively for the purpose of fighting the pandemic but there is no clarity on how much of this is being invested to strengthen and expand the public sector institutions at different levels, health personnel training institutions, research and government medical colleges and how much is subsidising the private sector via PPPs as in the case of PMJAY which now has a special component for COVID-19 treatment.[4] Despite the push to promote PMJAY, the cover provided comes to about 3% only of the diagnosed COVID-19 casesby June (Mathew & Singh, 2020). This 1.5 billion dollar loan is said to be invested in social security of migrant workers and emergency financing to support better screening, contact tracing, and laboratory diagnostics; procure personal protective equipment; and set up new isolation wards, surveillance, digital health, and strengthening hospitals: but its distribution over public and private sectors remains obfuscated. Even in the Press Information Bureau Report of September 2020, the health Minister claiming achievements over the year does not make this differentiation.[5]

Jayaprakash Muliyil, an eminent epidemiologist, commented that what we achieved by the lockdown is not commensurate with the damage from it. He opined that we need to put all our money in hospitals, and provide oxygen for patients; this will save more lives. Others commented on haphazard travel restrictions, shortage of emergency supplies, testing kits, low testing rates, delay in local production and red tapism. Lack of transparency in decision making and denial of community transmission of the virus were also critical (Pulla, 2020; Jose, 2020). These negative policy outcomes are closely linked to the state's commitment to depend heavily on the private sector at the cost of its public sector health services—wasting its strengths and potential. Comparing India and China, Baru argues, "The Chinese realized the need to strengthen primary level care and surveillance system after the SARS epidemic. In addition, they also sought to improve coverage of public insurance schemes for hospitalisation. This led to a fourteen-fold increase in the State expenditure between 2003 and 2018. The lessons from SARS hold true for COVID-19 as well". Even then in China, she argues that the link between primary level care and hospitals is weak and the commercialised public hospitals have led to a fragmented health system. A weak primary care system due to a hospital based legacy was the reason for the delayed response in controlling the COVID-19 outbreak (Baru Rama, 2020). This applies to Indiaeven more as evident by the declining public sector performance revealed by the post COVID data analysis of NHM 2019 April-2020 March. It reflected significant declines in non-COVID-19 services such as immunisation, ante natal care, emergency obstetric care, inpatient and OPD care and DOTs registration over the previous year in 627 districts. Similarly ICU beds were insufficient in states most affected (Ghosh & Qadeer, 2020). Whether the Loans were used to fill in this gap in public sector infrastructure, and how much remains is yet to be made explicit, though the Minister in the September PIB report, projects over all infrastructural improvement achievements.

Another feature of the post lockdown period is that the state, obsessed with international comparisons, fails to recognise the contextual differences and the fact that Indian innovative research and health infrastructure are intertwined. Shahid Jameel, India's foremost virologist suggests that the ICMR should allow access to the samples collected from COVID-19 patients to help the leading sequencing laboratories identify the new variants of SARS-CoV-2 virus from across the country to fill the gaps in our knowledge (Jameel, 2020). Unfortunately, far from involving the academic institutions, there are reports of lack of communication and coordination between ICMR, the National Centre for Communicable Diseases (NCDC) and the Health Ministry regarding COVID-19 related activities and data (Qadeer & Ghosh, 2020). Amirullah Khan, a Professor of economics with his vast experience of working with the Ministry of Finance and UNDP, comments on the poor research financing in India where only 0.6% of GDP is invested as against 2.1% by China. He points to the glaring public health challenges, despite which the budget for its apex medical research organisation is one of the lowest among government agencies for science research. Also, unlike other countries where research is funded in equal measure by the private sector, much of the R&D funding here is provided by the government (Khan, 2020). Instead of correcting this imbalance, the Finance Minister has granted Rs. 900 crore to the Department of Biotechnology in November under the COVID Suraksha Mission, for research and development of the Indian COVID vaccine.

The Present Policy Concern

Whether it is the removal of the vulnerable by deaths or the rising herd immunity, India hit the peak of the pandemic by mid-September 2020 when it reported a7 day rolling average of daily new confirmed cases of 93,198.6 and a 7 day rolling average daily deaths of 1166.6 on Sept. 19. These numbers declined to 21,312.4 (23% reduction) and 291.7 respectively (on Dec 28).[6] Some states still continue to struggle but the issue of building public sector infrastructure has been side lined. A parliamentary committee recently mooted the idea of a comprehensive Public Health Act at the national level with legal provisions for governmental checks and controls over private hospitals. It recognised their crass exploitation of COVID-19 patients and the exorbitant charges slapped on them (Nair Sobhana, 2020). Yet, the state's efforts to save its earlier strategy to tame the private sector while encouraging its participation is still being pursued.

Yet another diversion is publicising the hope of an accessible, effective and safe vaccine to be delivered by our public sector network for universal immunisation. A safe and effective vaccine is welcome but the problem lies in not following the due process of even the given norms of emergency use of a new product. Talk of vaccine availability started in political circles in August[7] and became louder with the celebration of August 15th; then before the Bihar election its free availability for the State was announced. Also, any questioning on such premature promises was considered un-Indian and a criticism of Indian scientists. Pfizer India was allowed to apply to the drug regulator for permission to import its vaccine for sale and distribution without the requirement for local clinical trials. Serum Institute of India Ltd. (AstraZeneca's Indian vaccine partner) applied for emergency use authorisation using data from Phase-III trials that are still going on locally, as well as in Brazil and the UK. Hyderabad-based Bharat Biotech sought the nod for Covaxin which is being indigenously developed in collaboration with the Indian Council of Medical Research (ICMR). The Subject Expert Committee (SEC) of the Central Drugs Standard Control Organisation (CDSCO) stopped vaccine use saying they need more data on efficacy, adverse events and safety (Ramachandran, 2020). However in the first week of January Covaxin and Covashield got the approved by the Controller General of India—the first under the trial mode and the second only for emergency use. The contradictions are several: first and foremost being absence of analysis of phase III study results; secondly, that Covaxin, cleared only for emergency use, is to be marketed commercially; thirdly, under the trial mode and emergency use labels, providers are taking consent, but not ensuring legal responsibility of the companies for adverse reactions—a common global practice. Other remaining issues are: do the phase III healthy volunteers necessarily represent the population characteristics, especially when the general population has significant undernutrition? Does immunogenicity necessarily mean protection? Do all vaccines prevent infection or only disease progression in individuals? Does unequal protection to older population, and the false sense of safety due to unknown period of protection make the vaccinated vulnerable? If its effectiveness is only 60–80 and 94% infected population recovers from disease as of now then, what is its utility when already the epidemic is receding due to natural causes in India? Or if mutated variants do cause mass re-infections, then can our poor primary care grassroots network support a time bound universal (or near universal) vaccination drive? Above all, now that almost 50% of the so called effective produce has been bought by the rich countries, what are the chances of the poor among the underdeveloped countries actually getting the vaccine when the companies are hoping to make their entry into the COVID market for profits? The share market around vaccine firms is already expanding.

A safe and effective vaccine may help even the descending limb of the pandemic as it accelerates the decline in disease incidence. That is why addressing and disseminating the above gaps in knowledge is critical as it points out how careful the state as well as people needs to be when yet another isolated, single protection strategy as a vertical programme is imposed. With poor preparedness, Universal Immunisation Programme can barely take this additional burden requiring very especial inputs for monitoring adverse effects, surveillance for efficacy, cold chain for storage and transportation, and an army of trained providers. It is not surprising then that a large proportion of the World Bank and AIIB loan money is being invested into production, purchase and distribution of vaccines. Yet again, will it be at the cost of treatment and prevention of non-COVID-19 ailments such as tuberculosis; and the rising scourge of child under nutrition? India's basic services, as they are, failed to provide full coverage with even the six basic immunisations beyond 61% of the under five children. The field workers are overstretched and the private sector does not believe in providing free preventive services. It will enter the scene only when the vaccine acquires high monetary value, as it did with the diagnostic tests.

Conclusions

The lessons of the initial months were, that lockdown can at best buy time to strengthen health services provided subsistence for people can be maintained. It alone does not break the chain of transmission. That testing rates must use cases examined as the denominator, and not total populations, in order to appreciate that rising levels of prevalence with increased testing indicates that the peak has yet to arrive; and inadequate number of tests with a slowly rising prevalence does not reflect control. Tracking cases, tracing contacts, quarantine, isolation and treatment is the only way to actually contain spread for which good infrastructural facilities and public participation and cooperation in surveillance and trust is the key. Strengthening basic services, supplies of PPEs and oxygen are critical as is not neglecting serious non-COVID-19 morbidities. When a lock down is used for containing social conflicts as well, it inevitably undermines trust and the possibility of citizen's cooperation. Finally, a prolonged and harsh lockdown becomes counterproductive as it undermines the economy, destroys subsistence of the vulnerable and their food security, trapping them into hunger, undernutrition and increased load of unattended non-COVID ailments. And this is what happened in India.

In the post lockdown period, officially its negative impact was never analysed despite its underestimated deaths and neglect of non-COVID-19 patients. Only the slow rise of the pandemic was talked about. Strengthening public sector infrastructure never acquired centre space in this debate nor was its fragmentation rectified. Efforts at regulating the private sector were not effective, permitting huge profits to be extracted from those who had deep pockets or insurance covers. The brunt of the crisis fell on the shoulders of the public sector providers who remained uncared for. The insured anyway constituted a very small proportion (68.2% less than the official claim of 109 million families as reported by the 75th round of NSS[8]). State support for cooperation and collaboration between Indian research organizations and health care institutions to develop clinical, population, and genetic epidemiology of COVID 19, to produce new knowledge, and effective therapies was also weak. The economic devastation leading to the poor state of nutrition, as reflected by the 5th National Family Health Survey (NFSH), called for the urgent need of strengthening PDS and feeding programmes. Thus, an important lesson was that the approach to

COVID control has to be systemic and within the national epidemiological context where endemic diseases like tuberculosis kill four times more people in a year even if their prevalence is one fourth of COVID-19. Only a multipronged long term strategy could be the answer, along with the tasks of rebuilding services and lives by providing livelihoods.

The government however, consistently refuses to acknowledge the writing on the wall—the multidimensionality of the problem and the urgency of investing in health service infrastructure. The lop sided financing of public sector health services continues with the public sector losing resources and shrinking, in the name of 'partnership'. Even the loans that came in the name of COVID-19 management support, are servicing those components that promote industrial production of consumables like ventilators, PPEs, vaccine production etc. which have not necessarily reached peripheral public hospitals including district hospitals. Institutions of primary health care and their personnel remain neglected. Thus, the techno-centric, market oriented, exclusionary strategy to deal with COVID-19 is propelled by international financing and brings to the fore the power of corporate institutions and their global links to policy and planning in India. Once again the people are being sold the dream of yet another silver bullet—a vaccine—which is neither universally available as promised by the PM[9] nor easy to deliver given the state of the infrastructure. The Niti Aayog even sought the help of the Election Commission for distributing the vaccine at the cost of further fragmentation of the service delivery system[10]. Technology then dominates and simplifies a complex situation. The peasants are questioning similar efforts at corporatisation of agriculture and the destruction of India's food security. In the clutches of the experts and officials and political leaders will public health find a way to clear the smog?

Notes

1. https://www.devex.com/news/shortage-of-health-care-workers-plagues-india-s-fight-against-covid-19-98108 accessed on 24.12.2020.
2. https://www.brookings.edu/blog/future-development/2020/07/02/how-well-is-india-responding-to-covid-19/ accessed on 24.12.2020.
3. https://www.hindustantimes.com/india-news/in-budget-2020-21-health-sector-allocations-witness-8-jump/story-OQWW8vQJ19Dbt23HZcToxN.html accessed on 25.12.2020.
4. https://economictimes.indiatimes.com/news/economy/finance/asian-infrastructure-investment-bank-approves-500-million-loan-to-support-indias-covid-19-operations/articleshow/75618374.cms accessed on 28.12.2020.
5. https://pib.gov.in/PressReleasePage.aspx?PRID=1653947 accessed 24.12.2020.
6. https://ourworldindata.org/coronavirus-data-explorer?country=~IND&region=World&casesMetric=true&interval=total&perCapita=true&smoothing=0&pickerMetric=location&pickerSort=asc accessed on 26.12.2020.
7. https://health.economictimes.indiatimes.com/news/industry/india-to-have-coronavirus-vaccine-by-2020-end-harsh-vardhan/77698942 accessed on 27.12.2020.

8. https://cegh.net/article/S2213-3984(20)30081-6/fulltext 30.12.2020.
9. https://economictimes.indiatimes.com/news/politics-and-nation/govt-making-u-turn-on-pms-assurance-that-every-citizen-will-get-covid-vaccine-congress/articleshow/79535558.cms accessed on 27. 12.2020.
10. https://economictimes.indiatimes.com/news/politics-and-nation/health-ministry-niti-aayog-officials-likely-to-meet-ec-top-brass-over-covid-vaccine-distribution-sources/articleshow/79782380.cms?from=mdr accessed on 30.12.2020.

References

Babu Nikhil, M. (2020, June 30). Coronavirus India lockdown Day 98 updates. *The Hindu*. https://www.thehindu.com/news/national/india-coronavirus-lockdown-june-30-2020-live-updates/article31950742.ece accessed on 26.12.2020

Baru Rama, V. (2020). Health systems preparedness during COVID-19 pandemic: China and India. *Indian Journal of Public Health, 64*(6), 96–98.

Bhargava, A., Benedetti, A., Oxlade, O., Pai, M., & Menziesthe, M. (2014). Undernutrition and the incidence oftuberculosis in India: National and subnational estimates of the population-attributable fraction related to undernutrition. *National Medical Journal of India, 27*(3), 128–133. Google Scholar I Medline I ISI.

Chatterjee, P. (2020, September 5). Is India missing COVID-19 deaths? *Lancet, 396*(10252), 657.

EDT. (2020, March 31). Indian Supreme Court denies government request for prior censorship of Covid-19 news. *Committee to Protect Journalists*. https://cpj.org/2020/03/indian-supreme-court-denies-government-request-for.php Google Scholar

Ellis-Petersen, H. & Azizur Rahman, S. (2020). Coronavirus conspiracy theories targeting Muslims spread in India. *The Guardian*. https://www.theguardian.com/world/2020/apr/13/coronavirus-conspiracy-theories-targeting-muslims-spread-in-india/ Accessed 20 April, 2020

Ganguly, A. (2020, May 6). Private hospitals have used the pandemic to profiteer. *Mumbai Mirror*. http://mumbaimmirror.Indiatimes.com/coronavirus/news/private-hospitals-have-used-the-pandemic-to-profiteer/articleshow/75566265.cms/ Google Scholar

Ghosh Sourindra, M., & Qadeer, I. (2020, September 5). Public good perspective of public health: Evaluating health systems response to COVID-19. *Economic &Political Weekly, LV*(36), 39–46.

Ghosh, A. (2015, May 21). NRHM 10 years on: Short of centres by 20–30%, of doctors by 70–80%. *The Indian Express*. https://indianexpress.com/article/india/india-others/nrhm-10-yrs-on-short-of-centres-by-20-30-of-doctor accessed on 19.1.2021

GoI (Government of India). (2020). *Enabling delivery of essential health services during the COVID-19 outbreak: Guidance note*. Ministry of Health and Family Welfare, New Delhi. https://www.mohfw.gov.in/pdf/EssentialservicesduringCOVID19updated0411201.pdf Google scholar

ILO (International Labour Organization). (2018). India wage report: Wage policy for decent work and inclusive growth. https://www.ilo.org/wcmsp5/groups/public/—asia/—ro-bangkok/—sro-new_delhi/documents/publication/wcms_638305.pdf

Jameel, S. (2020, December 28). Beware the UK mutant. *The Indian Express*, p. 11, https://indianexpress.com/article/explained/uk-mutant coronavirus-covid-death-covid-vaccine-7122548/ accessed 28.12.2020

Jha, V. (2020, January 15). Public sector healthcare is dying in India. How can we resurrect it? *The Wire*. https://thewire.in/health/public-sector-healthcare-niti-aayog accessed on 27.12.2020

Jose, S. (2020, April 11). Five mistakes India could have done without. *The Wire*. https://thewire.in/health/five-covid-19-policy-mistakes-india-could-have-done-without

Karnad, R. (2020, March 24). Farewell to ShaheenBagh, as political togetherness yields to social distance. *The Wire*. https://thewire.in/politics/farewell-to-shaheen-bagh-as-political-togetherness-yields-to-social-distance Google Scholar

Khan, A. (2020, April 28). Why India must take lead in COVID fight and boost R&D expenditure, *The Quint*. 2020, https://www.thequint.com/voices/opinion/coronavirus-pandemic-india-vaccine-research-and-develoment-health-infrastructure-govt-spending#read-more 29.12.2020

Koshy, J. (2020, April 9). Corona virus: ICMR study points to community spread. *The Hindu*. https://www.thehindu.com/news/national/coronavirus-icmr-study-points-to-community-transmission/article31303270.ece accessed on 29.12.2020.

Krishnan, V. (2020, May 12). Epidemiologists say India's centre of disease control withheld COVID data since pandemic began. *The Caravan*. https://caravanmagazine.in/health/epidemiologists-say-india-centre-disease-control-withheld-covid-19-data-since-pandemic-began Google Scholar

Kulkarni, S. (2020, March 28). COVID-19 exposes our public health system. *Deccan Herald*. https://www.deccanherald.com/specials/insight/covid-19-exposes-our-public-health-system-818767.html Google Scholar

Kundu, S. (2018). Rural wage dynamics in India: What role does inflation play? Working Paper Series No. 03. Reserve Bank of India.

Lakshmanan, R., & Nayyar, M. (2020, May 25). Personal protective equipment in India INR 7000 crore industry in the making. SIRU. https://www.investindia.gov.in/siru/personal-protective-equipment-india-INR-7000-cr-industry-in-the-making accessed on 24.12.2020.

Mathew, G., & Singh, S. (2020) Only 5600 health insurance claims—3% of total Covid cases. *The Indian Express*. https://indianexpress.com/article/business/only-5600-health-insurance-claims-coronavirus-6438004/ accessed on 27.12.2020

Nair Sobhana, K. (2020, December 22). House panel moots law to keep a check on private hospitals. *The Hindu*. https://myupsc.com/wp-content/uploads/2020/12/The-Hindu-HD-NewDelhii-22_12.pdf

Perappadan, B. S. (2020, April 15). Coronavirus longer lockdown essential to break chain of infection, says government. *The Hindu*. https://www.thehindu.com/news/national/coronavirus-india-says-longer-lockdown-essential-to-break-chain-of-infection/article31342597.ece Google Scholar

PTI. (2020a, November 15). Unaffected by deaths. *The Hindu*. https://www.thehindu.com/news/national/unaffected-by-deaths-rahul-attacks-govt-on-no-data-on-migrant-labourers-deaths/article32608944.ece

PTI. (2020b, April 9). Government announces Rs 15,000 crore package to ramp up health infra to fight COVID-19. *The New Indian Express*. https://www.newindianexpress.com/nation/2020/apr/09/government-announces-rs-15000-crore-package-to-ramp-up-health-infra-to-fight-COVID-19-2128035.html/ Google Scholar

PTI. (2020c, May 3). Coronavirus: Rise in COVID-19 cases expected to stabilise any time soon, says NitiAayog member V. K. Paul. *The Hindu*. https://www.thehindu.com/news/national/coronavirus-rise-in-COVID-19-cases-expected-to-stabilise-any-time-soon-says-niti-aayog-member-vk-aul/article31494186.ece Google Scholar

Pulla, P. (2020, June 26). The epidemic is growing very rapidly': Indian government adviser fears coronavirus crisis will worsen. *Nature*. https://www.nature.com/articles/d41586-020-01865-w accessed on 28.12.2020

Qadeer, I., & Ghosh, S. M. (2020, July 24). COVID-19: Beyond biological dynamics. *Social Change, 50*(3), 359–384.

Raghavan, P., Barnagarwala, T., & Ghosh, A. (2020, April 30). COVID fight: Govt. system in front, private hospitals do the distancing. *The Indian Express*. https://indianexpress.com/article/india/coronavirus-COVID-19-private-hospitals-6385631/

Ramachandran, R. (2020, January 01). Safety concerns delay vaccine approval in India. *The Frontline*. https://frontline.thehindu.com/the-nation/public-health/covid19-vaccine-update-safety-concerns-delay-coronavirus-vaccine-approval-in-india/article33319710.ece accessed on 29.12.2020

Sathish, D. (2020, April 21). Private players getting into manufacturing PPEs to cash in the opportunity. *Thenew Indian Express*. https://www.newindianexpress.com/states/tamil-nadu/2020/apr/21/private-players-getting-into-manufacturing-ppes-to-cash-in-the-opportunity-2133013.html accessed on 25.12.2020

Sharma, M. (2020, September 24). Coronavirus: 60,948 ventilators purchased but only 23,699 installed in hospitals across India, reveals govt. data. *India Today*. https://www.indiatoday.in/india/story/coronavirus-60-0963-purchased-but-only-23-699-installed-in-hospitals-across-india-reveals-govt-data-1724961-2020-09-24 accessed 22.12.2021

SNS Web. (2020, April 20). Surplus rice produced will be used to manufacture sanitisers': Govt. amid lockdown. *The Statesman*. https://www.thestatesman.com/coronavirus/surplus-rice-produced-will-be-used-to-manufacture-sanitisers-govt-amid-lockdown-1502879413.html

Vohra, R. (2020, April 21). Where do we go with our harvested wheat? *The Hindu BusinessLine*. https://www.thehindubusinessline.com/specials/india-file/where-do-we-go-with-our-harvested-wheat/article31393685.ece [accessed May 14, 2020]

Vyas, M. (2020, May 5). *The jobs bloodbath of April 2020*. Centre for Monitoring Indian Economy. https://www.cmie.com/kommon/bin/sr.php?kall=warticle&dt=2020-05-05%2008:22:21&msec=776 Google Scholar

Zurbrigg, S. (2019). *Epidemic malaria and hunger in colonial Punjab: Weakened by want (the social history of health and medicine in South Asia)*. Routledge.

Postscript

Reflecting upon the shift from a social democratic perspective to the current economic thrust of planning, the chapters in this book focus on two contrasting, though similar sounding visions of universality: the Universal Healthcare, which is now being offered as the panacea for the crisis of public health; and the Comprehensive Primary Healthcare (CPHC), which was not given its due in India. The authors offer insights into the limits of Universal Health Coverage (UHC) in handling the crisis that the health sector faces and its contemporary challenges. Investing in the health of citizens engaged in the economy increases revenues, through higher productivity of labour as well as taxation, and by way of pooling resources to expand appropriate health services as well as employment. Thus, there is a two-way relationship between the health of a people and their economy. However, capital is also generated when sections unable to purchase or pool resources are financed by the state, not to keep them healthy, but for their terminal and tertiary care, and these services are provided by private institutions—specially the fast growing corporate tertiary care institutions—which primarily serve sections that can pay substantive charges. By thus maximising their profits, these private institutions serve the interests of national and international finance. The revenues thus generated keep the global markets breathing, not necessarily the people.

The industrial revolutions, along with the wealth extracted from the Asian and African colonies had overcome the poverty hump in the imperial nations. The consequent experiment with universal provision of health over the 1940s starting from Britain and Saskatchewan district of Canada, funded by the state as a part of welfare services in the post-World War II reconstruction of Europe, had itself become the very basis of capitalist growth. Striving for equity in the distribution of services according to needs distinguished a situation where the required finances could be mobilised. Also, these experiments in UHC did not have to address absolute poverty. In proposing UHC as an alternative to countries with high levels of poverty and social deprivation today to primarily address financial risk protection through "revenue collection, pooling and purchasing" (World Health Organisation (WHO), 2005: 1) as well as external funding the WHO ignores welfare, social equality and, democratic participation as critical. It ignores that if the state does not fully support health

I. Qadeer et al. (eds.), *Universalising Healthcare in India*,
https://doi.org/10.1007/978-981-16-5872-3

interventions for all according to their ability to pay, a certain level of income must be in everyone's reach. It underplays the reality that, for the poorer countries, 'prevention' is not immunisation and health education alone, but addressing issues of food security, drinking water, work, housing and other welfare services which are systemic challenges. As these cannot be purchased by all, and as financial protection of the vulnerable for tertiary and secondary level care alone is an uneconomical way of handling diseases, all these must remain a state obligation. Even if we concede that, given its political constraints, the WHO did its best in suggesting a move from Out-of-Pocket Expenditure (OOPE) as the primary financing model to a mixed financing model (OOPE, insurances and revenues), and ultimately to revenue-based social insurance systems, which countries like Brazil and South Africa and many others are struggling for (People's Health Movement (PHM) et al., 2014), the case of India stands apart.

In India the commitment to the Alma Ata Declaration for Primary Healthcare has been side-lined without much ado since 1980. The explanations vary from resource scarcity to the long period required for a comprehensive approach, the inefficiency of the state health sector, the crisis of catastrophic OOPE, and an existing efficient private sector infrastructure. Hence, the state investment in public sector health has barely improved and supportive welfare services have declined. Also, over the years, direct taxes have declined and indirect taxation has risen pushing up service costs for all sections, making the poor even more vulnerable. Here we briefly explore the overall utility of a given model of UHC, the official attempts to justify it, and underline the need for an alternative strategy.

What Has UHC Contributed and for Whom?

The chapters reveal that UHC in India is not about addressing the complexity of epidemiological priorities through appropriate and affordable technologies; it is about building a demand based hi-tech medical care market for a small section, that also transforms the state into a client by promoting protection of the poor against 'catastrophic expenditure'. It maximises the operation of the medical industry and undermines public institutions in the process. Born out of the state's dependence on global corporate interests, UHC transforms medical care services into profitmaking commodities and changes the nature of public health itself. Within the frame work of neoliberal reforms, UHC is more amenable to working as an engine for economic growth. The logic of 'catastrophic expenditure' lends urgency and an impression of concern for the people, ignoring the issue of comprehensive health as a constitutional right.

The strategies to commoditise and commercialise health services over the 1990s were considered inadequate as introduction of user fees could not add sufficiently to institutional revenues and pushed the poor out (Prinja et al., 2012); private insurances were untenable for the majority; and Public Private Partnerships (PPPs) barely improved public institutions by casualisation of workers, contracting out services and locating private diagnostics in public institutions. Their quality of services, in fact, declined as the service ethos got undermined while private partners got away with huge concessions and unbridled profits. Prevention too has become the domain of unsafe technological interventions. At the turn of the new century then, the union government initiated its Janani Suraksha Yojana (JSY) in 2005 and Rashtriya Swasthya Bima Yojana (RSBY) in 2008. The first state-level insurance scheme (Chiranjivi Scheme in Gujarat) was rolled out in 2006. These so-called insurance schemes (now assurance) offered limited technology packages in new forms of PPPs. State-financed services were offered both by public and private institutions. These schemes empanel much higher proportions of private institutions compared to public institutions, indicating the latter's poor working conditions. The new monetary management strategies, based on prescribed conditions for empanelment and numbers of families registered, did not address the issue of years of resource depletion of public hospitals and their need for strengthening. It only added to the resource depletion and quality declines of public institutions. Their potential to become a cheaper, effective, efficient, ethical, institutional authority, that could compete with, and thus regulate the private sector providers, was thus compromised while the state-financed insurance schemes became a way to shift public resources to the private sector. The OOPE remains high given the insufficient monetary help for hospitalisation and the neglect of basic outpatient services, while the competition within the private sector itself marginalises its primary care providers.

Rising investment in new models of fragmented central and state- financed medical insurance schemes—without simultaneous increase in total investments in the health sector— negatively affected areas of public health other than medical care. Declining finances for the Integrated Child Development Scheme (ICDS), Public Distributive System (PDS), drinking water and National Rural Employees Guarantee Act (NREGA) were also not conducive to the health of the poor. The unregulated cost spirals of health services and basic food rose making more vulnerable those just above the poverty line and left out of health insurance. The poor economic and social conditions in which the diseases of poverty are embedded[1] did not concern the Indian model of UHC. Thus, pushing technology while ignoring the limits of medical care, concerns of equity or coverage, and even evidence, it left the responsibility of the less profitable but basic components of the health service system (maternity care, communicable disease control, training of paramedical personnel, monitoring, drugs, equipment, etc.), to the public sector. The value of people's participation, despite its demonstrated impact as in chapter 18 of this book, was also neglected. The public and private sectors remain functionally uncoordinated and cooperation between them regarding information pooling and running national disease control programmes, or regulation of standards, is conspicuous by its absence. A grave example of this neglect is the current handling of COVID-19 pandemic where vaccines—with trials that do not make their results public—are being pushed as a silver bullet at the cost of infrastructural strengthening, regulatory mechanisms as well as a rational strategy for similar epidemics in future. Clearly, the objectives of the two sectors conflict, and preferences of policy makers for revenue generation stand out as a strong force in the undermining of public institutions and contracting these out for private management.

This fast-transforming health sector is located in a larger context where the focus is on economic growth without much attention to redistribution or improving significantly the purchasing capacity of the people. When health-services become a commodity in such conditions and are brought into an unregulated market of sophisticated technologies, the majority of the working classes cannot access it until the state pays for them. The consequence of this is what we observe today. Political exigencies restrain the government from withdrawing the promise of providing health services. So UHC, by undermining the earlier approach of building a three-tier state health infrastructure or even National Rural Health Mission (NRHM) within district boundaries, pushes commoditisation of medical care services and forces a vast majority to fall into the net of the medical market or state-led insurance schemes for medical care run mostly by private institutions.

There have been improvements in average health and nutrition indicators over the past twenty years (1993–2012) and economic growth is important in this. But the model of development could not retain growth and be justified as is evident from the current experience of economic recession and fall in nutritional status of children as well as the lack of attention paid to caste and class differentials (Saikia et al., 2019). The major beneficiaries are the Indian elite and the upper middle class who support the prevailing state policies. This is reflected in the analyses of the stresses on purchasing power, urban governance of water supplies and the agricultural crisis—all so critical for health. The well-off however, having acquired welfare and basic facilities for themselves, see hi-tech medical care as desirable. The public overcrowding and inadequacy of public hospitals repels them and privatisation of care is welcome. This class is defined as the 'aspirational classes' (Visvanathan, 2015), as if aspirations are dependent only on money and social position. The historical advantages they have acquired are certainly not 'natural' or based on merit as they are rooted in their historical alliance with the power of the state. Their self-interest absolves the state of its responsibility towards those who live below, on, or just above the poverty line. They participate in proposing global help for UHC and achieving outcomes within the global directives of investing in health to achieve economic growth and freedom from disease (Lancet Commission, 2013). The state, in turn, helps by rejecting long term planning and pronounces that, 'India's middle class is unique in its size and purchasing power…and an important driver of growth…Our continued challenge is to ensure that this economically vibrant group, remains engaged and its potential is fully realised. The Non-Resident Indian (NRI) is a strength…Future national policies must incorporate this strength in order to broaden their participation in the new India…' (GoI, 2015).

The promotion of UHC at the cost of a systemic approach to health is rooted within this vision. Instead of strictly delineating shared objectives and elaborating on how the public and private could function as one system, the defence of the private sector is that its size cannot be ignored. What does get ignored, however, are the unregulated prices, profits and investment patterns within the private, especially corporate, sectors that ignore primary care. Their partnerships are being encouraged, and concessions and exemptions are awarded to them as industrial units contributing to revenues, rather than to the health of populations. These biases reflect state priorities which lie in faster growth rates and not in equity. The fact that slow infrastructural growth due to low investments over the past decades actually induced the growth of the corporate sector, is being overlooked in favour of a two hundred and eighty billion dollar health market by 2020 (Federation of Indian Chamber of Commerce and Industry (FICCI), 2015).

It is not very surprising then, that despite the evidence that average gains or declines, when broken into class averages indicate serious inequalities, not much attention is paid to real health needs of people living at different consumption levels.[2] The reality of rural lives reflected by the 2011 caste survey, where 73% of household live, of which 74% earn less than five thousand INR per month, 56% are landless, and 51% are casual labourers, is not debated in public fora (Mander, 2015), while clinical medical care of the UHC is projected as the panacea for their ill-health.

Justifying UHC and Carrying It Forward

PPP based state-led insurance has become the central thrust of the prevailing medicalised and targeted model of UHC (a contradiction in terms). These insurance schemes (now called assurance schemes) contradict the principles of insurance system—risk pooling and fair financing in health (where every member of society pays the same share of their disposable incomes to cover their health costs). By targeting the poor only the high risk populations are clustered and the elite who get the higher share of social welfare benefits falling sick less often and also demand a different set of services affecting the market- are free from the responsibility of social solidarity. For example, poor surveillance of communicable diseases (John et al., 2011) known as the diseases of the poor-hampers their monitoring and adds to the disadvantage of the poor. Similarly, increased indirect taxation and lowered direct taxation of the rich reduce the fund pool and increase the burden on the poor. So, in an effort to enhance decentralised district planning, the National Population Commission initiated the Annual Health Survey (GoI, n.d.(a)) for nine states (empowered action group and Assam), for information on vital health, caste and class composition of the population. Unfortunately, this data has not been used to show the health differentials among castes or classes, ignoring the distributive injustices. Unlike the NSS the unit data of these surveys are not freely accessible to researchers either!

Official financial accounting is another effort at rational planning. A National Health Accounting (NHA) system recording financial flows 'is meant to present resource mobilisation for investments to build productive infrastructure for a sector'. For example, revenue generated by taxes, equity, debentures, bonds, public deposits, self-financing, borrowing from global development finance institutions, indigenous bankers advancing finance and direct foreign capital, all are ways to finance industry. Similarly, in a NHA system concerned with financing strengthening of health services, the resources may be domestic or foreign, private or public in origin and in the form of direct investment, credit, charity, taxation, or, premium for insurances (Choudhury & Amar Nath, 2012). The emphasis here is on expenditures with an eye to future capital building and not for immediate utility (current expenditures) though even that is important to track.

The Tenth Plan proposed developing a NHA system for tracking resource flow into all components of health sector to rationalise and streamline this critical aspect of planning. It pointed out that, the high levels out-of-pocket expenditure come from both in and out patient care as the latter is primarily from private and the former from public sector which despite its much lower costs leads to OOPE due to poor availability of drugs in public hospitals (GoI, 2002: 135).The NHA was set up in 2005 and published its report in 2009 to present the details of health expenditure (NHA Cell, 2009). While it was clear that OOPE constitutes a substantial share of the private expenditure, NHA provided little clarity on any other form of private expenditure either as direct investment or as private equity (domestic or foreign). Unlike the Annual Budget documents, NHA only uses the term 'expenditure', it does not specify revenue or capital expenditure. So, the public, non-profit entrepreneurial expenditure, premiums of public and private firms, social insurance funds, external funds are all acknowledged as 'expenditure' without any complete accounting for the corporate or non-corporate private business investment in health. Even the basis of categorisation of expenditures are mixed with some categories based on functions (social security insurance and premiums giving firms in both public and private firms) and others on source of expenditure (public, private, NGO, local body and external funding). It is therefore difficult to separate 'public' from 'private' and capital from revenue expenditure.

As a consequence of the above practice, while at the policy level, cooperation with the public sector and aliening with national objectives is prescribed for the private sector, in matters of accounting it is left alone. Despite this significant information gap, the NHA projects OOPE as the main representative of private expenditure in the total expenditure! Even the private sector expenditure on employee premiums in firms and social insurances is mixed with public sector expenditures on the same, and cannot be delineated.

Irrespective of this flawed methodology of including price paid by individuals for treatment in private sector expenditures, the National Commission on Macroeconomics and Health (GoI, 2005; Rao et al., 2005), using the NHA cell data, estimated a total expenditure of 4.8% of Gross Domestic Product (GDP) for the year 2001–02. It emphasised the role of private sector expenditure and OOPE as a part of it while public expenditure on health was said to be one-fourth of the total. This was supported by the Eleventh Five Year Plan that projected the total private expenditure in health as 3.5% as against 0.96% public expenditure and an estimation of INR 76,094 crores as OOPE, including both premiums paid as well a cost of treatment (GoI, 2007: 105).Thus, an impression has been created of a key financial role played by the private sector. In reality a big chunk of it goes into profits that make medical market attractive. Interestingly, this accounting practice of including OOPE in private expenditure is promoted both by the World Bank (WB, n.d.) as well as the WHO (2008). This is contradictory as OOPE is also considered as a 'financial barrier' (Guy et al., 2008) to healthcare for millions of people.

The distinction between expenditure as price for services, current expenditure of the state and as investment in building infrastructure is thus lost by NHA. OOPE or the price of services is in fact the 'investment recovered' by investors and the 'profits they make'. It can be clubbed with private expenditure only at the cost of losing clarity regarding actual investment in the health sector. The irony lies in the fact that for most other commodities the buyer can withdraw from the market when under economic duress but the same is not possible if life is threatened. The choice of treatment is also not in the users hands. People incur this expenditure to save themselves, not as premiums or as security and solidarity to strengthen services. It is this vulnerability of the people that enables the 'steward' of the market economy, the state, to blur over the difference between expenditure as price and expenditure as investment! The distortion also lies in the fact that money recovered by providers as OOPE is not necessarily reinvested in building infrastructure as it may go to the state treasury or to the private investor as profit. Thus, without any theoretical clarity, explanations, or data on how OOPE is divided, it is assumed to be a part of the total private expenditure. This only artificially expands the latter's resource mobilisation capacity to 3.5% of the GDP.

The actual financial flows, when tracked, show an immense business potential for corporate medical company credits that flow into the private health sector and help pay the loans, dividends on shares as well as make profits out of the real investments that start to pay back in about 7–8 years of setting up a hospital (Alam & Khader, 2015; Itumalla & Acharyulu, 2012). It is not surprising then that the growth of the private hospital sector is the highest with a compound annual growth rate (CAGR) of 12–15%, and so is its capacity to attract foreign and domestic private investors. The attraction of India's medical market for financial institutions (both domestic and foreign is well recognised and is linked to its lax regulation, poor services, rising affordability, demographic shifts towards chronic diseases and policy support. Also, equity funds search for voting rights and management control to shape the sector to keep the rate of returns high (Kalyani & Lakshmi, 2015) and the directions of growth conducive to profit making. The size of medical market is expected to be around US$104 billion in 2014 and 280 billion by 2020 (HDFC Investment Advisory Group, 2015; Alam and Khader, 2015).

The NHA also treats the assured medical care schemes (direct payment for the poor), as state insurances and an investment. This is a perfect camouflage under the umbrella of partnerships where 50–80% of the empanelled hospitals across states happen to be private (GoI, n.d.(b)). They transform the state into a 'client', purchasing services not building or strengthening it. Like OOPE, this assurance price too is falsely presented as state's productive expenditure. While the poor continue to carry the burden of catastrophic expenditures, the financial benefits of these assurance/insurance schemes are shared by the insurance company, Third Party Administrators (TPAs), the hospital owners and the financial institutions- free to reinvest as they like. The eleventh chapter in this book illustrates the severe limitations of the much advertised PMJAY, the largest state led insurance scheme, and how its appropriation of state resources exhausts the funding of other subsectors in health. The National Health Agency with an independent CEO that oversees this scheme, makes it autonomous and deepens the fragmentation of an initially integrated health infrastructure of the 1980s.

In brief the NHA adds up capital and revenue expenditures and by adding a fraction of private expenditure to OOPE in its accounting, it absolves the private sector from any scrutiny. This jugglery helps camouflage the unaccounted private sector and obfuscates the vast gap in information regarding private investments. When we disassemble it, we find:

1. The way the data is presented a systematic analysis is not possible. For the US, Illich provided evidence of profits of the medical industry,[3] but we have no accounting of how much of the actual private investment is recovered, what part of it is private profit[4] and how much of the profit is actually reinvested in health by the private sector. Thus, there is a huge information gap which is covered by calling all of OOPE private expenditure.
2. If in the NHA data, we take out OOPE from the total health expenditure, the actual expenditure accounted for is only 1.25% of the GDP of which 0.86% is public sector expenditure and 0.39 is private.
3. The NHA also underestimates OOPE by families on sickness as it does not include expenses on travel, income loss, staying arrangements and food for attendants (NHA Cell, 2009).
4. In a situation where overall public investment in health has not improved and the state still continues to be responsible for disease control programmes, family welfare, PHC infrastructure, medical manpower education and training, health information, monitoring and regulation, it is but obvious that, due to the rising share of targeted direct payments to the providers (wrongly called state insurance), all these public functions will be undermined thereby creating more space for the private sector.[5,6,7]

This undermining of the public sector is clearly reflected in the slow but definite handing over of medical education to the private sector, declining investments in the NRHM, discontinuation of monitoring systems (such as National Nutrition Monitoring Bureau (NNMB), and constant emphasis on partnerships with private providers, even for national disease control programmes such as National Tuberculosis Programme (Unger et al., 2010). This blind faith in the business model for medical care is also reflected in the fact that, land costs almost 60–70% of the total cost of building hospitals (Dhawan, 2015). And of this total cost, the government policy is to give loans at throw away prices, and annuity loans up to 20% and viability gap funding of up to 40% as shown by Bijoya Roy in this volume (Roy, 2019), for the private projects, this in itself becomes an incentive to investment, given India's attractive medical market. This business model distorts health service system where health is peripheral to generating profits. The emphasis is on becoming self-sufficient and generating further profits without any accountability towards medical services. This underbelly of the reforms needs to be explored.

The Twelfth Five Year Plan 'against all public health rationale' split UHC, tertiary care, and National Health Mission (NHM) and made funding "an instrument of reforms and incentive" (GoI, 2012: 18). The funding for states is made conditional to force higher investments but the social responsibility of the corporate sector is emphasised without any conditions! While the public sector was to take care of residual services, the PPPs such as RSBY and PMJAY were to deliver UHC to protect against catastrophic expenditure. Its expansion thus became a priority while the funds for basic infrastructure shrank! This arrangement is in favour of perfect for the corporate sector, with rights to retain profits from an unregulated market without any risks through PPPs where the state assures payment for the poor who otherwise remain out of coverage. Yet, the very low level and fragmented risk pooling among the lowest 40% was not sufficient for profit-making. Thus, without even covering the poorest adequately, Niti Aayog is now proposing further reforms to perfect the arrangements for the market model. It hopes to consolidate the small providers (with less than 10 employees) through mergers in order to reduce inefficiencies and bring into the net families who are contributing 64% of the total expenditure on health—these are households with out-of-pocket expenditure on illness. This strategy will expand PMJAY (and shrink the public institutions) to capture the middle class that will be forced to pay higher premiums for some degree of security. The 150,000 Primary Health Care Centres (now called Wellness Centres) in rural areas will be picking up non-communicable diseases and cases for tertiary care for referral under PMJAY (Niti Aayog, 2019).

At the Crossroad

OOPE in India has declined by 11% according to the WHO.[8] This is commendable and matches the 55% coverage of the targeted BPL families, but has it contributed to better health and equity of welfare for the poor? The evidence from official sources itself speaks otherwise. It calls for a relook at NITI Aayog's advocacy for, greater dependence on insurance-based models, with the private sector playing a central role (Sethi, 2015), and UHC needs to be redefined in a way that suits the needs of the majority. While it is true that we cannot hope to go back in time and the private sector cannot be ignored, it is equally true that the thinking professionals from public and private sectors must face the dilemmas facing a model of UHC reduced to medical care based on a system of two-tier care—one for those with means and a voice and the other for the voiceless and indigent (Ibid.). All other components of public health are considered irrational in this model as they require 'subsidies' that are considered to be a chimera and irrational, while state funds when demanded by the corporations are called 'incentives' and are rational. The underlying emphasis here again is revenue generation, not wellbeing.

Firstly, this model is not able to provide full coverage to the needy. Secondly, even those who are covered continue to pay heavily as their primary expenditures of Out Patient Department (OPD) and excess OOPEs in hospitalisation are not covered. Thirdly, when the state directly pays the private providers at a higher rates as compared to the public sector (Choudhury & Amar Nath, 2012), it is using an inefficient strategy. Fourthly, this diversion of resources impedes investments in strengthening and rebuilding the weakened public sector. With rising demands from the private providers for higher 'incentives', and the crisis within primary and secondary level care due to lack of institutional sufficiency, as in NRHM, this model may become unsustainable as happened in Venezuela (Lohman, 2015). Fifthly, state-led insurances are targeted schemes; herding of the poor together seriously impacts the quality of tertiary services being provided (Vasan et al., 2015). Last, but not the least, in this process the broader vision of comprehensive, integrated public health exits the national vision.

This crisis is fuelled by increasing dependence on hi-tech and spiralling costs which lead to shrinking markets and sucking in of state funding through rising premiums as in Central Government Health Services (CGHS) (Mukherjee, 2012).The Annual Union Budget 2016–17 (GoI, 2016) has pushed the proportion of state health insurance to 9.5% of the health budget from 7.3% of the total health expenditure in 2014–15, while the total investment has declined from 0.256% to 0.254 over this period, affecting negatively disease control programmes, drug availability, and manpower for basic care. If the 73,144,919 targeted BPL families are to be covered by the RSBY— of which at present only 55% is covered (40,430,279 families) (GoI, n.d.(b))—then, this expenditure will continue to increase (Qadeer & Ghosh, 2016) and yet the country will be nowhere near universal care, as equal numbers sit on the BPL line while the rest pay for services. This in fact, will lead us from crisis to chaos in the absence of an increase in the health budget.

Instead of ignoring market failures in the distribution of healthcare services for the sake of high economic growth rates, the need is to recognise that: (i) public health service is inclusive of medical care and, only when provided as an organised systemic intervention based on epidemiological needs, can it begin to assure health. The manpower, technological and managerial needs of such a system should be affordable and responsive to all sections; (ii) expenditures on personnel and drugs should be considered an integral element of such a system, and not redundant or dispensable; (iii) the state must take the responsibility and begin to increase its investment in infrastructure over time; (iv) the cycle of declining investment in infrastructure and increasing cash payment to private hospitals needs to be reversed by actually including private primary care providers for partnerships while secondary and tertiary care for priority diseases of the BPL must be strengthened over time in public hospitals; (v) strengthen the NRHM and its urban component and use traditional systems and local health traditions; (vi) use of technology needs to be rationalised; along with (vii) addressing issues of food security and agriculture, safe drinking water (not just its sufficiency and access), healthy and safe environment, housing and transport are no less important. This means controlling medical markets and monitoring its revenues for the purposes of regulating it.

Can the private sector play a role in this reorganisation as a self-disciplined partner sharing objectives and mutually agreed responsibilities within a legal framework? Or would it prefer to stay in the free market space without incentives? This question must be posed if India is to move towards covering its citizens with basic services. Partnerships, if any, have to be well defined and well-regulated with level playing fields ensured to public institutions. This calls for the state to free itself of the shackles of dependence on global policies and for strategic experiments with management designs for PPPs. In other words, there is a need to re-examine the notions of social responsibility of both the state as well as the corporate sector. Corporate responsibility, we have argued elsewhere, should not only mean the right to partnership and subsidies but good and ethical business (Qadeer, 2014) where the boundaries of the health markets are not unduly stretched or profits are redefined by adding health benefits; the small and single private primary providers are not squeezed out; and effective regulation is created for both sectors. This is not possible without organisational and professional rejuvenation, market regulation, adequate state financing and recognising state responsibility for the public sector and social participation. The role of democratic processes cannot be overemphasised in this alternative model. If the state chooses to, or is compelled to, attempt a midway correction by addressing these issues and learn from the democratic low-cost experiments that are going on within the country in making drugs and healthcare available with people's participation, it may surprise itself by finding within the country experiments that indicate some desirable directions for the future.

Notes

1. The WHO estimates 25% deaths each year due to environment related deaths (Prüss-Üstün & Corvalán, 2006).
2. The differentials in calorie intakes across expenditure groups are highlighted in Qadeer et al. (2016).
3. According to Ivan (1975), 8.4% of American GNP was due to medical industry compared to 4.5% in 1962, there was a 74% rise in general price index over past 20 years but the price of treatment had escalated by 330%. This has lessons for India.
4. Indian industry claims contributing 4–5% of the GDP and its medical market as one hundred and four billion US dollars in 2014, but no estimates of profits or reinvestments of the industry are known while the number of equity shares rises! (HDFC Bank Investment Advisory Group, 2015).
5. The last three years annual budgets show an increase in state financing of insurances and tertiary care while the finances for NRHM, basic services, and human resources have come down (Annual budgets of 2014–15, 15–16 and 2016–17 GOI, Ministry of Finance http://www.unionbudget.nic.in/vol2.asp?pageid=4 accessed on 12 April 2017.
6. The financial pressure is evident as the RSBY estimate of 29 percent BPL families is much lower than the Tendulkar Committee's estimates of 37.6 percent BPL families as pointed out by (Dror & Vellakkal, 2012). At the same time household OOPE on health as share of total expenditure has increased (Krishnan, 2015).
7. It is also evident that the steps suggested for resource mobilisation by the Working group of Planning Commission for the Eleventh Plan on financing healthcare, have remained on paper except for private partnerships (GoI, 2006).
8. The decline in OOPE between 2005 and 2009 is 11% (estimated as 60% of total health expenditure in 2009) (WHO, 2014).

References

Alam, M. I., & Khader J. A. (2015, April–June). An analysis of foreign direct investment inflows in healthcare system in India. *Pezzottatite Journals, 4*(2), 1669–1674.

Choudhury, M., & Amar Nath, H. K. (2012, May). *An estimate of public expenditure on health in India*. National Institute of Public Finance and Policy (NIPFP). Accessed May 26, 2016. http://nipfp.in/org/in/medicalibrary/2013/08/healthcare+estimate_report.pdf

Dhawan, A. (2015). 2015 healthcare outlook: India. *Deloitte India* (e-document). Accessed March 1, 2016. http://www.2.deloictte.com/content/dam/deloitte/global/Documents/Life-Science-Health-care/gx-Ische-2015-health-care-outlook-india.pdf.

Dror, D. M., & Vellakkal, S. (2012). Is RSBY India's platform to implementing universal hospital insurance? *The Indian Journal of Medical Research, 135*(1), 56–63.

FICCI. (2015). Healthcare: The neglected GDP driver—Need for paradigm shift. KPMG.

Government of Canada, Health Canada. (2011). Canada's healthcare system [Health Canada, 2011]. Accessed May 4, 2018. http://www.hc-sc.gc.ca/hcs-sss/pubs/system-regime/2011-hcs-sss/index-eng.php

Government of India, Office of the Registrar General & Census. (2002). *Tenth five year plan 2002–2007* (Vol. II). Planning Commission.

Government of India, Office of the Registrar General & Census. (2005). *Report of the national commission on macroeconomics and health*. Ministry of Health and Family Welfare. Accessed May 25, 2016. http://www.who.int/macrohealth/action/Report%20of%20the%20National%20Commission.pdf

Government of India, Office of the Registrar General & Census. (2006). *Planning commission, report of the working group on healthcare financing including health insurance for the eleventh five year plan*. Accessed March 22, 2016. http://planningcommission.nic.in/aboutus/committee/wrkgrp11/wg11_rphfw3.pdf

Government of India, Office of the Registrar General & Census. (2007). *Eleventh five year plan, 2007–2012*. Planning Commission of India.

Government of India, Office of the Registrar General & Census. (2012). *Twelfth five year plan 2012–2017* (Vol. III) Planning Commission of India.

Government of India, Office of the Registrar General & Census. (2015). *Government constitutes National Institution for Transforming India (NITI) Aayog*. Press Information Bureau, Cabinet Press Release January 1, 2015. March 26, 2016 http://pib.nic.in/newsite/PrintRelease.aspx?relid=114268

Government of India, Office of the Registrar General & Census. (2016). *Union Budget 2016–17, 2015–16, 2014–15*. Ministry of Finance. Accessed March 22, 2016. http://www.unionbudget.nic.in/vol2.asp?pageid=4

Government of India, Office of the Registrar General & Census, n.d.a. *Census of India: Annual health survey 2010–11 fact sheet*. Commissioner, Ministry of Home Affairs.

I. Qadeer et al. (eds.), *Universalising Healthcare in India*,
https://doi.org/10.1007/978-981-16-5872-3

Government of India, Office of the Registrar General & Census. (n.d.b). Rashtriya Swasthya Bima Yojana: India Portal. Accessed March 20, 2016. https://india.gov.in/spotlight/rashtriya-swasthya-bima-yojana

Guy, C., Mathauer, I., Xu, K., & Evans, D. B. (2008, November). Universal coverage of health services: Tailoring its implementation. *Bulletin of the World Health Organisation* 86(11), 857–863.

HDFC Bank Investment Advisory Group. (2015, March 11). Indian healthcare industry—Hospitals sector sector update. Accessed April 2, 2016. https://www.hdfcbank.com/assets/pdf/privatebanking/Sector_Update_Indian_Health_care_Industry_March_2015.pdf.

Itumalla, R., & Acharyulu, G. V. R. K. (2012, October). Indian healthcare and foreign direct investment: Challenges and opportunities. *Asia Pacific Journal of Marketing and Management Review, 1*(2), 57–69.

Ivan, I. (1975). *Medical Nemesis: The expropriation of health.* Calder and Boyars Ltd.

John, T. J., Dandona, L., Sharma, V. P., & Kakkar, M. (2011). Continuing challenge of infectious diseases in India. *The Lancet,377*(9761), 252–269.

Kalyani, B., Girija, & Lakshmi, V. B. (2015, December). Private equity in India: A special reference to healthcare sector. *Global Journal for Research Analysis, 4*(12), 306–308.

Krishnan, V. (2015, October 23). Poor risk cover under govt. health scheme. *The Hindu.*

Lancet Commission. (2013). Global health 2035: A world converging within a generation. Accessed May 15, 2015. http://globalhealth2035.org/

Lohman, D. (2015, April 29). Venezuela's health-care crisis. *The Washington Post.*

Mander, H. (2015, July 30). Many degrees of hopelessness in India's villages. *Hindustan Times.*

Mukherjee, W. (2012, March 13). India Inc cuts down on employees' medical reimbursements as healthcare costs rise. *The Economic Times.*

National Health Account (NHA) Cell. (2009). *National Health Accounts India (2004–05).* Ministry of Health and Family Welfare, Government of India.

NITI Aayog. (2019, November). *Health system for a new India: "Building blocks potential pathways to reforms"* (pp. 3–11). GoI.

People's Health Movement (PHM), Medact, Medico International, Third World Network, Health Action Network, and Asociacion Latinoamericana de Medicina Social. (2014). *Global health watch 4: An alternative world health report.* Zed Books.

Prinja, S., Aggarwal, A. K., Kumar, R., & Kanavos, P. (2012, November). User charges in healthcare: Evidence of effect on service utilisation and equity from North India. *The Indian Journal of Medical Research, 136*(5), 868–876.

Prüss-Üstün, A., & Corvalán, C. (2006). *Preventing disease through healthy environments: Towards an estimate of the environmental burden of disease.* The WHO.

Qadeer, I., & Ghosh, S. M. (2016, April 17). Public health's in the infirmary. *The Hindu Businessline.*

Qadeer, I., Ghosh, S. M., & Arathi P. M. (2016, March). India's declining calorie intake: Development or distress? *Social Change, 46*(1), 1–26.

Qadeer, I. (2014). Universal healthcare and social responsibility of the private sector. In *India infrastructure report 2013/14: The road to universal health coverage.* Orient BlackSwan.

Rao, S. K., Selvaraju, S., Nagpal, S., & Sakthivel, S. (2005). Financing and delivery of healthcare services in India National Commission on macroeconomics and health, financing and delivery of healthcare services in India. NCMH Background Papers: 239-255. Ministry of Health & Family Welfare, Government of India.

Roy, B. (2019). The role of public private partnerships in ensuring healthcare in India. In I. Qadeer, K. B. Saxena, & P. M. Arathi (Eds.), *Universalising healthcare in India from care to coverage.* Aakar Books.

Saikia, N., Bora, J. K., & Luy, M. (2019). Socioeconomic disparity in adult mortality in India: Estimations using the orphanhood method. *Journal of Population Sciences. Genus, 75*(7). https://doi.org/10.1186/s41118-019-0054-1 Accessed on 25.1.2021.

Sethi, N. (2015, August 25). NITI Aayog aagainst free healthcare, bats for more private sector role. *Business Standard.*

Unger, J.-P., De Paepe, P., Ghilbert, P., Zocchi, W., van Dessel, P., Qadeer, I., & Sen, K. (2010). Privatisation (PPM-DOTS) strategy for tuberculosis control: How evidence-based is it? In Unger, J.-P., De Paepe, P., Ghilbert, P., Zocchi, W., van Dessel, P., Qadeer, I., & Sen, K. (Eds.), *International health and aid policies*. Cambridge University Press.

Vasan, A., Karpagam, S., & Seethappa, V. (2015). Design, implementation, and patient experiences of the Rashtriya Swasthbima Yojana and Vajpayee Arogyashree Scheme: A qualitative study from Bangalore District, Karnataka. In I. Qadeer (Ed.), *India social development report 2014: Challenges of public health*. Oxford University Press.

Visvanathan, S. (2015, September 28). Revolt of the aspirational class. *The Hindu*. Accessed April 6, 2016. http://www.thehindu.com/opinion/lead/patel-next-door-revolt-of-the-aspirational-clats/article76950-57.ece.

WHO. (2005). *Technical briefs for policy makers number 1: Achieving universal health coverage: Developing the health financing system*. The WHO. Accessed January 10, 2016. http://www.who.int/health_financing/pb_1.pdf

WHO. (2008, June). *Health systems financing: Toolkit on monitoring health systems strengthening* (draft).

WHO. (2014). *Global health expenditure database: Health system financing profile by country (India)*. Accessed March 31, 2016. http://apps.who.int/nha/database/Country_Profile/Index/en.

World Bank. (n.d.) Health systems-financing. Accessed March 23, 2016. http://web.worldbank.org/WEBSITE/EXTERNAL/TOPICS/EXTHEALTHNUTRITIONANDPOPULATION/EXTHSD/0,contentMDK:22523961~menuPK:6485082~pagePK:148956~piPK:216618~theSitePK:376793,00.html#Out_of_Pocket_Payments_&_User_Fees.